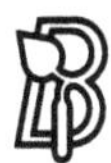

Progress in Inflammation Research

Series Editor

Prof. Dr. Michael J. Parnham
PLIVA
Research Institute
Prilaz baruna Filipovica 25
10000 Zagreb
Croatia

Forthcoming titles:

Disease-modifying Therapy in Vasculitides, C.G.M. Kallenberg, J.W. Cohen Tervaert (Editors), 2001

Mechanisms and Mediators of Neuropathic Pain, A.B. Malmberg, S.R. Chaplan (Editors), 2001

Inflammation and Stroke, G. Feuerstein (Editor), 2001

NMDA Antagonists as Potential Analgesic Drugs, R.G. Hill, D.J.S. Sirinathsinghji (Editors), 2001

The Hereditary Basis of Allergic Disorders, J.Holloway, S. Holgate (Editors), 2001

Migraine: A Neuroinflammatory Disease?, E.L.H. Spierings, M. Sanchez del Rio (Editors), 2002

(Already published titles see last page)

Neuroinflammatory Mechanisms in Alzheimer's Disease
Basic and Clinical Research

Joseph Rogers

Editor

Springer Basel AG

Editor

Dr. Joseph Rogers
Sun Health Research Institute
10515 West Santa Fe Drive
Sun City, AZ 85372
USA

A CIP catalogue record for this book is available from the Library of Congress, Washington D.C., USA

Deutsche Bibliothek Cataloging-in-Publication Data
Neuroinflammatory mechanisms in Alzheimer's disease : basic and clinical research /
Joseph Rogers ed.. - Basel ; Boston ; Berlin : Birkhäuser, 2001
(Progress in inflammation research)
ISBN 978-3-7643-6074-0 ISBN 978-3-0348-8350-4 (eBook)
DOI 10.1007/978-3-0348-8350-4

The publisher and editor can give no guarantee for the information on drug dosage and administration contained in this publication. The respective user must check its accuracy by consulting other sources of reference in each individual case.

Originally published by Birkhäuser Verlag in 2001

Printed on acid-free paper produced from chlorine-free pulp. TCF ∞
Cover design: Markus Etterich, Basel
Cover illustration: Accumulation of astrocytes in neuritic plaques in an AD brain (p. 95ff).

ISBN 978-3-7643-6074-0

9 8 7 6 5 4 3 2 1

Contents

List of contributors

Haruhiko Akiyama, Tokyo Institute of Psychiatry, 2-1-8 Kamikitazawa, Setagaya-ku, Tokyo, 156-8585, Japan; e-mail: akiyama@prit.go.jp

Steven W. Barger, Geriatric Research Education Clinical Center, Central Arkansas Veterans Healthcare System, Little Rock, AR 72205, USA;
e-mail: bargerstevenw@uams.edu

Bonnie M. Bradt, Department of Internal Medicine, University of California Davis Medical Center, 1508 Alhambra Blvd., Sacramento, CA 95816, USA;
e-mail: bonnie.bradt@ucdmc.ucdavis.edu

Neil R. Cooper, Department of Immunology, The Scripps Research Institute, 10550 North Torrey Pines Road, La Jolla, CA 92037, USA; e-mail: nrcooper@scripps.edu

Piet Eikelenboom, Research Institute Neurosciences Vrije Universiteit, Department of Psychiatry, PCA Valeriuskliniek, Valeriusplein 9, 1075 BG Amsterdam, The Netherlands; e-mail: piete@ggzba.nl

Caleb E. Finch, Andrus Gerontology Center and Department of Biological Sciences, University of Southern California, Los Angeles, CA 90089-0191, USA;
e-mail: cefinch@usc.edu

C. Erik Hack, Department of Autoimmune Diseases, Central Laboratory of the Netherlands Red Cross Bloodtransfusion Service, Plesmanlaan 125, 1066 CX Amsterdam, The Netherlands; e-mail: e_hack@clb.nl

Harald Hampel, Dementia Research Section, Department of Psychiatry, Ludwig-Maximilian University, Nussbaumstr. 7, 80336 Munich, Germany;
e-mail: hampel@psy.med.uni-muenchen.de

Andreas Haslinger, Dementia Research Section, Department of Psychiatry, Ludwig-Maximilian University, Nussbaumstr. 7, 80336 Munich, Germany

Andis Klegeris, Kinsmen Laboratory of Neurological Research, University of British Columbia, 2255 Wesbrook Mall, Vancouver, B.C., V6T IZ3 Canada;
e-mail: aklegeri@interchange.ubc.ca

Valter D. Longo, Andrus Gerontology Center and Department of Biological Sciences, University of Southern California, Los Angeles, CA 90089-0191, USA;
e-mail: vlongo@usc.edu

Lih-Fen Lue, Sun Health Research Institute, 10515 West Santa Fe Drive, Sun City, AZ 85351, USA; e-mail: llue@sunhealth.org

Ian R.A. Mackenzie, Department of Pathology and Laboratory Medicine, University of British Columbia, Vancouver, B.C., V6T 2B5 Canada;
e-mail: imackenz@vanhosp.bc.ca

Edith G. McGeer, Kinsmen Laboratory of Neurological Research, Department of Psychiatry, University of British Columbia, 2255 Wesbrook Mall, Vancouver, B.C., V6T 1Z3 Canada; e-mail: mcgeer@interchange.ubc.ca

Patrick L. McGeer, Kinsmen Laboratory of Neurological Research, Department of Psychiatry, University of British Columbia, 2255 Wesbrook Mall, Vancouver, B.C., V6T 1Z3 Canada; e-mail: mcgeerpl@interchange.ubc.ca

Stephen A. O'Barr, College of Pharmacy, Western University of Health Sciences, 309 East Second Street, Pomona, CA 91766-1854, USA

Giulio Maria Pasinetti, Neuroinflammation Research Laboratories, Department of Psychiatry, Mount Sinai School of Medicine, One Gustave L. Levy Place, New York, NY 10029, USA; e-mail: gp2@doc.mssm.edu

Harry E. Peery, Department of Pharmacology and Toxicology, College of Pharmacy, Arizona Health Sciences Center, University of Arizona, Tucson, AZ 85721, USA

Joseph Rogers, Sun Health Research Institute, 10515 West Santa Fe Drive, Sun City, AZ 85351, USA; e-mail: jrogers@mail.sunhealth.org

Michael Scheloske, Dementia Research Section, Department of Psychiatry, Ludwig-Maximilian University, Nussbaumstr. 7, 80336 Munich, Germany

Michael Schulzer, Kinsmen Laboratory of Neurological Research, Departments of Medicine and Statistics, University of British Columbia, 2255 Wesbrook Mall, Vancouver, B.C., V6T 1Z3 Canada; e-mail: michael@stat.ubc.ca

Ron W. Strohmeyer, Sun Health Research Institute, 10515 West Santa Fe Drive, Sun City, AZ 85351, USA

Ikuo Tooyama, Molecular Neuroscience Research Center, Shiga University of Medical Science, Otsu 520-2192, Japan; e-mail: kinchan@sums.shiga-med.ac.jp

Freek L. Van Muiswinkel, Research Institute Neurosciences Vrije Universiteit, Department of Pharmacology, Van der Boechorststraat 7, 1081 BT Amsterdam, The Netherlands; e-mail: flv.muiswinkel.pharm@med.vu.nl

Robert Veerhuis, Research Institute Neurosciences Vrije Universiteit, Department of Pathology, De Boelelaan 1117, 1081 HV Amsterdam, The Netherlands;
e-mail: r.veerhuis@azvu.nl

Douglas G. Walker, Sun Health Research Institute, 10515 West Santa Fe Drive, Sun City, AZ 85351, USA; e-mail: dgwalker@altavista.net

Scott D. Webster, Department of Molecular Biology and Biochemistry, 3205 Biological Sciences II, University of California, Irvine, CA 92697, USA;
e-mail: swebster@uci.edu

Jack X. Yu, Department of Immunology, The Scripps Research Institute, 10550 North Torrey Pines Road, La Jolla, CA 92037, USA

Preface

Research into inflammatory mechanisms that may cause damage to the Alzheimer's disease (AD) brain has now been ongoing for nearly two decades. Some two dozen clinical studies have strongly suggested that conventional anti-inflammatory drugs may be useful to delay the onset or slow the progression of the disorder. Moreover, virtually all the major systems of the innate immune response appear to be present, and most are upregulated, in pathologically-vulnerable regions of the AD brain. These new findings are described in this volume – first in overview form, followed by chapters on topics of special interest.

In many ways, to understand AD brain inflammation, one need only review a text on peripheral inflammation biology, leaving out the chapters on humoral mediators and substituting microglia for macrophages. In several other key respects, however, AD brain inflammation is unique, due primarily to idiosyncratic interactions of inflammatory mediators and mechanisms with classical AD pathology: amyloid β peptide (Aβ) deposits and neurofibrillary tangles (NFTs). For this reason, some key concepts about the inflammation that occurs in AD may warrant discussion in preparation for the more detailed chapters that follow.

AD brain inflammation does not appear to be humorally mediated. Although CD4- and CD8-immunoreactive T cells are easily demonstrated in the AD brain, no rigorously measured quantitative difference with T cells in the non-demented elderly (ND) brain has been reported. Immunoreactivity for antibodies is also similar in AD and ND cortical samples, and the staining itself is equivocal. Assays for serum antibodies directed at Aβ reveal that approximately half of AD patients and half of ND patients have equivalent, low titers. B cells and natural killer cells appear to be absent from the AD brain parenchyma. As negative results, these observations (J. Rogers, unpublished observations) have never been formally reported, but may warrant re-examination in light of the success of a vaccination approach to removing Aβ, implying some form of humoral mediation.

The fact that AD inflammation uses innate rather than humoral mechanisms does not mean that it is unimportant. Neuroimmunology has become progressively dominated by lymphocyte biology, and remarkable progress has been made thereby in understanding humorally-mediated neuroinflammatory disorders such as multiple sclerosis. Nonetheless, innate inflammatory mechanisms are present and are of profound physiological significance throughout phylogeny. When they are misdirected, and especially when they are chronically misdirected, innate inflammatory mechanisms are known to cause secondary damage to affected tissues. Indeed, innate inflammatory mechanisms may be more prone to misdirected, pathogenic actions precisely because they lack the fascinating-to-study specificity of antibody-antigen responses.

Though unique to AD, the elements that stimulate AD brain inflammation are similar in type to those that stimulate peripheral inflammation. Damaged tissue and the chronic presence of highly insoluble, abnormal materials are classical stimulants of peripheral inflammation. It should therefore not be surprising that damaged neurons and neurites and the chronic presence of highly insoluble, abnormal Aβ deposits and NFTs stimulate inflammation in the brain. The surprising thing is that it took so long to notice the obvious parallels between the classical stimulants of innate inflammatory responses and the classical elements of AD pathology.

Mediators of the innate inflammatory system exhibit unusual interactions with classical AD pathology. Not only do the classical elements of AD pathology bear obvious parallels to classical stimulants of inflammation, they also exhibit unusual interactions with the classical elements of AD pathology. Aβ and neurofibrillary tangles, for example, are potent antibody-independent activators of the classical complement pathway. Certain of the cytokines appear to induce the Aβ precursor protein and are, in turn, induced by Aβ (see subsequent chapters). Because the classical elements of AD pathology are present from pre-symptomatic to terminal stages of the disorder, their general inflammagenic properties and their amplifying interactions with innate inflammatory mediators insure a state of localized, chronic inflammation in the AD brain throughout the disease course. Even very weak, highly localized AD inflammation should become pathophysiologically relevant when cumulated over the many years of AD progression.

Most of the inflammatory mediators found in the AD brain appear to be endogenously produced. For decades, the blood-brain barrier was thought to provide a nearly impenetrable shield against inflammation within the brain. How such a dogma arose when many of the same people espousing it were treating their multiple sclerosis and meningitis patients with anti-inflammatory drugs remains a mystery. Nonetheless, an overwhelming amount of research has demonstrated mRNA and proteins for virtually all classes of inflammatory mediators, including complement, cytokines, and acute phase reactants, co-localized with endogenous brain cells.

Prevention versus intervention trials of anti-inflammatory drugs in AD. The physician to a patient who is about to play his first touch football game in two decades will advise the patient to take anti-inflammatory drugs before the game, not afterwards when he is lying immobilized from stiffness and pain on his couch. This prevention rather than intervention strategy may be particularly cogent to AD therapeusis if we take seriously the idea that AD inflammation is chronic and only cumulates to significant damage over the course of many years.

Which anti-inflammatory drugs should be given for AD remains uncertain. Like most investigators in biomedicine, the scientists who perform research on AD inflammation tend to believe that the mechanisms they study are more important than the mechanisms others study. Although minor examples may be seen in the present volume, this phenomenon has increasingly been inhibited in AD inflammation research by the growing recognition that the many mechanisms involved in the innate inflammatory response are so tightly coupled that to have one is virtually to have them all. As such, there is little information from basic research concerning which anti-inflammatory or class of anti-inflammatories might be most useful for AD. The clinical studies to date are also not terribly helpful, as most only cover epidemiological data where specific anti-inflammatory drugs are seldom singled out. Moreover, the three prospective, placebo-controlled trials that have been done with specific agents were intervention trials on patients who already had AD, a time point that, as previously noted, is likely to be less than optimum for discerning beneficial effects of anti-inflammatory drugs. For these reasons, we presently have very little to go on with respect to choice of anti-inflammatory agent. This does not mean, however, that we should wait to conduct trials, particularly prevention trials with commonly available non-steroidal anti-inflammatory drugs, as the costs of such studies, high though they may be, are still far less than the enormous economic and social costs of AD.

February 2001 Joseph Rogers

Basic Research Overview

Cellular and molecular mechanisms of Alzheimer's disease inflammation

Harry E. Peery[1,2], Ron W. Strohmeyer[1] and Joseph Rogers[1]

[1]Sun Health Research Institute, 10515 West Santa Fe Drive, Sun City, AZ 85351, USA, and [2]Department of Pharmacology and Toxicology, College of Pharmacy, Arizona Health Sciences Center, University of Arizona, Tucson, AZ 85721, USA

Introduction

Over the last two decades, many of the peripheral mechanisms and mediators of the innate inflammatory response have been identified as endogenously-mediated, localized reactions in pathologically vulnerable regions of the Alzheimer's disease (AD) brain (for previous reviews see [1–5]). The fine details of these processes are considered in subsequent chapters of this volume. Here, we summarize broadly what the mechanisms and mediators are, the evidence for their endogenous production in the AD brain, and the mounting evidence of their significance to AD pathology. We also provide a brief summary of the clinical and pathological features of AD for those readers who are not already familiar with this disorder. Conversely, we have attempted to provide a simplified description of several key inflammatory mechanisms such as the complement cascade for those readers who do not have expertise in immunology.

Clinical and pathological features of AD

AD is a progressive neurological disorder leading to dementia. It is the most common form of dementia in the elderly, accounting for 70% or more of senile dementia cases at autopsy worldwide [6], and affecting an estimated 4–5 million people in the US in the year 2000 [7, 8] and 37 million or more people worldwide by 2020 [6]. Frequently encountered clinical abnormalities include problems with recent memory, calculation, and executive function. These difficulties progress to frank dementia over an average course of eight to nine years. Motor function is generally spared, although in the terminal stages of AD most patients gradually cease to walk or feed themselves [9].

The pathological antecedents of AD are believed to begin as much as several decades before overt clinical symptoms are manifest [10]. The hallmark pathologies of the disorder, known since Alois Alzheimer's first characterization in 1907 [11], are neuronal loss, profuse extracellular deposition of amyloid β peptide (Aβ), and

Neuroinflammatory Mechanisms in Alzheimer's Disease: Basic and Clinical Research,
edited by Joseph Rogers

widespread formation of intraneuronal neurofibrillary tangles. These changes occur primarily in higher order cortical regions, including frontal, parietal, and temporal cortex and the limbic system, and are relatively rare in primary motor or sensory areas except for olfaction [12], hence the clinical manifestation of AD as a cognitive rather than motor disorder [9].

Autosomally dominant inheritance of AD is known to occur in 1–5% of cases and is generally believed to be due to mutations in genes involved in Aβ production and metabolism. A genetic basis for enhanced susceptibility to AD has also been demonstrated, particularly for the E4 isoform of the apolipoprotein E gene. Varying susceptibility for risk of AD has been found for polymorphisms of several pro-inflammatory genes as well, including interleukin-1 (IL-1) [13–18] and interleukin-6 (IL-6) ([19–21], reviewed in [22]).

Neurodegeneration is the clear underlying cause of AD dementia, with particular recent emphasis on synapse loss as the best correlate of AD disease state [23]. In turn, AD neurodegeneration is undoubtedly caused by Aβ and neurofibrillary tangles, although the primacy of one or the other as a pathogenetic factor is still occasionally debated, and other processes are likely to contribute as well. In particular, it is still incompletely understood how Aβ and neurofibrillary tangles cause neurodegeneration and synapse loss. Aβ, for example, is known to act on a multitude of receptors and pathogenic mechanisms. Perhaps not surprisingly, many of these receptors and mechanisms are tied to the innate inflammatory response.

Basic principles of AD inflammation

Based on principles elucidated from more than a century of studies of the peripheral innate inflammatory response, many of the innate inflammatory mechanisms underlying AD inflammation can now be described with some confidence. Cell death and the deposition of highly inert and insoluble deposits, aggregated Aβ and neurofibrillary tangles, are the most likely sources of AD inflammation, just as cell death and the deposition of highly insoluble, inert deposits are common causes of peripheral innate inflammatory responses. Because these inflammatory stimuli are micro-localized and chronically present in the AD brain from its earliest to its terminal stages (reviewed in [22]), AD inflammation is likely to be similarly micro-localized and chronic. Also as in the periphery, the innate inflammatory response of AD is characterized by amplification and a high degree of interaction among the inflammatory elements (reviewed in [22]). Finally, as a further parallel, AD inflammation appears to be capable of causing bystander damage to healthy cells [24–27].

Because of the unique anatomy and physiology of the brain as an organ system, and its unique shielding from the rest of the body through the blood-brain barrier, several critical differences in AD and peripheral inflammation also exist. In the brain, for example, the post mitotic state of neurons makes bystander pathology a significant problem, whereas it may not be in peripheral tissues that display much greater regenerative capacities. It has also been noted that AD inflammation, like that observed in such other central nervous system inflammatory disorders as multiple sclerosis, does not meet the classical standards for peripheral inflammation laid down by the Roman physician Cornelius Celsius almost 2,000 years ago, *rubor et tumor cum calor et dolor* (redness and swelling with heat and pain), though AD inflammation and multiple sclerosis certainly do meet the additional criterion described by Rudoph Virchow in 1858, *functio laesa* (loss of function) [28, 29]. In addition, Aβ, a hallmark pathogen of AD, appears to have multiple idiosyncratic actions on various inflammatory mechanisms. Aβ, for example, binds to C1q and activates the classical complement pathway [30–32]; it is a ligand for several inflammation-related receptors (e.g. the formyl peptide receptor) [33–35]; and several inflammatory mediators (e.g. IL-1) have been reported to induce Aβ (reviewed in [22]). Finally, humorally-mediated inflammatory responses involving lymphocytes have not so far been found to play a role in AD pathology, although the possibility remains open to more rigorous testing, particularly in light of recent findings concerning a vaccination approach to AD therapy [36].

In summary, in so far as the basic antecedents, mechanisms, and mediators go, there is little about AD inflammation that could not be gleaned from a graduate-level text on the peripheral innate immune response. What makes AD inflammation novel is that it occurs chronically in the brain and features multiple interactions with the AD pathology that engendered the inflammation in the first place.

The cellular mediators of AD inflammation

Astrocytes

Astrocytes are essential for the normal function of neurons in that they rapidly take up potassium after neuronal depolarization and process the excitatory neurotransmitter glutamate and inhibitory neurotransmitter gamma aminobutyric acid (GABA) after its release by neurons [37]. Astrocyte foot processes provide a component of the blood-brain barrier [38].

In the AD cortex, astrocytes typically have a hypertrophied, reactive morphology characterized by enhanced expression of glial fibrillary acidic protein (GFAP) [39, 40]. They may also divide (hyperplasia), with some estimates giving a four-fold increase in their numbers in AD [41]. They also exhibit a characteristic peri-plaque localization around Aβ deposits, interdigitating the neuritic halo that surrounds the Aβ core of the plaque [42–47]. Interestingly, astrocytes may inhibit microglial clearance of Aβ by depositing peptidoglycans on the plaque [48, 49]. Astrocytes can also be found surrounding ghost tangles, the extracellular remnants of cells that presumably once contained neurofibrillary tangles [50–52].

Astrocyte responses in the AD brain include the expression of early response genes, adhesion proteins, cytokines, proteases, eicosanoids, and other cytotoxic products (Tab. 1) [53]. They may also secrete ectoenzymes in an attempt to break down the Aβ in plaques [54] or, possibly, the paired helical filaments that are the main constituent of neurofibrillary tangles [55, 56].

Microglia

Microglia are likely to be part of the mononuclear phagocyte system, a system of tissue macrophages and their immature blood precursor cells, the monocytes, found throughout the body [57–61]. Microglia constitute 10–15% of the cells in brain [59, 62, 63], and have neurotrophic functions in the normal central nervous system [59, 64].

First noticed by their profuse expression of major histocompatibility complex type II (MHCII) cell surface glycoprotein, the microglia in AD cortical gray matter become highly activated [22, 59–61, 65]. As such, they produce a wide range of inflammatory mediators (reviewed in [22]) including complement, cytokines, chemokines (see Tab. 1), reactive oxygen intermediates, secreted proteases, excitatory amino acids including glutamate [66] and quinolinic acid [67], and nitric oxide (NO). Notably, some of these inflammatory factors (e.g. complement) have only been shown in isolated culture systems, and have not been observed with *in situ* hybridization techniques, perhaps because of the relatively small size of microglia (and the hybridization signal they generate) compared to neurons, which also express these proteins.

Many of the inflammation-related secretory responses of microglia appear to be stimulated by Aβ. For example, it has been reported that microglia activated by plaque Aβ exhibit increases in intracellular signaling cascades as manifested by an increase in phosphotyrosine. In this pathway, tyrosine kinases Syk, Lyn, are activated, which causes calcium to be liberated from the ryanodyne receptors [68] and IP_3 calcium receptors on the endoplasmic reticulum [69–71]. The release of calcium activates tyrosine kinases FAK and Pyk2 pathways [72], which cause morphological alterations in the cells and the activation of two microtubule-associate protein (MAP) kinase cascades, ERKs and p38 MAP kinases [69, 72]. These kinases are responsible for the phosphorylation of transcription factors that are involved in activation of several inflammation-related genes.

Neurons

Neurons are also capable of producing inflammatory mediators, including complement [73–76], cyclooxygenase (COX) [77–82], pro-inflammatory cytokines [83–

90], the IL-6 receptor signal transducing component gp130 [91], macrophage colony-stimulating factor (M-CSF) [92], and others (Tab. 1).

The molecular mediators of AD inflammation

Complement

In vertebrates, complement is an ancient antibacterial system. During evolution, it also became associated at several points with the humoral immune system, which is found only in vertebrates [93]. In the periphery, 90% of the complement proteins are produced by the liver, with the remaining 10% produced by the intestinal epithelium and by members of the mononuclear phagocyte system, which includes macrophages [24, 94]. In the brain, however, little or no peripherally-derived complement should be present, as most of these proteins are unlikely to cross the blood-brain barrier. The dramatically upregulated levels of complement in pathologically vulnerable areas of the AD brain are therefore believed to derive from endogenous sources, and multiple studies have confirmed this possibility (reviewed in [22]).

Complement consists of over 30 plasma or membrane proteins organized into three different cascades [24, 93]. Two of these, the classical and the alternative pathways, have been intensively studied in AD [5, 22, 73, 75, 95–99], as both are activated by and highly co-localized with Aβ. Activation of the classical pathway begins with the binding of Aβ to a site on the first classical pathway component, C1q . The binding site is a 13–15 amino acid residue on the C1q A chain collagen tail, a consensus region for binding of several different antibody-independent activators of C1q [30–32]. Exposed neurofilaments [100] and DNA [30], the products of AD neurodegeneration, also are likely to be antibody-independent sources of complement activation in the AD brain [101, 102].

Complement activation has several pathogenic consequences: it generates the anaphylatoxins C3a, C4a, and C5a, complement activation fragments that further trigger local inflammatory reactions; it generates opsonins, complement activation fragments that help target inflammatory responses; and it generates the membrane attack complex (MAC), the terminal product of all the complement cascades (reviewed in [24–27]). When fixed to cell membranes, the MAC opens a transmembrane channel permitting free entry of ions, particularly calcium. Cell lysis, including lysis of healthy bystander cells [24–27] follows if sufficient MAC binding has occurred.

In addition to these classical mechanisms for complement toxicity, several unusual interactions of complement with AD pathology have been reported. For example, among the many inflammatory mediators that have been suggested to enhance the aggregation of Aβ into the highly insoluble fibrils characteristic of plaques, C1q appears to be the most potent. Conversely, C1q may also act as an "anti-opsonin" that blocks microglial clearance of Aβ deposits.

Cytokines and chemokines

Phylogenetically, cytokines are one of the oldest surveillance systems of the immune system, being present in invertebrates [103]. Cytokines and chemokines are intercellular and intracellular signaling factors that presumably serve the same purpose in microglia and astrocytes as they do in peripheral macrophages and other cells of the immune system. In AD, a number of cytokines and chemokines have been found to be upregulated when compared to ND samples (Tab. 1), especially the major pro-inflammatory mediators IL-1, IL-6, and TNFα (Tab. 1) (reviewed in [22, 104]). Cytokines and chemokines activate a large number of inflammatory response genes in AD and the resulting proteins are synthesized by astrocytes, microglia, and, in some cases, neurons.

Cytokines and chemokines are often detected in Aβ plaques, and Aβ itself appears to induce the synthesis of cytokines and chemokines in microglia, astrocytes, and in some neurons. At the same time, high levels of cytokines reportedly stimulate increased expression of Aβ precursor protein (APP) and Aβ. The production of cytokines and chemokines has been suggested to rise and fall in concurrence with plaque deposition, so that the highest production occurs in early diffuse and dense-core neuritic plaques. In addition, when studied *in vitro* or in knockout preparations, many of the cytokines and chemokines seem to play a functional role in the evolution of plaques, as they appear to have a dystrophic effect on neurites within and neurons around Aβ plaques. Paradoxically, a few of these factors have also been suggested to play a neuroprotective role. Confirmation of these findings, however, must await studies done on cytokine interactions in systems that are not limited to a single cell type (e.g. isolated neuron cultures) and that permit interactions with the vasculature and other essential components of brain (reviewed in [22]). Over-expression of pro-inflammatory cytokines in transgenic mice under the control of brain-specific promoters consistently results in inflammatory pathology, with little or no neuroprotective responses observed [105–108].

Cyclooxygenase

Cyclooxygenase (COX) is a key enzyme in the pathway from arachidonic acid to prostaglandin. Once initiated, COX synthesis is autoregulated by feedback mechanisms emanating from the inflammation mediators it produces. Within the past few years, two COX isoforms, COX-1 and COX-2, have been identified in both the periphery and brain (reviewed in [109]). COX-1 is a constitutively expressed enzyme throughout the body that produces pro- and anti-inflammatory products, whereas COX-2 is induced primarily at sites of inflammation. For this reason, selective COX-2-inhibiting anti-inflammatory drugs have the significant advantage of working primarily at sites of inflammation, sparing adverse reactions in uninvolved organ systems such as the gastrointestinal tract.

The proteins produced by COX-2 isoenzyme are increased in several locations of the AD brain and may correlate with levels of Aβ and plaque density [77, 110, 111]. Moreover, in Down's syndrome and AD there is one report of the COX-2 protein co-localizing with neurons containing tangles [80].

In the periphery, high levels of COX stimulate multiple downstream mechanisms of inflammation. These same processes may also occur in the AD brain. In astrocyte and microglia cultures, there is increased synthesis of cytokines and other inflammatory mediators in response to PGE_2 [112–118]. In AD neuroinflammation, COX-2 may also be involved in the development of glutamate excitotoxicity [119], free radicals [120], and PPARγ synthesis [22, 121–124]. Because of its relationship to inflammation, and the availability of a wide range of efficacious antagonistic products for short-term use, the application of COX inhibitors for chronic use in AD treatment has become a recent focus of several clinical studies (see the chapter by McGeer and colleagues, this volume).

Coagulation and fibrinolysis systems

Several proteins of the coagulation cascade have been either found in Aβ plaques or are upregulated in the AD brain (Tab. 1). The actions of several of these proteins are enhanced by heparin binding [125, 126]. Heparan sulfate proteoglycan, a component of basement membranes and a peripheral adhesion molecule for acetylcholinesterase, is found in greater quantities in Aβ plaques and in neurofibrillary tangles [127, 128].

Adhesion molecules

A number of intercellular adhesion molecules, whose upregulation is induced by cytokines (reviewed in [99, 129–132]), are upregulated in AD (Tab. 1). The β_2-integrins, complement receptor 3, complement receptor 4, and LFA-1, an astrocyte ligand for ICAM-1 [133], are also upregulated in AD [134] and may play roles in activating microglia and astrocytes at sites of inflammation.

Other acute phase proteins and inflammatory agents

Acute phase proteins are produced early in the inflammatory process as part of the acute phase response. Many of these molecules have been found associated with senile plaques and extracellular neurofibrillary tangles (Tab. 1), α1-antichymotrypsin (α1-ACT), for example, is found co-localized with Aβ plaques and may enhance their formation by assisting in the conversion of non-fibrillar to fibrillar Aβ [135–138].

α2 macroglobulin (α2-MAC) acts as a substrate for a large number of proteases [139, 140], and is another acute phase protein that has been intensely studied in AD. Combination of α2-MAC with a protease exposes a receptor-binding domain. This domain is then bound to low density lipoprotein receptor-related protein (LRP) and the whole complex (α2-MACR/LRP) is removed by endocytosis. Both α2-MAC and α2-MACR/LRP inhibit proteases and also remove proteases and inflammatory proteins [139, 141–144] as well as inhibit Aβ plaque formation [145]. Both α2-MAC and α2-MACR/LRP have been found in Aβ plaques and neurofibrillary tangles [146–150]. Particular polymorphisms of α1-ACT [138], α2-MAC [151–154], and α2-MAC/LRP [153] genes have been reported to be risk factors for AD.

Apolipoprotein E allele 4 (ApoE4) is another major susceptibility factor for AD, shortening on average the age of onset of AD by some five to ten years [155]. ApoE is increased at sites of peripheral inflammation and peripheral amyloidosis [156]. Increased congophilic amyloid angiopathy is found in AD patients who possess one ApoE4 allele, and is increased further in patients who are homozygous for ApoE4 [157]. In addition, ApoE4 has been reported to influence microglial expression of several inflammatory factors [158, 159].

Free radicals

Oxidative damage has been demonstrated in the AD brain [160–163], including the modification of proteins with advanced glycation end products (AGEs) [164], malondialdehyde, 8-hydroxy-deoxyguanosine, 4-hydronoenenal [163, 165], nitrotyrosine [166–168], nitrotyrosine-modified proteins [166–169], and increased amounts of lipid peroxidation [163]. Free radicals cause cellular injury, cell death, and may reduce neuronal integrity by triggering redox-sensitive NF-κB-mediated transcription of pro-inflammatory genes [170].

The relationship between free radicals and inflammation has been known for many years in the periphery, where the production of reactive nitrogen and oxygen molecules by immune cells is a major method of attacking opsonized targets. In the brain, microglia activated by Aβ have the capacity to produce large amounts of reactive oxygen species via NADPH oxidase and can thus serve as an alternative source of free radicals [70, 171–175]. Recent data have also indicated that some microglia associated with plaques in the AD brain may produce myeloperoxidase (MPO) [176]. MPO produces hypochlorous acid, which can proceed further to form a number of other reactive oxygen species.

Table 1 - Inflammatory markers in AD

Protein mediator	**Δ in AD**	**Where located**	**Cell**
Complement proteins			
Classical pathway			
Clr	↑	Plaques [76], neurons [76], homogenates [98] mRNAs [98]	N
Cls	↑	Plaques [76], neurons [76], homogenates [98] mRNAs [98, 177]	N
Clq	↑	3.6X in superior frontal gyrus [178]	N
	↑	Plaques [73, 76, 179–186], NFTs [181, 182, 187], neurons [76, 179], dystrophic neurites [181, 182], homogenates [76, 98]	N
	↑	mRNAs [75, 95, 98, 186]	M,N
	↑	mRNAs [177]	
		mRNAs – 3.5X in frontal cortex [97, 188]	
C2	↑	Plaques [76], neurons [76], homogenates [76, 98]	N
	↑	mRNAs [75, 98]	
	↑	Plaques [76, 181, 182, 184, 185, 189–192]	
C3	↔	mRNAs [73]	
	↑	mRNAs [75, 97, 98, 188]	N
	↑	Homogenates [76, 98]	
	↑	Plaques [184]	
C3a	↑	Plaques [183, 193]	
C3b	↑	Plaques [182–184, 186, 193]	
C3c	↑	Plaques [182, 184, 186]	
C3d	↑	NFTs, dystrophic neurites [181–183, 185, 194, 195]	
	↑	Homogenates [98]	
	↑	Oligodendroglial fibers [196]	O
	↑	Plaques [76, 181, 183–185, 191, 197]	
C4	↑	mRNAs [75, 95, 198]	N
	↑	mRNAs [97, 98]	
	↑	NFTs [181], neurons [76]	N
	↑	Homogenates [76, 98]	
	↑	Plaques [182]	
C4d	↑	Homogenates [98]	
	↑	NFTs [182, 199], dystrophic neurites [181, 182, 187]	
	↑	Degenerating myelin sheaths [196]	O

Table 1 - Inflammatory markers in AD (continued)

Protein mediator	Δ in AD	Where located	Cell
Complement proteins (continued)			
Terminal pathway			
C5	↑	mRNAs [75, 98]	N
	↑	Plaques [76], neurons [76]	N
	↑	Homogenates [76, 98]	
C6	↑	Plaques [76, 193], neurons [76]	N
	↑	mRNAs [75, 98]	N
	↑	Homogenates [76, 98]	
C7	↑	Plaques [76], neurons [76], NFTs [200]	N
	↑	mRNAs [75, 98]	N
	↑	Homogenates [76, 98]	
C8	↑	Plaques [76], neurons [76]	N
	↑	mRNAs [75, 98]	N
	↑	Homogenates [76, 98]	
C9	↑	Plaques [76, 201], neurons [76]	N
	↑	Homogenates [76, 98, 201]	
	↑	mRNAs [75, 98, 201, 202]	N
	↑	NFTs, dystrophic neurites [201]	
C5b-9 (MAC)	↑	Myelinated and unmyelinated neurons (endocytic vesicles) [203]	N
	↑	Plaques [181, 182, 201]	
	↑	NFTs, dystrophic neurites [181, 182, 201]	
	↑	Homogenates [98, 201]	
Alternative pathway			
Factor B, Ba, Bb	↑	Plaques, frontal cortex [96]	N
	↑	Serum AD vs ND [204]	
Properdin	↑	Serum AD vs ND [204]	
Complement defense proteins			
Factor H, FHL-1	↑	Plaques, frontal cortex [96, 205]	N, M, A
Factor I	↑	Plaques, frontal cortex [96]	N
CD59 (Protectin, MIRL)	↑	Plaques [202, 206]	
	↑	Tangled neurons, dystrophic neurites [206]	
	↑	RNA extracts from brain [206]	
	↑	Slightly increased in AD vs ND brains [207]	
	↓	Deficiency in AD brain vs ND [208]	

Table 1 - Inflammatory markers in AD (continued)

Protein mediator	**Δ in AD**	**Where located**	**Cell**
Complement proteins (continued)			
Complement defense proteins			
Clusterin (APOJ, SP40, 40)	↑	Plaques [202, 209–212], pyramidal neurons	N, A
	↑	[202, 210, 213], dystrophic neurites [202],	
	↑	neuropil threads [202, 210], NFTs [202, 210],	
	↑	CAA [214], astrocytes [213]	
	↑	CSF [209]	
	↑	homogenates [213]	
	↑	mRNAs [210, 215]	N
Vitronectin (S-protein)	↑	Plaques [189, 202, 216, 217], NFTs [202, 216]	M
	↑	Dystrophic neurites, neuropil threads [202]	
C4-binding protein (C4BP)	↑	Plaques, CSF, cerebral cortex and microvessels [218–220]	
C1-inhibitor (C1-INH)	↑	Plaques, dystrophic neurites, neuropil threads, pyramidal neurons, astrocytes, [177, 207, 221, 222]	N, M, A
Complement receptors			
Complement receptor 3 (CR3)	↑	Activated microglia [189, 190, 223]	M
Complement receptor 4 (CR4)	↑	Activated microglia [223]	M
C3a receptor	↑	[224, 225]	N, M, A
C5a receptor	↑	[225, 226]	N, M, A
Vitronectin receptor	↑	Activated microglia in classical plaques [189, 190, 216]	M
Cytokines			
Interleukin-1α (IL-1α)	↑	Plaque associated microglia [227–229]	M
Interleukin-1β (IL-1β)	↑	Homogenates from frontal cortex, parietal cortex, temporal cortex, hypothalamus, thalamus and hippocampus [190, 230]	
	↑	NFTs associated microglia [231]	M
	↑	Activated microglia and astrocytes in AD [232]	M, A
	↑	Plasma [233], CSF [234]	
ICE caspase	↑	Hippocampus and parahippocampus [235]	

Table 1 - Inflammatory markers in AD (continued)

Protein mediator	Δ in AD	Where located	Cell
Cytokines (continued)			
S100β	↑	Reactive astrocytes around plaques [47, 236–240], around NFT [231]	A
	↑	Activated microglia and astrocytes in AD [232]	M, A
	↑	Hippocampus and temporal cortex [236]	
Interleukin-2 (IL-2)	↑	AD cortex [99, 241], Hippocampus [240]	M
Interleukin-6 (IL-6)	↑	Plaques [146, 148, 242–244]	
	↑	mRNA [245, 246]	M
	↑	Temporal cortex AD vs ND [247]	
	↑	Neurons [148]	N
	↑	Plasma [233, 233, 248, 249], CSF [234]	
	↑	CSF [250]	
Tumor necrosis factor	↑	Serum AD vs ND [251, 252]	
(TNFα)	↑	Serum AD vs ND [253]	
	↑	CSF AD vs ND [252, 254]	
IFNα	↑	Subset of neurons [255, 256]	N
	↑	White matter and activated microglia [255–257]	M
M-CSF	↑	Microglia [258] and neurons [92] around plaques	M, N
	↑	CSF (5X) [92]	
Pleiotrophin (PTN or HB-GAM)	↑	Plaques with dystrophic neurites [259]	
TGFβ	↑	Serum [260, 261], CSF [261]	
TGFβ1	↑	Plaques [262, 263]	
	↑	NFT [262, 263]	
TGFβ2	↑	NFT [264]	
	↑	Neurites, astrocytes, microglia [262]	A, M
	↑	Cortex (3.2X) [264]	
TGFβ3	↑	Hirano bodies [262]	
Midkine	↑	Plaques and homogenates [265]	
FGF-a (acidic)	↑↓	Entorhinal cortex neurons [266]	N
	↑	Plaque associated astrocytes [267]	A
FGF-b (basic)	↑	Plaques [268, 269], NFTs [270], neurons and astrocytes [268, 270], mRNAs [270]	N, A
FGF-9	↑	Dystrophic neurites, neurons, astrocytes [271]	N, A
IGF (insulin-like growth	↑	Subpopulation of astrocytes [272]	A
factor)	↑	Serum and CSF [273]	

Table 1 - Inflammatory markers in AD (continued)

Protein mediator	Δ in AD	Where located	Cell
Cytokines (continued)			
HGF (hepatocyte growth factor)	↑	Astrocyte, microglia, some neurons [274]	A, M, N
VEGF	↑	Astrocytes, vessels, perivascular deposits [275]	A
PDGF-AA and BB	↑	Neurons (AA, BB), vessels (AA), NFTs (BB) [276]	N
NGF (nerve growth factor)	↑	Hippocampus [277, 278]	
	↑	Frontal cortex [277–280]	
	↑	Temporal cortex [278, 279]	
	↑	Dentate Gyrus [281]	
	↑	Parietal Cortex [278, 282]	
	↑	Superior frontal gyrus [278]	
	↑	Occipital cortex [278, 280]	
	↑	Amygdala [278]	
	↑	Putamen [278]	
Decreased in these structures due	↓	Nucleus basalis of Meynert [278]	
to failure of retrograde transport of	↓	Nucleus basalis of Meynert [283]	N
NGF in cholinergic neurons	↓	Cholinergic basal forebrain neurons [284]	N
	↑	CSF [285]	
BDNF (brain derived	↓	Hippocampus and parietal cortex [277]	
neurotrophic factor)	↓	Entorhinal cortex [281]	
	↓	mRNA parietal lobe [286], hippocampus [287, 288]	N
	↓	Hippocampus and neocortex neurons [289–291]	N
	↑	Plaques [292]	
	↑	Dystrophic neurites [291]	
Trk-A (NGF receptor)	↓	mRNAs 2X in parietal cortex [293]	N
	↓	Nucleus Basalis cholinergic neur. [294–297]	N
	↓	Nucleus Basalis and frontal cortex [294]	N
	↓	mRNAs in cholinergic neurons of nucleus basalis, ventral striatum, and putamen [298, 299]	N
	↑	mRNAs in hippocampus [300]	
	↑	Plaques associated hippocampal astrocytes [300]	A
	↑	Plaques in hippocampus and temporal cortex [300]	
Trk-B (catalytic p145)	↓	Temporal and frontal cortex [301]	
(BDNF receptor)	NC	Neuronal perikarya of hippocampus and cortex [289]	N
	↓	Frontal cortex [291]	
	↓	Frontal cortex neurons [291]	N

Table 1 - Inflammatory markers in AD (continued)

Protein mediator	Δ in AD	Where located	Cell
Cytokines (continued)			
Trk-B (catalytic p145)	↑	Glial cells (especially around plaques) [291, 300]	M, A
(BDNF receptor)	↓	Nucleus basalis cholinergic neurons [296]	N
	↑	Plaques in hippocampus and temporal cortex [300]	
Trk-C (NGF receptor)	↓	Nucleus basalis cholinergic neurons [296]	N
Cytokine receptors			
sIL-1RII	↑	CSF [302]	
IL-1RA	↔	Temporal cortex homogeneates [247]	
	↑	Plaques, neurons, some microglia and NFTs [303]	M, N
CSFR-1 (rec. for M-CSF)	↑	Plaque associated and reactive microglia [258]	M
IL-6R	↓	CSF AD vs ND [304]	
sIL-6R	↓	CSF AD vs ND [304, 305]	
gü130	↓	CSF AD vs ND [305]	
TβR I (type I ser/thr kin.rec.)	↑	Microglia and neurons [306]	M, N
TβR II (type II ser/thr kin.rec.)	↑	Microglia and neurons [306]	M, N
FAS (CD95)	↑	Frontal and temporal lobe homogenates [307]	
	↑	Neurons and dystrophic neurites [307, 308]	N
	↑	Plaques and associated astrocytes [308]	
EGFR	↑	Neuritic plaques [309], endothelial cells [310]	E
FGFR-1	↑	Plaque associated astrocytes, neurons, mRNAs [311]	A, N
FGFR-3	↑	Plaque associated astrocytes [312]	
Chemokines and receptors			
Chemokines		In AD: Reviewed in [104]	
IP-10	↑	Astrocytes (especially around plaques) [313]	A
MIP-1α (CCβ)	↑	Neurons, microglia (weakly) [314]	N, M
MIP-1β (CCβ)	↑	Astrocytes (especially around plaques) [313, 314]	A
MIP-1 (CCβ)	↑	Plaques, microglia [315]	M
Chemokine receptors		In AD: Reviewed in [104]	
CXCR3 (IP-10 receptor)	↑	Neurons [313]	N
CXCR2 (IL-8RB)	↑	Plaques [316, 317]	
	↑	Neurons and dystrophic neurites [317]	N
CCR3	↑	Microglia (especially in plaques) [314]	M
	↑	Microglia (especially in plaques) [314]	M

Table 1 - Inflammatory markers in AD (continued)

Protein mediator	Δ in AD	Where located	Cell
Cell surface markers			
MHCI	↑	Endothelial cells [182, 318], microglia [318, 319]	E, M
MHCII – HLA-DR	↑	Activated microglia (concentrated in plaques) [99, 182, 190, 193, 223, 241, 318–323]	M
	↑	[324]	M
MHCII – HLA-DP	↑	[241]	M
MHCII – HLA-DQ	↑	[241]	M
LCA	↑	Activated microglia [223]	M
Cyclooxygenase (COX) and eicosanoids			
Cyclooxygenase		COX in AD: Reviewed in [109]	
PLA_2 (phospholipase A_2)	↓	Cerebral cortex (multiple areas) [325–327]	
$cPLA_2$ (cytosolic PLA_2)	↑	Cerebral cortex protoplasmic astrocytes [328]	A
COX-1	↑	Cortical homogenates [110, 329]	
	↑	Hippocampus and neocortex neurons [329, 330]	N
	↑	Microglia (especially in plaques) [330]	M
	↑	mRNAs [329, 331]	
COX-2	↑	Frontal [111], hippocampal [77], and temporal	N
	↑	cortex [110], neurons [80, 329] and NFTs [80]	
	↑	mRNAs [329, 331, 332]	
PGHS-2 (COX-2)	↓	mRNAs [333, 334]	
Eicosanoids			
Prostaglandin D2 (PGD2)	↓	Cortex AD vs ND [335, 336]	
Prostaglandin E2 (PGE2)	↓	Frontal cortex AD vs ND [335]	
	↑	5X in CSF [337]	
Prostaglandin F1α (PGF1α)	↓	4X in CSF [337]	
Prostaglandin F2α (PGF2α)	↓	Frontal cortex AD vs ND [335]	
Isoprostanes	↑	CSF [337–339], cortex [339, 340]	
Thromboxane B2 (TXB2)	↓	Cortex AD vs ND [335, 336]	
Coagulation and fibrinolysis systems			
Prothrombin	↑	In areas of vascular damage [341]	
Thrombin	↑	Plaques, tangles [342–345]	
Antithrombin	↑	Plaques, tangles, paired helical filaments, dystrophic neurites, some astrocytes, mRNAs [346]	A

Table 1 - Inflammatory markers in AD (continued)

Protein mediator	Δ in AD	Where located	Cell
Coagulation and fibrinolysis systems (continued)			
Tissue factor (thromboplastin)	↑	Plaques [347]	
Tissue factor pathway inhibitor-1	↑	Plaques and microglia [348]	M
Hageman factor	↑	Plaques, mRNAs [349]	
TPA	↑	Plaques [350]	
UPA	↑	Plaques [350], Serum activity and conc. [351]	
PAI I	↑	Plaques [350], CSF [352]	
PAI II	↑	Activated microglia [353]	M
Protease nexin-1 (PN-1)	↓	Activity decreased ≈85%, AD homogenates [354]	
	↓	Immunoreactivity and number of blood vessels [355]	
	↓	Cortical homogenates and immunoreactivity [356]	
	↑	Plaques, NFTs [354, 357]	
Protease nexin-1/ thrombin complex	↑	AD homogenates [354] (increased complexes but decreased free PN-1)	
Protease nexin-2 (PN2 or AβPP)	↓	Cortical homogenates and immunoreactivity [356]	
XIIIa	↑	Expressed in AD microglia [358]	M
Adhesion molecules			
ICAM-1	↑	Plaques [134, 189, 320, 359]	
	↑	Cerebrovascular endothelial cells [320]	E
	↑	Plaques and associated astrocytes [133]	A
ICAM-2	↑	Activated microglia [359]	M
NCAM	↔	Astrocytes, Cortical homogenates [360]	A
	↓	Frontal cortex neurons [361]	N
PSA-NCAM	↑	Hippocampal formation	
LFA-1 (CD11a)	↑	Activated microglia [134, 223, 320, 342]	M
VLA (very late antigen) α3	↑	Plaque corona [189]	
VLA α6	↑	Plaque corona [189]	
VLA β1	↑	Plaque corona [189]	
LeuCAM (β2 integrin)	↑	Activated microglia [189]	M
CD44	↑	Astrocytes AD vs ND [362]	A

Table 1 - Inflammatory markers in AD (continued)

Protein mediator	Δ in AD	Where located	Cell
Acute phase and other proteins		In AD: Reviewed in [363]	
α1-antichymotrypsin	↑	Plaques [197, 220, 364–367], tangles [197]	
(α1-ACT)	↑	Astrocytes [197, 365] , some neurons [365]	A, N
	↑	Serum [233, 368, 369], CSF [369]	
	↑	Serum [370]	
α2-macroglobulin (α2-MAC)	↑	Plaques [146, 148, 350, 371], microglia bordering plaques [371], hippocampal neurons [146, 148]	N, M
	↑	2X in AD vs ND [247]	
ApoE (apolipoprotein E)	↑	Plaques [211, 212, 220, 350]	
LRP (ApoE and α2-MAC receptors	↑	Plaques [350], NFTs [149], neurons [149, 150, 350], glia [149, 150]	N,M,A
α1-antitrypsin	↑	Plaques, tangles, astrocytes [197]	A
	↑	Serum [204, 372]	
Serum amyloid A	↑	Homogenates [373], mRNAs [373], serum [374]	
Serum amyloid P (pentraxin)	↑	Plaques, CAA [218, 375–377], NFTs [199, 376, 377]	
C-reactive protein (pentraxin)	↑	3X in AD vs ND [247]	
	↑	Plaques [148, 378], NFTs [379]	
Ceruloplasmin	↑	CSF [380]	
	↑	Homogenates, plaques, neurons, astrocytes [381]	N, A
	↓	Temporal cortex [382]	
ApoA-I	↑	Plaques [211]	
ApoA-IV	↑	Plaques [211]	
ApoD	↑	Plaques [211]	
Receptor associated protein	↑	Neuronal soma (inhibitor of LRP) [350]	N
Lipoprotein lipase	↑	Plaques [350]	
Lactoferrin/lactotransferrin	↑	Plaques [350]	
	↑	Plaques, neurons, NFTs, glia [378, 383, 384]	N,M,A
Free radicals and by-products		In AD: Reviewed in [160, 162, 163]	
AGEs	↑	Colocalized with astrocytes and microglia [164]	A, M
Malondialdehyde	↑	[163]	
8-hydroxy-deoxyguanosine	↑	mtDNA of parietal cortex [385], CSF [386]	
4-hydroxynonenal	↑	Plaques [165], ventricular fluid [387]	
	↑	Multiple brain regions [388]	
Glutathione S transferase	↓	Multiple brain regions and CSF [389]	
Nitrotyrosine (& derivatives)	↑	NFTs [166]	
	↑	Hippocampus, cortical regions, and CSF [169]	

Table 1 - Inflammatory markers in AD (continued)

Protein mediator	Δ in AD	Where located	Cell
Free radicals and by-products			
Peroxynitrite	↑	Neurons and NFT bearing neurons [167, 168]	N
Nitrotyrosine-modified prot.	↑	[166–169]	
p22-phox (NADPH subunit)	↑	[390]	
MPO (myeloperoxidase)	↑	Plaques and associated microglia [176]	M
Iron (Fe)	↑	Multiple brain regions [391–393]	
	↑	NFTs neurons vs non-NFT neurons in AD [394]	N
	↑	Plaques and associated microglia [395]	M
Ferritin	↑	Plaque associated microglia [395]	M
	↑	Ferritin has more Fe in AD [396]	
Melanotransferin	↑	Serum, CSF, plaque associated microglia [397, 398]	M
Lipid peroxidation	↑	Multiple brain regions [399–402]	
iNOS	↑	Hirano bodies, plaques, NFTs [403]	N
Transcription factors			
NF-κB	↑	Parallel increase with COX-2 mRNA [332]	
	↑	Hippocampus, entorhinal, temporal, and visual cortex neurons [170, 404–406]	N
	↑	Nucleus basalis cholinergic neurons [407]	N
PPAR-γ	↑	Temporal cortex [110]	
pCREB	↓	Phosphorylated CREB in hippocampus [408]	
ATF	↑	Cortical neurons [409]	N
c-fos	↑	Hippocampus neurons [410]	N
	↑	Hippocampus neurons [411]	N
	↑	Cortical and plaque associated astrocytes [412]	A
	↑	PHF-1 expressing neurons [412]	N
c-jun	↑	Hippocampus neurons [411, 413]	N
	↑	Cortical and plaque associated astrocytes [412, 414]	A
	↑	PHF-1 expressing neurons [412]	N
	↑	Meningeal and cerebral vessels with CAA [414]	
Krox24	↑	Hippocampus neurons [413]	N
STAT1	↑	Temporal cortex [406]	

Table 1 - Inflammatory markers in AD (continued)

Protein mediator	Δ in AD	Where located	Cell
Miscellaneous receptors			
Aβ-binding receptors			
RAGE	↑	Upregulated on neurons and microglia [35, 92]	N, M
MSR (macrophage	↑	Expressed on AD microglia [34, 415–417]	M
scavenger receptor)	↑	Plaques [417], (review [418])	
FPR (fMLP receptor)	↑	Chemotactic for Aβ [33] (expressed on AD microglia – D. Lorton, personal communication)	M
Other receptors			
FcγR1	↑	Activated microglia [193, 342]	M
FcγR2	↑	Activated microglia [193]	M

This table represents those factors that have been specifically detected in the AD brain or related material. It should be noted that many more inflammatory factors have been observed in cell culture and animal models. Thus, this list, without doubt, will continue to grow.

Abbreviations: WB, western blot; IHC, immunohistochemistry; ISH, in situ *hybridization; ELISA or EIA, enzyme linked immunosorbent assay; PCR, (reverse transcriptase) polymerase chain reaction; EM, electron microscopy; RIA, radio immunoassay; BA, bioassay; NB, northern blot; GC/MS, gas chromatography/mass spectroscopy; HPLC, high pressure liquid chromatography; EMSA, electrophoretic mobility shift assay; N, neuron; A, astrocyte; M, microglia; E, endothelia; O, oligodendroglia; NFTs, neurofibrillary tangles; ND, non-demented; AD, Alzheimer's disease; CSF, cerebral spinal fluid; MAC, membrane attack complex; ↑, increased in AD compared to ND; ↓, decreased in AD compared to ND; ↔, no difference between AD and ND; NC, not compared.*

References

1 Aisen PS, Davis KL (1994) Inflammatory mechanisms in Alzheimer's disease: implications for therapy. *Am J Psychiatry* 151: 1105–1113
2 McGeer PL, McGeer EG (1995) The inflammatory response system of brain: implications for therapy of Alzheimer and other neurodegenerative diseases. *Brain Res Rev* 21: 195–218
3 Rogers J, Webster S, Lue L-F, Brachova L, Civin WH, Emerling M, Shivers B, Walter D, McGeer PL (1996) Inflammation and Alzheimer's disease pathogenesis. *Neurobiol Aging* 17: 681–686
4 Rogers J, Griffin WST (1998) Inflammatory mechanisms of Alzheimer's disease. In: PL Wood (ed): *Neuroinflammation: mechanisms and management.* Humana Press Inc, Totowa, NJ, 177–193
5 Rogers J, O'Barr S (1996) Inflammatory mediators in Alzheimer's disease. In: RE Tanzi, W Wasco (eds): *Molecular approaches to Alzheimer's disease.* Humana Press, Totawa, N.J., 177–197
6 Esiri MM, Hyman BT, Beyreuther K, Masters CL (1997) Ageing and dementia. In: DI Graham, PL Lantos (eds): *Greenfield's neuropathology.* Arnold Press, London, 153–177
7 Nakawatase TV, Cummings JL (2000) Alzheimer's disease and related dementias. In: L Goldman, JC Bennet (eds): *Cecil textbook of medicine.* WB Saunders, Philadelphia, 2043–2045
8 Price DL (2000) Aging of the brain and dementia of the Alzheimer type. In: ER Kandel, JH Schwartz, TM Jessel (eds): *Principles of neural science.* McGraw-Hill, New York
9 Solodkin A, Van Hoesen GW (1997) Neuropathology and functional anatomy of Alzheimer's disease. In: J Brioni, M Decker (eds): *Pharmacological treatment of Alzheimer's disease: Molecular and neurobiological foundations.* Wiley-Liss, New York, 151–177
10 Katzman R (1994) Apolipoprotein E and Alzheimer's disease. *Curr Opin Neurobiol* 4: 703–707
11 Alzheimer A (1907) Über eine eigenartige Erkankung der Hirnrinde. *Allgemeine Zeitschrift für Psychiatrie und Gerichtliche Medizin* 64: 146–148
12 Warner MD, Peabody CA, Flattery JJ, Tinklenberg JR (1986) Olfactory deficits and Alzheimer's disease. *Biol Psychiatry* 21: 116–118
13 Du Y, Dodel RC, Eastwood BJ (2000) Association of an interleukin-1α polymorphism with Alzheimer's disease. *Neurology* 55: 480–483
14 Rogers J (2000) An IL-1 alpha susceptibility polymorphism in Alzheimer's disease:new fuel for the inflammation hypothesis. *Neurology* 55: 464–465
15 Griffin WS, Nicoll JA, Grimaldi LM, Sheng JG, Mrak RE (2000) The pervasiveness of interleukin-1 in Alzheimer pathogenesis: a role for specific polymorphisms in disease risk. *Exp Gerontol* 35: 481–487
16 Mrak RE, Griffin WS (2000) Interleukin-1 and the immunogenetics of Alzheimer disease. *J Neuropathol Exp Neurol* 59: 471–476
17 Nicoll JA, Mrak RE, Graham DI, Stewart J, Wilcock G, MacGowan S, Esiri MM, Mur-

ray LS, Dewar D, Love S et al (2000) Association of interleukin-1 gene polymorphisms with Alzheimer's disease. *Ann Neurol* 47: 365–368
18 Grimaldi LM, Casadei VM, Ferri C, Veglia F, Licastro F, Annoni G, Biunno I, De Bellis G, Sorbi S, Mariani C et al (2000) Association of early-onset Alzheimer's disease with an interleukin-1alpha gene polymorphism. *Ann Neurol* 47: 361–365
19 Papassotiropoulos A, Bagli M, Jessen F, Bayer TA, Maier W, Rao ML, Heun R (1999) A genetic variation of the inflammatory cytokine interleukin-6 delays the initial onset and reduces the risk for sporadic Alzheimer's disease. *Ann Neurol* 45: 666–668
20 Bhojak TJ, DeKosky ST, Ganguli M, Kamboh MI (2000) Genetic polymorphisms in the cathespin D and interleukin-6 genes and the risk of Alzheimer's disease. *Neurosci Lett* 288: 21–24
21 Bagli M, Papassotiropoulos A, Knapp M, Jessen F, Luise RM, Maier W, Heun R (2000) Association between an interleukin-6 promoter and 3' flanking region haplotype and reduced Alzheimer's disease risk in a German population. *Neurosci Lett* 283: 109–112
22 Neuroinflammation Working Group, Akiyama H, Barger S, Barnum S, Bauer J, Bradt B, Cole GM, Cooper NR, Eikelenboom P, Emmerling M et al (2000) Inflammation and Alzheimer's disease. *Neurobiol Aging* 21: 383–421
23 Terry RD, Masliah E, Salmon DP, Butters N, DeTeresa R, Hill R, Hansen LA, Katzman R (1991) Physical basis of cognitive alterations in Alzheimer's disease: synapse loss is the major correlate of cognitive impairment. *Ann Neurol* 30: 572–580
24 Kuby J (1994) The complement system. In: *Immunology*, W.H. Freeman and Company, New York, 393–415
25 Pangburn MK, Muller-Eberhard HJ (1984) The alternative pathway of complement. *Springer Semin Immunopathol* 7: 163–192
26 Whaley K, Schwaeble W (1997) Complement and complement deficiencies. *Semin Liver Dis* 17: 297–310
27 Muller-Eberhard HJ (1988) Molecular organization and function of the complement system. *Annu Rev Biochem* 57: 321–347
28 Majno G (1975) *The healing hand*. Harvard University Press
29 Kuby J (1994) Overview of the immune system. In: *Immunology*, W.H. Freeman and Company, New York, 1–21
30 Gewurz H, Ying SC, Jiang H, Lint TF (1993) Nonimmune activation of the classical complement pathway. *Behring Inst Mitt* 138–147
31 Jiang H, Burdick D, Glabe CG, Cotman CW, Tenner AJ (1994) β-Amyloid activates complement by binding to a specific region of the collagen-like domain of the C1q a chain. *J. Immunol* 152: 5050–5059
32 Webster S, Glabe C, Rogers J (1995) Multivalent binding of complement protein C1Q to the amyloid beta-peptide (A beta) promotes the nucleation phase of A beta aggregation. *Biochem Biophys Res Commun* 217: 869–875
33 Lorton D, Schaller J, Lala A, De Nardin E (2000) Chemotactic-like receptors and Abeta peptide induced responses in Alzheimer's Disease. *Neurobiol Aging* 21: 463–473
34 El Khoury J, Hickman SE, Thomas CA, Cao L, Silverstein SC, Loike JD (1996) Scav-

enger receptor-mediated adhesion of microglia to beta-amyloid fibrils. *Nature* 382: 716–719

35 Yan SD, Chen X, Fu J, Chen M, Zhu H, Roher A, Slattery T, Zhao L, Nagashima M, Morser J et al (1996) RAGE and amyloid-beta peptide neurotoxicity in Alzheimer's disease. *Nature* 382: 685–691

36 Schenk D, Barbour R, Dunn W, Gordon G, Grajeda H, Guido T, Hu K, Huang J, Johnson-Wood K, Khan K et al (1999) Immunization with amyloid-beta attenuates Alzheimer-disease-like pathology in the PDAPP mouse. *Nature* 400: 173–177

37 Kandal ER, Schwartz JH, Jessel TM (2000) *Principles of neural science*. McGraw-Hill, New York

38 Andriezen WL (1893) On a system of fibre-like cells surrounding the blood vessels of the brain of man and mammals and its physiological significance. *Int Monatsschr Anat Physiol* 10: 532–540

39 Montgomery DL (1994) Astrocytes: form, functions, and roles in disease. *Vet Pathol* 31: 145–167

40 Malhotra SK, Shnitka TK, Elbrink J (1990) Reactive astrocytes – a review. *Cytobios* 61: 133–160

41 Schechter R, Yen SH, Terry RD (1981) Fibrous Astrocytes in senile dementia of the Alzheimer type. *J Neuropathol Exp Neurol* 40: 95–101

42 Wisniewski HM, Wegiel J, Wang KC, Kujawa M, Lach B (1989) Ultrastructural studies of the cells forming amyloid fibers in classical plaques. *Can J Neurol Sci* 16: 535–542

43 Mandybur TI, Ormsby I, Zemlan FP (1989) Cerebral aging: a quantitative study of gliosis in old nude mice. *Acta Neuropathol (Berlin)* 77: 507–513

44 Dickson DW, Farlo J, Davies P, Crystal H, Fuld P, Yen SH (1988) Alzheimer's disease. A double-labeling immunohistochemical study of senile plaques. *Am J Pathol* 132: 86–101

45 Mandybur TI (1989) Cerebral amyloid angiopathy and astrocytic gliosis in Alzheimer's disease. *Acta Neuropathol (Berlin)* 78: 329–331

46 Wisniewski HM, Sinatra RS, Iqbal K, Grunde-Iqbal I (1981) Neurofibrillary and synaptic pathology in the aged brain. In: AE Johnson (ed): *Aging and cell structure*. Plenum Publishing, New York, 105–142

47 Mrak RE, Sheng JG, Griffin WS (1996) Correlation of astrocytic S100 beta expression with dystrophic neurites in amyloid plaques of Alzheimer's disease. *J Neuropathol Exp Neurol* 55: 273–279

48 DeWitt DA, Perry G, Cohen M, Doller C, Silver J (1998) Astrocytes regulate microglial phagocytosis of senile plaque cores of Alzheimer's disease. *Exp Neurol* 149: 329–340

49 Shaffer LM, Dority MD, Gupta-Bansal R, Frederickson RC, Younkin SG, Brunden KR (1995) Amyloid beta protein (Aβ) removal by neuroglial cells in culture. *Neurobiol Aging* 16: 737–745

50 Johnson AB, Blum NR (1970) Nucleoside phosphatase activities associated with the tangles and plaques of alzheimer's disease: a histochemical study of natural and experimental neurofibrillary tangles. *J Neuropathol Exp Neurol* 29: 463–478

51 Braak E, Braak H, Mandelkow EM (1994) A sequence of cytoskeleton changes related

to the formation of neurofibrillary tangles and neuropil threads. *Acta Neuropathol (Berlin)* 87: 554–567

52 Bancher C, Brunner C, Lassmann H, Budka H, Jellinger K, Wiche G, Seitelberger F, Grundke-Iqbal I, Iqbal K, Wisniewski HM (1989) Accumulation of abnormally phosphorylated tau precedes the formation of neurofibrillary tangles in Alzheimer's disease. *Brain Res* 477: 90–99

53 Eddleston M, Mucke L (1993) Molecular profile of reactive astrocytes – implications for their role in neurologic disease. *Neuroscience* 54: 15–36

54 Wegiel J, Wisniewski HM (1998) Astrocyte pathology in Alzheimer's Disease. In: HM Schipper (ed): *Astrocytes in brain aging and neurodegeneration.* R.G. Landes Company, Austin, TX, 91–109

55 Probst A, Ulrich J, Heitz PU (1982) Senile dementia of Alzheimer type: astroglial reaction to extracellular neurofibrillary tangles in the hippocampus. An immunocytochemical and electron-microscopic study. *Acta Neuropathol (Berlin)* 57: 75–79

56 Yamaguchi H, Morimatsu M, Hirai S, Takahashi K (1987) Alzheimer's neurofibrillary tangles are penetrated by astroglial processes and appear eosinophilic in their final stages. *Acta Neuropathol (Berlin)* 72: 214–217

57 Perry VH, Hume DA, Gordon S (1985) Immunohistochemical localization of macrophages and microglia in the adult and developing mouse brain. *Neuroscience* 15: 313–326

58 Perry VH, Bell MD, Anthony DC (1999) Unique aspects of inflammation in the central nervous system. In: RR Ruffolo, GZ Feuerstain, AJ Hunter, G Poste, BW Metcalf (eds): *Inflammatory cells and mediators in CNS diseases.* Harwood Academic Publishers, Canada, 21–38

59 Barron KD (1995) The microglial cell. A historical review. *J Neurol Sci* 134 (Suppl): 57–68

60 Kreutzberg GW (1996) Microglia: a sensor for pathological events in the CNS. *Trends Neurosci* 19: 312–318

61 Giulian D (1987) Ameboid microglia as effectors of inflammation in the central nervous system. *J Neurosci Res* 18: 155–3

62 McGeer PL, McGeer EG (1995) Central nervous system immune reactions in Alzheimer's disease. In: NJ Rothwell (ed): *Immune responses in the nervous system.* Bios Scientific Publishers, Manchester, UK, 143–157

63 Chao CC, Hu S, Sheng WS, Kravitz FH, Peterson PK (1999) Inflammation-mediated neuronal cell injury. RR Ruffolo, GZ Feuerstain, AJ Hunter, G Poste, BW Metcalf (eds): *Inflammatory cells and mediators in CNS diseases.* Harwood Academic Publishers, Canada, 483–495

64 Streit WJ, Walter SA, Pennell NA (1999) Reactive microgliosis. *Prog Neurobiol* 57: 563–581

65 Walker DG (1998) Inflammatory markers in chronic neurodegenerative disorders with emphasis on Alzheiemer's disease. In: PL Wood (ed): *Neuroinflammation: mechanisms and management.* Humana Press Inc, Totowa, NJ, 61–90

66 Piani D, Spranger M, Frei K, Schaffner A, Fontana A (1992) Macrophage-induced cytotoxicity of N-methyl-D-aspartate receptor positive neurons involves excitatory amino acids rather than reactive oxygen intermediates and cytokines. *Eur J Immunol* 22: 2429–2436
67 Espey MG, Chernyshev ON, Reinhard JFJ, Namboodiri MA, Colton CA (1997) Activated human microglia produce the excitotoxin quinolinic acid. *Neuroreport* 8: 431–434
68 Leist M, Nicotera P (1999) Calcium and cell death. In: VE Koliatsos, RR Ratan (eds): *Cell death and diseases of the nervous system.* Humana Press, Totowa, NJ, 69-90
69 McDonald DR, Bamberger ME, Combs CK, Landreth GE (1998) beta-Amyloid fibrils activate parallel mitogen-activated protein kinase pathways in microglia and THP1 monocytes. *J Neurosci* 18: 4451–4460
70 McDonald DR, Brunden KR, Landreth GE (1997) Amyloid fibrils activate tyrosine kinase-dependent signaling and superoxide production in microglia. *J Neurosci* 17: 2284–2294
71 Wood JG, Zinsmeister P (1991) Tyrosine phosphorylation systems in Alzheimer's disease pathology. *Neurosci Lett* 121: 12–16
72 Combs CK, Johnson DE, Cannady SB, Lehman TM, Landreth GE (1999) Identification of microglial signal transduction pathways mediating a neurotoxic response to amyloidogenic fragments of beta-amyloid and prion proteins. *J Neurosci* 19: 928–939
73 Fischer B, Schmoll H, Riederer P, Bauer J, Platt D, Popa-Wagner A (1995) Complement C1q and C3 mRNA expression in the frontal cortex of Alzheimer's patients. *J Mol Med*73: 465–471
74 Pasinetti GM, Johnson SA, Rozovsky I, Lampert-Etchells M, Morgan DG, Gordon MN, Morgan TE, Willoughby D, Finch CE (1992) Complement C1qB and C4 mRNAs responses to lesioning in rat brain. *Exp Neurol* 118: 117–125
75 Shen Y, Li R, McGeer EG, McGeer PL (1997) Neuronal expression of mRNAs for complement proteins of the classical pathway in Alzheimer brain. Brain Res. 769: 391–395
76 Terai K, Walker DG, McGeer EG, McGeer PL (1997) Neurons express proteins of the classical complement pathway in Alzheimer disease. *Brain Res* 769: 385–390
77 Ho L, Pieroni C, Winger D, Purohit DP, Aisen PS, Pasinetti GM (1999) Regional distribution of cyclooxygenase-2 in the hippocampal formation in Alzheimer's disease. *J Neurosci Res* 57: 295–303
78 Nakayama M, Uchimura K, Zhu RL, Nagayama T, Rose ME, Stetler RA, Isakson PC, Chen J, Graham SH (1998) Cyclooxygenase-2 inhibition prevents delayed death of CA1 hippocampal neurons following global ischemia. *Proc Natl Acad Sci USA* 95: 10954–10959
79 Nogawa S, Zhang F, Ross ME, Iadecola C (1997) Cyclo-oxygenase-2 gene expression in neurons contributes to ischemic brain damage. *J Neurosci* 17: 2746–2755
80 Oka A, Takashima S (1997) Induction of cyclo-oxygenase 2 in brains of patients with Down's syndrome and dementia of Alzheimer type: specific localization in affected neurones and axons. *Neuroreport* 8: 1161–1164

81 Tocco G, Freire-Moar J, Schreiber SS, Sakhi SH, Aisen PS, Pasinetti GM (1997) Maturational regulation and regional induction of cyclooxygenase-2 in rat brain: implications for Alzheimer's disease. *Exp Neurol* 144: 339–349

82 Yamagata K, Andreasson KI, Kaufmann WE, Barnes CA, Worley PF (1993) Expression of a mitogen-inducible cyclooxygenase in brain neurons: regulation by synaptic activity and glucocorticoids. *Neuron* 11: 371–386

83 Botchkina GI, Meistrell ME, Botchkina IL, Tracey KJ (1997) Expression of TNF and TNF receptors (p55 and p75) in the rat brain after focal cerebral ischemia. *Mol Med* 3: 765–781

84 Breder CD, Tsujimoto M, Terano Y, Scott DW, Saper CB (1993) Distribution and characterization of tumor necrosis factor-alpha-like immunoreactivity in the murine central nervous system. *J Comp Neurol* 337: 543–567

85 Gong C, Qin Z, Betz AL, Liu XH, Yang GY (1998) Cellular localization of tumor necrosis factor alpha following focal cerebral ischemia in mice. *Brain Res* 801: 1–8

86 Murphy PG, Borthwick LS, Johnston RS, Kuchel G, Richardson PM (1999) Nature of the retrograde signal from injured nerves that induces interleukin-6 mRNA in neurons. *J Neurosci* 19: 3791–3800

87 Orzylowska O, Oderfeld-Nowak B, Zaremba M, Januszewski S, Mossakowski M (1999) Prolonged and concomitant induction of astroglial immunoreactivity of interleukin-1beta and interleukin-6 in the rat hippocampus after transient global ischemia. *Neurosci Lett* 263: 72–76

88 Suzuki S, Tanaka K, Nagata E, Ito D, Dembo T, Fukuuchi Y (1999) Cerebral neurons express interleukin-6 after transient forebrain ischemia in gerbils. *Neurosci Lett* 262: 117–120

89 Tchelingerian JL, Vignais L, Jacque C (1994) TNF alpha gene expression is induced in neurones after a hippocampal lesion. *Neuroreport* 5: 585–588

90 Yan SD, Yan SF, Chen X, Fu J, Chen M, Kuppusamy P, Smith MA, Perry G, Godman GC, Nawroth P (1995) Non-enzymatically glycated tau in Alzheimer's disease induces neuronal oxidant stress resulting in cytokine gene expression and release of amyloid beta-peptide. *Nat Med* 1: 693–699

91 Ip NY, Nye SH, Boulton TG, Davis S, Taga T, Li Y, Birren SJ, Yasukawa K, Kishimoto T, Anderson DJ (1992) CNTF and LIF act on neuronal cells via shared signaling pathways that involve the IL-6 signal transducing receptor component gp130. *Cell* 69: 1121–1132

92 Yan SD, Zhu H, Fu J, Yan SF, Roher A, Tourtellotte WW, Rajavashisth T, Chen X, Godman GC, Stern D et al (1997) Amyloid-beta peptide-receptor for advanced glycation endproduct interaction elicits neuronal expression of macrophage-colony stimulating factor: a proinflammatory pathway in Alzheimer disease. *Proc Natl Acad Sci USA* 94: 5296–5301

93 Prodinger WM, Wurzner R, Erdei A, Dierich M (1999) Complement. In: WE Paul (ed): *Fundamental immunology.* Lippincott/Raven, Philadelphia, 967–995

94 Morgan BP, Gasque P (1997) Extrahepatic complement biosynthesis: where, when and why? *Clin Exp Immunol* 107: 1–7
95 Johnson SA, Lampert-Etchells M, Pasinetti GM, Rozovsky I, Finch CE (1992) Complement mRNA in the mammalian brain: responses to Alzheimer's disease and experimental brain lesioning. *Neurobiol Aging* 13: 641–648
96 Strohmeyer R, Shen Y, Rogers J (2000) Detection of complement alternative pathway mRNA and proteins in Alzheimer's disease brain. *Mol Brain Res* 81: 7–18
97 Walker DG, McGeer PL (1992) Complement gene expression in human brain: comparison between normal and Alzheimer disease cases. *Mol Brain Res* 14: 109–116
98 Yasojima K, Schwab C, McGeer EG, McGeer PL (1999) Up-regulated production and activation of the complement system in Alzheimer's disease brain. *Am J Pathol* 154: 927–936
99 Rogers J, Luber-Narod J, Styren SD, Civin WH (1988) Expression of immune system-associated antigens by cells of the human central nervous system: relationship to the pathology of Alzheimer's disease. *Neurobiol Aging* 9: 339–349
100 Linder E, Lehto VP, Stenman S (1979) Activation of complement by cytoskeletal intermediate filaments. *Nature* 278: 176–178
101 Finch CE (1999) *Clusterin in normal brain functions and during neurodegeneration.* RG Landes, Austin, TX
102 Johns TG, Bernard CC (1997) Binding of complement component C1q to myelin oligodendrocyte glycoprotein: a novel mechanism for regulating CNS inflammation. *Mol Immunol* 34: 33–38
103 Abbas A, Lichtman A, Pober JS (2000) *Cellular and molecular immunology.* WB Saunders, Philadelphia
104 Xia MQ, Hyman BT (1999) Chemokines/chemokine receptors in the central nervous system and Alzheimer's disease. *J Neurovirol* 5: 32–41
105 Akwa Y, Hassett DE, Eloranta ML, Sandberg K, Masliah E, Powell H, Whitton JL, Bloom FE, Campbell IL (1998) Transgenic expression of IFN-alpha in the central nervous system of mice protects against lethal neurotropic viral infection but induces inflammation and neurodegeneration. *J Immunol* 161: 5016–5026
106 Stalder AK, Carson MJ, Pagenstecher A, Asensio VC, Kincaid C, Benedict M, Powell HC, Masliah E, Campbell IL (1998) Late-onset chronic inflammatory encephalopathy in immune-competent and severe combined immune-deficient (SCID) mice with astrocyte-targeted expression of tumor necrosis factor. *Am J Pathol* 153: 767–783
107 Heyser CJ, Masliah E, Samimi A, Campbell IL, Gold LH (1997) Progressive decline in avoidance learning paralleled by inflammatory neurodegeneration in transgenic mice overexpressing interleukin 6 in the brain. *Proc Natl Acad Sci* 94: 1500–1505
108 Brett FM, Mizisin AP, Powell HC, Campbell IL (1995) Evolution of neuropathologic abnormalities associated with blood-brain barrier breakdown in transgenic mice expressing interleukin-6 in astrocytes. *J Neuropathol Exp Neurol* 54: 766–775
109 O'Banion MK (1999) Cyclooxygenase-2: molecular biology, pharmacology, and neurobiology. *Crit Rev Neurobiol* 13: 45–82

110 Kitamura Y, Shimohama S, Koike H, Kakimura J, Matsuoka Y, Nomura Y, Gebicke-Haerter PJ, Taniguchi T (1999) Increased expression of cyclooxygenases and peroxisome proliferator-activated receptor-gamma in Alzheimer's disease brains. *Biochem Biophys Res Commun* 254: 582–586

111 Pasinetti GM, Aisen PS (1998) Cyclooxygenase-2 expression is increased in frontal cortex of Alzheimer's disease brain. *Neuroscience* 87: 319–324

112 Bauer MK, Lieb K, Schulze-Osthoff K, Berger M, Gebicke-Haerter PJ, Bauer J, Fiebich BL (1997) Expression and regulation of cyclooxygenase-2 in rat microglia. *Eur J Biochem* 243: 726–731

113 Minghetti L, Polazzi E, Nicolini A, Creminon C, Levi G (1996) Interferon-gamma and nitric oxide down-regulate lipopolysaccharide- induced prostanoid production in cultured rat microglial cells by inhibiting cyclooxygenase-2 expression. *J Neurochem* 66: 1963–1970

114 O'Banion MK, Miller JC, Chang JW, Kaplan MD, Coleman PD (1996) Interleukin-1 beta induces prostaglandin G/H synthase-2 (cyclooxygenase- 2) in primary murine astrocyte cultures. *J Neurochem* 66: 2532–2540

115 Blom MA, van Twillert MG, de Vries SC, Engels F, Finch CE, Veerhuis R, Eikelenboom P (1997) NSAIDS inhibit the IL-1 beta-induced IL-6 release from human post- mortem astrocytes: the involvement of prostaglandin E2. *Brain Res.* 777: 210–218

116 Fiebich BL, Hull M, Lieb K, Gyufko K, Berger M, Bauer J (1997) Prostaglandin E2 induces interleukin-6 synthesis in human astrocytoma cells. *J Neurochem* 68: 704–709

117 Janabi N, Hau I, Tardieu M (1999) Negative feedback between prostaglandin and alpha- and beta-chemokine synthesis in human microglial cells and astrocytes. *J Immunol* 162: 1701–1706

118 Lee RK, Knapp S, Wurtman RJ (1999) Prostaglandin E2 stimulates amyloid precursor protein gene expression: inhibition by immunosuppressants. *J Neurosci* 19: 940–947

119 Kelley KA, Ho L, Winger D, Freire-Moar J, Borelli CB, Aisen PS, Pasinetti GM (1999) Potentiation of excitotoxicity in transgenic mice overexpressing neuronal cyclooxygenase-2. *Am J Pathol* 155: 995–1004

120 Pasinetti GM (1998) Cyclooxygenase and inflammation in Alzheimer's disease: experimental approaches and clinical interventions. *J Neurosci Res.* 54: 1–6

121 Jiang C, Ting AT, Seed B (1998) PPAR-gamma agonists inhibit production of monocyte inflammatory cytokines. *Nature* 391: 82–86

122 Lehmann JM, Lenhard JM, Oliver BB, Ringold GM, Kliewer SA (1997) Peroxisome proliferator-activated receptors alpha and gamma are activated by indomethacin and other non-steroidal anti-inflammatory drugs. *J Biol Chem* 272: 3406–3410

123 Lemberger T, Desvergne B, Wahli W (1996) Peroxisome proliferator-activated receptors: a nuclear receptor signaling pathway in lipid physiology. *Annu Rev Cell Dev Biol* 12: 335–363

124 Ricote M, Li AC, Willson TM, Kelly CJ, Glass CK (1998) The peroxisome proliferator-activated receptor-gamma is a negative regulator of macrophage activation. *Nature* 391: 79–82

125 Schmaier AH, Dahl LD, Rozemuller AJ, Roos RA, Wagner SL, Chung R, Van Nostrand WE (1993) Protease nexin-2/amyloid beta protein precursor. A tight-binding inhibitor of coagulation factor IXa. *J Clin Invest* 92: 2540–2545
126 Smith RP, Higuchi DA, Broze GJJ (1990) Platelet coagulation factor XIa-inhibitor, a form of Alzheimer amyloid precursor protein. *Science* 248: 1126–1128
127 Snow AD, Mar H, Nochlin D, Kimata K, Kato M, Suzuki S, Hassell J, Wight TN (1988) The presence of heparan sulfate proteoglycans in the neuritic plaques and congophilic angiopathy in Alzheimer's disease. *Am J Pathol* 133: 456–463
128 Iozzo RV (1998) Matrix proteoglycans: from molecular design to cellular function. *Annu Rev Biochem* 67: 609–652
129 Munoz-Fernandez MA, Fresno M (1998) The role of tumour necrosis factor, interleukin 6, interferon-gamma and inducible nitric oxide synthase in the development and pathology of the nervous system. *Prog Neurobiol* 56: 307–340
130 Cotman CW, Hailer NP, Pfister KK, Soltesz I, Schachner M (1998) Cell adhesion molecules in neural plasticity and pathology: similar mechanisms, distinct organizations? *Prog Neurobiol* 55: 659–669
131 Arvin B, Neville LF, Barone FC, Feuerstein GZ (1996) The role of inflammation and cytokines in brain injury. *Neurosci Biobehav Rev* 20: 445–452
132 Benveniste EN, Huneycutt BS, Shrikant P, Ballestas ME (1995) Second messenger systems in the regulation of cytokines and adhesion molecules in the central nervous system. *Brain Behav Immun* 9: 304–314
133 Akiyama H, Kawamata T, Yamada T, Tooyama I, Ishii T, McGeer PL (1993) Expression of intercellular adhesion molecule (ICAM)-1 by a subset of astrocytes in Alzheimer disease and some other degenerative neurological disorders. *Acta Neuropathol (Berlin)* 85: 628–634
134 Rozemuller JM, Eikelenboom P, Pals ST, Stam FC (1989) Microglial cells around amyloid plaques in Alzheimer's disease express leucocyte adhesion molecules of the LFA-1 family. *Neurosci Lett* 101: 288–292
135 Eriksson S, Janciauskiene S, Lannfelt L (1995) Alpha 1-antichymotrypsin regulates Alzheimer beta-amyloid peptide fibril formation. *Proc Natl Acad Sci USA* 92: 2313–2317
136 Fraser PE, Nguyen JT, McLachlan DR, Abraham CR, Kirschner DA (1993) Alpha 1-antichymotrypsin binding to Alzheimer A beta peptides is sequence specific and induces fibril disaggregation *in vitro*. *J Neurochem* 61: 298–305
137 Ma J, Yee A, Brewer HBJ, Das S, Potter H (1994) Amyloid-associated proteins alpha 1-antichymotrypsin and apolipoprotein E promote assembly of Alzheimer beta-protein into filaments. *Nature* 372: 92–94
138 Kamboh MI, Sanghera DK, Ferrell RE, DeKosky ST (1995) APOE*4-associated Alzheimer's disease risk is modified by alpha 1-antichymotrypsin polymorphism. *Nat Genet* 10: 486–488
139 Borth W (1992) α2-macroglobulin, a multifunctional binding protein with targeting characteristics. *FASEB J* 6: 3345–3353

140 Sottrup-Jensen L (1989) Alpha-macroglobulins: structure, shape, and mechanism of proteinase complex formation. *J Biol Chem* 264: 11539–11542
141 Kounnas MZ, Moir RD, Rebeck GW, Bush AI, Argraves WS, Tanzi RE, Hyman BT, Strickland DK (1995) LDL receptor-related protein, a multifunctional ApoE receptor, binds secreted beta-amyloid precursor protein and mediates its degradation. *Cell* 82: 331–340
142 Williams SE, Kounnas MZ, Argraves KM, Argraves WS, Strickland DK (1994) The alpha 2-macroglobulin receptor/low density lipoprotein receptor- related protein and the receptor-associated protein. An overview. *Ann NY Acad Sci* 737: 1–13
143 Du Y, Ni B, Glinn M, Dodel RC, Bales KR, Zhang Z, Hyslop PA, Paul SM (1997) alpha2-Macroglobulin as a beta-amyloid peptide-binding plasma protein. *J Neurochem* 69: 299–305
144 Hughes SR, Khorkova O, Goyal S, Knaeblein J, Heroux J, Riedel NG, Sahasrabudhe S (1998) Alpha2-macroglobulin associates with beta-amyloid peptide and prevents fibril formation. *Proc Natl Acad Sci USA* 95: 3275–3280
145 Du Y, Bales KR, Dodel RC, Liu X, Glinn MA, Horn JW, Little SP, Paul SM (1998) Alpha2-macroglobulin attenuates beta-amyloid peptide 1–40 fibril formation and associated neurotoxicity of cultured fetal rat cortical neurons. *J Neurochem* 70: 1182–1188
146 Bauer J, Strauss S, Schreiter-Gasser U, Ganter U, Schlegel P, Witt I, Yolk B, Berger M (1991) Interleukin-6 and alpha-2-macroglobulin indicate an acute-phase state in Alzheimer's disease cortices. *FEBS Lett* 285: 111–114
147 Rebeck GW, Reiter JS, Strickland DK, Hyman BT (1993) Apolipoprotein E in sporadic Alzheimer's disease: allelic variation and receptor interactions. *Neuron* 11: 575–580
148 Strauss S, Bauer J, Ganter U, Jonas U, Berger M, Volk B (1992) Detection of interleukin-6 and alpha 2-macroglobulin immunoreactivity in cortex and hippocampus of Alzheimer's disease patients. *Lab Invest* 66: 223–230
149 Tooyama I, Kawamata T, Akiyama H, Moestrup SK, Gliemann J, McGeer PL (1993) Immunohistochemical study of alpha 2 macroglobulin receptor in Alzheimer and control postmortem human brain. *Mol Chem Neuropathol* 18: 153–160
150 Wolf BB, Lopes MB, VandenBerg SR, Gonias SL (1992) Characterization and immunohistochemical localization of alpha 2- macroglobulin receptor (low-density lipoprotein receptor-related protein) in human brain. *Am J Pathol* 141: 37–42
151 Blacker D, Wilcox MA, Laird NM, Rodes L, Horvath SM, Go RC, Perry R, Watson BJ, Bassett SS, McInnis MG et al (1998) Alpha-2 macroglobulin is genetically associated with Alzheimer disease. *Nat Genet* 19: 357–360
152 Poller W, Faber JP, Klobeck G, Olek K (1992) Cloning of the human alpha 2-macroglobulin gene and detection of mutations in two functional domains: the bait region and the thiolester site. *Hum Genet* 88: 313–319
153 Kang DE, Saitoh T, Chen X, Xia Y, Masliah E, Hansen LA, Thomas RG, Thal LJ, Katzman R (1997) Genetic association of the low-density lipoprotein receptor-related protein gene (LRP), an apolipoprotein E receptor, with late-onset Alzheimer's disease. *Neurology* 49: 56–61

154 Liao A, Nitsch RM, Greenberg SM, Finckh U, Blacker D, Albert M, Rebeck GW, Gomez-Isla T, Clatworthy A, Binetti G et al (1998) Genetic association of an alpha2-macroglobulin (Val1000lle) polymorphism and Alzheimer's disease. *Hum Mol Genet* 7: 1953–1956
155 Strittmatter WJ, Weisgraber KH, Huang DY, Dong LM, Salvesen GS, Pericak-Vance M, Schmechel D, Saunders AM, Goldgaber D, Roses AD (1993) Binding of human apolipoprotein E to synthetic amyloid beta peptide: isoform-specific effects and implications for late-onset Alzheimer disease. *Proc Natl Acad Sci USA* 90: 8098–8102
156 Kisilevsky R (1992) Proteoglycans, glycosaminoglycans, amyloid-enhancing factor, and amyloid deposition. *J Intern Med* 232: 515–516
157 Lue LF, Kuo YM, Roher AE, Brachova L, Shen Y, Sue L, Beach T, Kurth JH, Rydel RE, Rogers J (1999) Soluble amyloid beta peptide concentration as a predictor of synaptic change in Alzheimer's disease. *Am J Pathol* 155: 853–862
158 Laskowitz DT, Goel S, Bennett ER, Matthew WD (1997) Apolipoprotein E suppresses glial cell secretion of TNF alpha. *J Neuroimmunol* 76: 70–74
159 Laskowitz DT, Matthew WD, Bennett ER, Schmechel D, Herbstreith MH, Goel S, McMillian MK (1998) Endogenous apolipoprotein E suppresses LPS-stimulated microglial nitric oxide production. *Neuroreport* 9: 615–618
160 Behl C (1999) Alzheimer's disease and oxidative stress: implications for novel therapeutic approaches. *Prog Neurobiol* 57: 301–323
161 Liu H, Bowes RC, van de Water B, Sillence C, Nagelkerke JF, Stevens JL (1997) Endoplasmic reticulum chaperones GRP78 and calreticulin prevent oxidative stress, Ca^{2+} disturbances, and cell death in renal epithelial cells. *J Biol Chem* 272: 21751–21759
162 Markesbery WR (1997) Oxidative stress hypothesis in Alzheimer's disease. *Free Radic Biol Med* 23: 134–147
163 Markesbery WR, Carney JM (1999) Oxidative alterations in Alzheimer's disease. *Brain Pathol* 9: 133–146
164 Takeda A, Yasuda T, Miyata T, Goto Y, Wakai M, Watanabe M, Yasuda Y, Horie K, Inagaki T, Doyu M et al (1998) Advanced glycation end products co-localized with astrocytes and microglial cells in Alzheimer's disease brain. *Acta Neuropathol (Berlin)* 95: 555–558
165 Ando Y, Brannstrom T, Uchida K, Nyhlin N, Nasman B, Suhr O, Yamashita T, Olsson T, El Salhy M, Uchino M et al (1998) Histochemical detection of 4-hydroxynonenal protein in Alzheimer amyloid. *J Neurol Sci* 156: 172–176
166 Good PF, Werner P, Hsu A, Olanow CW, Perl DP (1996) Evidence of neuronal oxidative damage in Alzheimer's disease. *Am J Pathol* 149: 21–28
167 Smith MA, Richey HP, Sayre LM, Beckman JS, Perry G (1997) Widespread peroxynitrite-mediated damage in Alzheimer's disease. *J Neurosci* 17: 2653–2657
168 Su JH, Deng G, Cotman CW (1997) Neuronal DNA damage precedes tangle formation and is associated with up-regulation of nitrotyrosine in Alzheimer's disease brain. *Brain Res* 774: 193–199
169 Hensley K, Maidt ML, Yu Z, Sang H, Markesbery WR, Floyd RA (1998) Electrochem-

ical analysis of protein nitrotyrosine and dityrosine in the Alzheimer brain indicates region-specific accumulation. *J Neurosci* 18: 8126–8132

170 Kaltschmidt B, Uherek M, Volk B, Baeuerle PA, Kaltschmidt C (1997) Transcription factor NF-kappaB is activated in primary neurons by amyloid beta peptides and in neurons surrounding early plaques from patients with Alzheimer disease. *Proc Natl Acad Sci USA* 94: 2642–2647

171 Della-Bianca V, Dusi S, Bianchini E, Dal-Pra I, Rossi F (1999) β amyloid activates the O_2 forming NADPH oxidase in microglia, monocytes and neutrophils. A possible inflammatory mechanism of neuronal damage in Alzheimer's disease. *J Biol Chem* 274: 15493–15499

172 Klegeris A, McGeer PL (1997) β-amyloid protein enhances macrophage production of oxygen free radicals and glutamate. *J Neurosci Res* 49: 229–235

173 Klegeris A, Walker DG, McGeer PL (1994) Activation of macrophages by Alzheimer beta amyloid peptide. *Biochem Biophys Res Commun* 199: 984–991

174 Van Muiswinkel FL, Raupp SF, de Vos NM, Smits HA, Verhoef J, Eikelenboom P, Nottet HS (1999) The amino-terminus of the amyloid-beta protein is critical for the cellular binding and consequent activation of the respiratory burst of human macrophages. *J Neuroimmunol* 96: 121–130

175 Van Muiswinkel FL, Veerhuis R, Eikelenboom P (1996) Amyloid beta protein primes cultured rat microglial cells for an enhanced phorbol 12-myristate 13-acetate-induced respiratory burst activity. *J Neurochem* 66: 2468–2476

176 Reynolds WF, Rhees J, Maciejewski D, Paladino T, Sieburg H, Maki RA, Masliah E (1999) Myeloperoxidase polymorphism is associated with gender specific risk for Alzheimer's disease. *Exp Neurol* 155: 31–41

177 Veerhuis R, Janssen I, Hack CE, Eikelenboom P (1996) Early complement components in Alzheimer's disease brains. *Acta Neuropathol (Berlin)* 91: 53–60

178 Brachova L, Lue LF, Schultz J, el Rashidy T, Rogers J (1993) Association cortex, cerebellum, and serum concentrations of C1q and factor B in Alzheimer's disease. *Brain Res Mol Brain Res* 18: 329–334

179 Afagh A, Cummings BJ, Cribbs DH, Cotman CW, Tenner AJ (1996) Localization and cell association of C1q in Alzheimer's disease brain. *Exp Neurol* 138: 22–32

180 Rogers J, Cooper NR, Webster S, Schultz J, McGeer PL, Styren SD, Civin WH, Brachova L, Bradt B, Ward P et al (1992) Complement activation by beta-amyloid in Alzheimer disease. *Proc Natl Acad Sci USA* 89: 10016–10020

181 McGeer PL, Akiyama H, Itagaki S, McGeer EG (1989) Activation of the classical complement pathway in brain tissue of Alzheimer patients. *Neurosci Lett* 107: 341–346

182 McGeer PL, Akiyama H, Itagaki S, McGeer EG (1989) Immune system response in Alzheimer's disease. *Can J Neurol Sci* 16: 516–527

183 Eikelenboom P, Stam FC (1982) Immunoglobulins and complement factors in senile plaques. An immunoperoxidase study. *Acta Neuropathol (Berlin)* 57: 239–242

184 Eikelenboom P, Stam FC (1984) An immunohistochemical study on cerebral vascular

and senile plaque amyloid in Alzheimer's dementia. *Virchows Arch B Cell Pathol* 47: 17–25

185 Ishii T, Haga S (1984) Immuno-electron-microscopic localization of complements in amyloid fibrils of senile plaques. *Acta Neuropathol* 63: 296–300

186 Eikelenboom P, Hack CE, Rozemuller JM, Stam FC (1989) Complement activation in amyloid plaques in Alzheimer's dementia. *Virchows Arch B Cell Pathol Incl Mol Pathol* 56: 259–262

187 Rogers J, Lue LF, Yang LB, Roher A, Kuo YM, Brachova L, Strohmeyer R, Goux WJ, Lee VM, Johnson GVW et al (2000) Complement activation by neurofibrillary tangles in Alzheimer's disease. *Proc Natl Acad Sci USA*

188 Fischer B, Popa-Wagner A (1996) [Alzheimer disease: involvement of the complement system in cell death. Gene expression of C1q and C3 in the frontal cortex of patients with Alzheimer disease and control probands] Morbus Alzheimer: Beteiligung des Komplementsystems am Zelluntergang. Genexpression von Komplement C1q und C3 im frontalen Kortex von Alzheimer-Patienten und Kontrollpersonen. *Fortschr Med* 114: 161–163

189 Eikelenboom P, Zhan SS, Kamphorst W, van d, V, Rozemuller JM (1994) Cellular and substrate adhesion molecules (integrins) and their ligands in cerebral amyloid plaques in Alzheimer's disease. *Virchows Arch* 424: 421–427

190 Eikelenboom P, Rozemuller JM, Kraal G, Stam FC, McBride PA, Bruce ME, Fraser H (1991) Cerebral amyloid plaques in Alzheimer's disease but not in scrapie-affected mice are closely associated with a local inflammatory process. *Virchows Arch B Cell Pathol Incl Mol Pathol* 60: 329–336

191 Ishii T, Haga S, Kametani F (1988) Presence of immunoglobulins and complements in the amyloid plaques in the brain of patients with Alzheimer's disease. In: A Pouplard-Bathelaix, J Emile, Y Christen (eds): *Immunology and Alzheimer's disease*. Springer-Verlag, Berlin, 17–29

192 Veerhuis R, van der Valk P, Janssen I, Zhan SS, Van Nostrand WE, Eikelenboom P (1995) Complement activation in amyloid plaques in Alzheimer's disease brains does not proceed further than C3. *Virchows Arch* 426: 603–610

193 McGeer PL, Itagaki S, Boyes BE, McGeer EG (1988) Reactive microglia are positive for HLA-DR in the substantia nigra of Parkinson's and Alzheimer's disease brains. *Neurology* 38: 1285–1291

194 Broe GA, Henderson AS, Creasey H, McCusker E, Korten AE, Jorm AF, Longley W, Anthony JC (1990) A case-control study of Alzheimer's disease in Australia. *Neurology* 40: 1698–1707

195 Castano A, Lawson LJ, Fearn S, Perry VH (1996) Activation and proliferation of murine microglia are insensitive to glucocorticoids in Wallerian degeneration. *Eur J Neurosci* 8: 581–588

196 Yamada T, Akiyama H, McGeer PL (1990) Complement-activated oligodendroglia: a new pathogenic entity identified by immunostaining with antibodies to human complement proteins C3d and C4d. *Neurosci Lett* 112: 161–166

197 Gollin PA, Kalaria RN, Eikelenboom P, Rozemuller A, Perry G (1992) Alpha 1-antitrypsin and alpha 1-antichymotrypsin are in the lesions of Alzheimer's disease. *Neuroreport* 3: 201–203
198 Dickson DW, Lee SC, Mattiace LA, Yen SH, Brosnan C (1993) Microglia and cytokines in neurological disease, with special reference to AIDS and Alzheimer's disease. *Glia* 7: 75–83
199 Schwab C, Steele JC, McGeer EG, McGeer PL (1997) Amyloid P immunoreactivity precedes C4d deposition on extracellular neurofibrillary tangles. *Acta Neuropathol (Berlin)* 93: 87–92
200 Itagaki S, McGeer PL, Akiyama H, Zhu S, Selkoe D (1989) Relationship of microglia and astrocytes to amyloid deposits of Alzheimer disease. *J Neuroimmunol* 24: 173–182
201 Webster S, Lue LF, Brachova L, Tenner AJ, McGeer PL, Terai K, Walker DG, Bradt B, Cooper NR, Rogers J (1997) Molecular and cellular characterization of the membrane attack complex, C5b-9, in Alzheimer's disease. *Neurobiol Aging* 18: 415–421
202 McGeer PL, Kawamata T, Walker DG (1992) Distribution of clusterin in Alzheimer brain tissue. *Brain Res* 579: 337–341
203 Knuckey NW, Finch P, Palm DE, Primiano MJ, Johanson CE, Flanders KC, Thompson NL (1996) Differential neuronal and astrocytic expression of transforming growth factor beta isoforms in rat hippocampus following transient forebrain ischemia. *Brain Res Mol Brain Res* 40: 1–14
204 Giometto B, Argentiero V, Sanson F, Ongaro G, Tavolato B (1988) Acute-phase proteins in Alzheimer's disease. *Eur Neurol* 28: 30–33
205 Honda S, Itoh F, Yoshimoto M, Ohno S, Hinoda Y, Imai K (2000) Association between complement regulatory protein factor H and AM34 antigen, detected in senile plaques. *J Gerontol A Biol Sci Med Sci* 55: M265–M269
206 McGeer PL, Walker DG, Akiyama H, Kawamata T, Guan AL, Parker CJ, Okada N, McGeer EG (1991) Detection of the membrane inhibitor of reactive lysis (CD59) in diseased neurons of Alzheimer brain. *Brain Res* 544: 315–319
207 Yasojima K, McGeer EG, McGeer PL (1999) Complement regulators C1 inhibitor and CD59 do not significantly inhibit complement activation in Alzheimer disease. *Brain Res* 833: 297–301
208 Yang LB, Li R, Meri S, Rogers J, Shen Y (2000) Deficiency of complement defense protein CD59 may contribute to neurodegeneration in Alzheimer's disease. *J Neurosci* 20: 7505–7509
209 Choi-Miura NH, Ihara Y, Fukuchi K, Takeda M, Nakano Y, Tobe T, Tomita M (1992) SP-40,40 is a constituent of Alzheimer's amyloid. *Acta Neuropathol (Berlin)* 83: 260–264
210 Giannakopoulos P, Kovari E, French LE, Viard I, Hof PR, Bouras C (1998) Possible neuroprotective role of clusterin in Alzheimer's disease: a quantitative immunocytochemical study. *Acta Neuropathol (Berlin)* 95: 387–394
211 Harr SD, Uint L, Hollister R, Hyman BT, Mendez AJ (1996) Brain expression of apolipoproteins E, J, and A-I in Alzheimer's disease. *J Neurochem* 66: 2429–2435

212 Kida E, Choi-Miura NH, Wisniewski KE (1995) Deposition of apolipoproteins E and J in senile plaques is topographically determined in both Alzheimer's disease and Down's syndrome brain. *Brain Res* 685: 211–216
213 Lidstrom AM, Bogdanovic N, Hesse C, Volkman I, Davidsson P, Blennow K (1998) Clusterin (apolipoprotein J) protein levels are increased in hippocampus and in frontal cortex in Alzheimer's disease. *Exp Neurol* 154: 511–521
214 Verbeek MM, Otte-Holler I, Veerhuis R, Ruiter DJ, de Waal RM (1998) Distribution of A beta-associated proteins in cerebrovascular amyloid of Alzheimer's disease. *Acta Neuropathol (Berlin)* 96: 628–636
215 May PC, Lampert-Etchells M, Johnson SA, Poirier J, Masters JN, Finch CE (1990) Dynamics of gene expression for a hippocampal glycoprotein elevated in Alzheimer's disease and in response to experimental lesions in rat. *Neuron* 5: 831–839
216 Akiyama H, Kawamata T, Dedhar S, McGeer PL (1991) Immunohistochemical localization of vitronectin, its receptor and beta-3 integrin in Alzheimer brain tissue. *J Neuroimmunol* 32: 19–28
217 McGeer PL, McGeer EG, Kawamata T, Yamada T, Akiyama H (1991) Reactions of the immune system in chronic degenerative neurological diseases. Can.*J Neurol Sci* 18: 376–379
218 Kalaria RN, Kroon SN (1992) Complement inhibitor C4-binding protein in amyloid deposits containing serum amyloid P in Alzheimer's disease. *Biochem Biophys Res Commun* 186: 461–466
219 Tuohy JM, Schultz JJ, Brachova L, Lue LF, Rogers J (1993) Evidence of increased levels of C4 binding protein in Alzheimer's disease. *Neurosci Abstr* (Abstract) 19: 834
220 Zhan SS, Veerhuis R, Kamphorst W, Eikelenboom P (1995) Distribution of beta amyloid associated proteins in plaques in Alzheimer's disease and in the non-demented elderly. *Neurodegeneration* 4: 291–297
221 Walker DG, Yasuhara O, Patston PA, McGeer EG, McGeer PL (1995) Complement C1 inhibitor is produced by brain tissue and is cleaved in Alzheimer disease. *Brain Res* 675: 75–82
222 Veerhuis R, Janssen I, Hoozemans JJ, De Groot CJ, Hack CE, Eikelenboom P (1998) Complement C1-inhibitor expression in Alzheimer's disease. *Acta Neuropathol* 96: 287–296
223 Akiyama H, McGeer PL (1990) Brain microglia constitutively express beta-2 integrins. *J Neuroimmunol* 30: 81–93
224 Davoust N, Jones J, Stahel PF, Ames RS, Barnum SR (1999) Receptor for the C3a anaphylatoxin is expressed by neurons and glial cells. *Glia* 26: 201–211
225 Nataf S, Stahel PF, Davoust N, Barnum SR (1999) Complement anaphylatoxin receptors on neurons: new tricks for old receptors? *Trends Neurosci* 22: 397–402
226 Gasque P, Singhrao SK, Neal JW, Gotze O, Morgan BP (1997) Expression of the receptor for complement C5a (CD88) is up-regulated on reactive astrocytes, microglia, and endothelial cells in the inflamed human central nervous system. *Am J Pathol* 150: 31–41
227 Griffin WS, Sheng JG, Roberts GW, Mrak RE (1995) Interleukin-1 expression in differ-

ent plaque types in Alzheimer's disease: significance in plaque evolution. *J Neuropathol Exp Neurol* 54: 276–281
228 Sheng JG, Mrak RE, Griffin WS (1995) Microglial interleukin-1 alpha expression in brain regions in Alzheimer's disease: correlation with neuritic plaque distribution. *Neuropathol Appl Neurobiol* 21: 290–301
229 Sheng JG, Griffin WS, Royston MC, Mrak RE (1998) Distribution of interleukin-1-immunoreactive microglia in cerebral cortical layers: implications for neuritic plaque formation in Alzheimer's disease. *Neuropathol Appl Neurobiol* 24: 278–283
230 Cacabelos R, Alvarez XA, Fernandez-Novoa L, Franco A, Mangues R, Pellicer A, Nishimura T (1994) Brain interleukin-1 beta in Alzheimer's disease and vascular dementia. *Methods Find Exp Clin Pharmacol* 16: 141–151
231 Sheng JG, Mrak RE, Griffin WS (1997) Glial-neuronal interactions in Alzheimer disease: progressive association of IL-1alpha+ microglia and S100beta+ astrocytes with neurofibrillary tangle stages. *J Neuropathol Exp Neurol* 56: 285–290
232 Griffin WS, Stanley LC, Ling C, White L, MacLeod V, Perrot LJ, White CL, Araoz C (1989) Brain interleukin 1 and S-100 immunoreactivity are elevated in Down syndrome and Alzheimer disease. *Proc Natl Acad Sci USA* 86: 7611–7615
233 Licastro F, Pedrini S, Caputo L, Annoni G, Davis LJ, Ferri C, Casadei V, Grimaldi LM (2000) Increased plasma levels of interleukin-1, interleukin-6 and alpha-1-antichymotrypsin in patients with Alzheimer's disease: peripheral inflammation or signals from the brain? *J Neuroimmunol* 103: 97–102
234 Blum-Degen D, Muller T, Kuhn W, Gerlach M, Przuntek H, Riederer P (1995) Interleukin-1 beta and interleukin-6 are elevated in the cerebrospinal fluid of Alzheimer's and de novo Parkinson's disease patients. *Neurosci Lett* 202: 17–20
235 Zhu SG, Sheng JG, Jones RA, Brewer MM, Zhou XQ, Mrak RE, Griffin WS (1999) Increased interleukin-1beta converting enzyme expression and activity in Alzheimer disease. *J Neuropathol Exp Neurol* 58: 582–587
236 Sheng JG, Mrak RE, Griffin WS (1994) S100 beta protein expression in Alzheimer disease: potential role in the pathogenesis of neuritic plaques. *J Neurosci Res* 39: 398–404
237 Sheng JG, Mrak RE, Rovnaghi CR, Kozlowska E, Van Eldik LJ, Griffin WS (1996) Human brain S100 beta and S100 beta mRNA expression increases with age: pathogenic implications for Alzheimer's disease. *Neurobiol Aging* 17: 359–363
238 Marshak DR, Pesce SA, Stanley LC, Griffin WS (1992) Increased S100 beta neurotrophic activity in Alzheimer's disease temporal lobe. *Neurobiol Aging* 13: 1–7
239 Van Eldik LJ, Griffin WS (1994) S100 beta expression in Alzheimer's disease: relation to neuropathology in brain regions. *Biochim Biophys Acta* 1223: 398–403
240 Araujo DM, Lapchak PA (1994) Induction of immune system mediators in the hippocampal formation in Alzheimer's and Parkinson's diseases: selective effects on specific interleukins and interleukin receptors. *Neuroscience* 61: 745–754
241 Luber-Narod J, Rogers J (1988) Immune system associated antigens expressed by cells of the human central nervous system. *Neurosci Lett* 94: 17–22
242 Huell M, Strauss S, Volk B, Berger M, Bauer J (1995) Interleukin-6 is present in early

stages of plaque formation and is restricted to the brains of Alzheimer's disease patients. *Acta Neuropathol (Berlin)* 89: 544–551

243 Hull M, Berger M, Volk B, Bauer J (1996) Occurrence of interleukin-6 in cortical plaques of Alzheimer's disease patients may precede transformation of diffuse into neuritic plaques. *Ann NY Acad Sci* 777: 205–212

244 Hull M, Strauss S, Berger M, Volk B, Bauer J (1996) The participation of interleukin-6, a stress-inducible cytokine, in the pathogenesis of Alzheimer's disease. *Behav Brain Res* 78: 37–41

245 Zarow C, Schlueter KE, Zhang Q (1996) Interleukin-6 mRNA is elevated in Alzheimer disease brain. *Soc Neurosci Abstr* 22: 214

246 Walker DG, Kim SU, McGeer PL (1995) Complement and cytokine gene expression in cultured microglia derived from postmortem human brains. *J Neurosci Res.* 40: 478–493

247 Wood JA, Wood PL, Ryan R, Graff-Radford NR, Pilapil C, Robitaille Y, Quirion R (1993) Cytokine indices in Alzheimer's temporal cortex: no changes in mature IL-1 beta or IL-1RA but increases in the associated acute phase proteins IL-6, alpha 2-macroglobulin and C-reactive protein. *Brain Res* 629: 245–252

248 Kalman J, Juhasz A, Laird G, Dickens P, Jardanhazy T, Rimanoczy A, Boncz I, Parry-Jones WL, Janka Z (1997) Serum interleukin-6 levels correlate with the severity of dementia in Down syndrome and in Alzheimer's disease. *Acta Neurol Scand* 96: 236–240

249 Singh VK (1997) Circulating cytokines in Alzheimer's disease. *J Psychiatr Res* 31: 657–660

250 Yamada K, Kono K, Umegaki H, Iguchi A, Fukatsu T, Nakashima N, Nishiwaki H, Shimada Y, Sugita Y (1995) Decreased interleukin-6 level in the cerebrospinal fluid of patients with Alzheimer-type dementia. *Neurosci Lett* 186: 219–221

251 Fillit H, Ding WH, Buee L, Kalman J, Altstiel L, Lawlor B, Wolf-Klein G (1991) Elevated circulating tumor necrosis factor levels in Alzheimer's disease. *Neurosci Lett* 129: 318–320

252 Tarkowski E, Blennow K, Wallin A, Tarkowski A (1999) Intracerebral production of tumor necrosis factor-alpha, a local neuroprotective agent, in Alzheimer disease and vascular dementia. *J Clin Immunol* 19: 223–230

253 Cacabelos R, Alvarez XA, Franco-Maside A, Fernandez-Novoa L, Caamano J (1994) Serum tumor necrosis factor (TNF) in Alzheimer's disease and multi-infarct dementia. *Methods Find Exp Clin Pharmacol* 16: 29–35

254 Tarkowski E, Liljeroth AM, Nilsson A, Ricksten A, Davidsson P, Minthon L, Blennow K (2000) TNF gene polymorphism and its relation to intracerebral production of TNFalpha and TNFbeta in AD. *Neurology* 54: 2077–2081

255 Kawaguchi N, Yamada T, Yoshiyama Y (1997) Expression of interferon-alpha mRNA in human brain tissues. *No To Shinkei* 49: 69–73

256 Yamada T, Horisberger MA, Kawaguchi N, Moroo I, Toyoda T (1994) Immunohisto-

chemistry using antibodies to alpha-interferon and its induced protein, MxA, in Alzheimer's and Parkinson's disease brain tissues. *Neurosci Lett* 181: 61–64
257 Akiyama H, Ikeda K, Katoh M, McGeer EG, McGeer PL (1994) Expression of MRP14, 27E10, interferon-alpha and leukocyte common antigen by reactive microglia in postmortem human brain tissue. *J Neuroimmunol* 50: 195–201
258 Akiyama H, Nishimura T, Kondo H, Ikeda K, Hayashi Y, McGeer PL (1994) Expression of the receptor for macrophage colony stimulating factor by brain microglia and its upregulation in brains of patients with Alzheimer's disease and amyotrophic lateral sclerosis. *Brain Res* 639: 171–174
259 Wisniewski T, Lalowski M, Baumann M, Rauvala H, Raulo E, Nolo R, Frangione B (1996) HB-GAM is a cytokine present in Alzheimer's and Down's syndrome lesions. *Neuroreport* 7: 667–671
260 Chao CC, Ala TA, Hu S, Crossley KB, Sherman RE, Peterson PK, Frey WH (1994) Serum cytokine levels in patients with Alzheimer's disease. *Clin Diagn Lab Immunol* 1: 433–436
261 Chao CC, Hu S, Frey WH, Ala TA, Tourtellotte WW, Peterson PK (1994) Transforming growth factor beta in Alzheimer's disease. *Clin Diagn Lab Immunol* 1: 109–110
262 Peress NS, Perillo E (1995) Differential expression of TGF-beta 1, 2 and 3 isotypes in Alzheimer's disease: a comparative immunohistochemical study with cerebral infarction, aged human and mouse control brains. *J Neuropathol Exp Neurol* 54: 802–811
263 van der Wal EA, Gomez-Pinilla F, Cotman CW (1993) Transforming growth factor-beta 1 is in plaques in Alzheimer and Down pathologies. *Neuroreport* 4: 69–72
264 Flanders KC, Lippa CF, Smith TW, Pollen DA, Sporn MB (1995) Altered expression of transforming growth factor-beta in Alzheimer's disease. *Neurology* 45: 1561–1569
265 Yasuhara O, Muramatsu H, Kim SU, Muramatsu T, Maruta H, McGeer PL (1993) Midkine, a novel neurotrophic factor, is present in senile plaques of Alzheimer disease. *Biochem Biophys Res Commun* 192: 246–251
266 Thorns V, Masliah E (1999) Evidence for neuroprotective effects of acidic fibroblast growth factor in Alzheimer disease. *J Neuropathol Exp Neurol* 58: 296–306
267 Kimura H, Tooyama I, McGeer PL (1994) Acidic FGF expression in the surroundings of senile plaques. *Tohoku J Exp Med* 174: 279–293
268 Cummings BJ, Su JH, Cotman CW (1993) Neuritic involvement within bFGF immunopositive plaques of Alzheimer's disease. *Exp Neurol* 124: 315–325
269 Gomez-Pinilla F, Cummings BJ, Cotman CW (1990) Induction of basic fibroblast growth factor in Alzheimer's disease pathology. *Neuroreport* 1: 211–214
270 Stopa EG, Gonzalez AM, Chorsky R, Corona RJ, Alvarez J, Bird ED, Baird A (1990) Basic fibroblast growth factor in Alzheimer's disease. *Biochem Biophys Res Commun* 171: 690–696
271 Nakamura S, Arima K, Haga S, Aizawa T, Motoi Y, Otsuka M, Ueki A, Ikeda K (1998) Fibroblast growth factor (FGF)-9 immunoreactivity in senile plaques. *Brain Res* 814: 222–225
272 Connor B, Beilharz EJ, Williams C, Synek B, Gluckman PD, Faull RL, Dragunow M

(1997) Insulin-like growth factor-I (IGF-I) immunoreactivity in the Alzheimer's disease temporal cortex and hippocampus. *Brain Res Mol Brain Res* 49: 283–290

273 Tham A, Nordberg A, Grissom FE, Carlsson-Skwirut C, Viitanen M, Sara VR (1993) Insulin-like growth factors and insulin-like growth factor binding proteins in cerebrospinal fluid and serum of patients with dementia of the Alzheimer type. *J Neural Transm Park Dis Dement Sect* 5: 165–176

274 Fenton H, Finch PW, Rubin JS, Rosenberg JM, Taylor WG, Kuo-Leblanc V, Rodriguez-Wolf M, Baird A, Schipper HM, Stopa EG (1998) Hepatocyte growth factor (HGF/SF) in Alzheimer's disease. *Brain Res* 779: 262–270

275 Kalaria RN, Cohen DL, Premkumar DR, Nag S, LaManna JC, Lust WD (1998) Vascular endothelial growth factor in Alzheimer's disease and experimental cerebral ischemia. *Brain Res Mol Brain Res* 62: 101–105

276 Masliah E, Mallory M, Alford M, DeTeresa R, Saitoh T (1995) PDGF is associated with neuronal and glial alterations of Alzheimer's disease. *Neurobiol Aging* 16: 549–556

277 Hock C, Heese K, Hulette C, Rosenberg C, Otten U (2000) Region-specific neurotrophin imbalances in Alzheimer disease: decreased levels of brain-derived neurotrophic factor and increased levels of nerve growth factor in hippocampus and cortical areas. *Arch Neurol* 57: 846–851

278 Scott SA, Mufson EJ, Weingartner JA, Skau KA, Crutcher KA (1995) Nerve growth factor in Alzheimer's disease: increased levels throughout the brain coupled with declines in nucleus basalis. *J Neurosci* 15: 6213–6221

279 Hellweg R, Gericke CA, Jendroska K, Hartung HD, Cervos-Navarro J (1998) NGF content in the cerebral cortex of non-demented patients with amyloid-plaques and in symptomatic Alzheimer's disease. *Int J Dev Neurosci* 16: 787–794

280 Crutcher KA, Scott SA, Liang S, Everson WV, Weingartner J (1993) Detection of NGF-like activity in human brain tissue: increased levels in Alzheimer's disease. *J Neurosci* 13: 2540–2550

281 Narisawa-Saito M, Wakabayashi K, Tsuji S, Takahashi H, Nawa H (1996) Regional specificity of alterations in NGF, BDNF and NT-3 levels in Alzheimer's disease. *Neuroreport* 7: 2925–2928

282 Fahnestock M, Scott SA, Jette N, Weingartner JA, Crutcher KA (1996) Nerve growth factor mRNA and protein levels measured in the same tissue from normal and Alzheimer's disease parietal cortex. *Brain Res Mol Brain Res* 42: 175–178

283 Higgins GA, Mufson EJ (1989) NGF receptor gene expression is decreased in the nucleus basalis in Alzheimer's disease. *Exp Neurol* 106: 222–236

284 Mufson EJ, Conner JM, Kordower JH (1995) Nerve growth factor in Alzheimer's disease: defective retrograde transport to nucleus basalis. *Neuroreport* 6: 1063–1066

285 Hock C, Heese K, Muller-Spahn F, Huber P, Riesen W, Nitsch RM, Otten U (2000) Increased CSF levels of nerve growth factor in patients with Alzheimer's disease. *Neurology* 54: 2009–2011

286 Holsinger RM, Schnarr J, Henry P, Castelo VT, Fahnestock M (2000) Quantitation of BDNF mRNA in human parietal cortex by competitive reverse transcription-polymerase

chain reaction: decreased levels in Alzheimer's disease. *Brain Res Mol Brain Res.* 76: 347–354
287 Phillips HS, Hains JM, Armanini M, Laramee GR, Johnson SA, Winslow JW (1991) BDNF mRNA is decreased in the hippocampus of individuals with Alzheimer's disease. *Neuron* 7: 695–702
288 Phillips HS, Hains JM, Armanini M, Laramee GR, Johnson SA, Winslow JW (1991) BDNF mRNA is decreased in the hippocampus of individuals with Alzheimer's disease. *Neuron* 7: 695–702
289 Soontornniyomkij V, Wang G, Pittman CA, Hamilton RL, Wiley CA, Achim CL (1999) Absence of brain-derived neurotrophic factor and trkB receptor immunoreactivity in glia of Alzheimer's disease. *Acta Neuropathol (Berlin)* 98: 345–348
290 Connor B, Young D, Yan Q, Faull RL, Synek B, Dragunow M (1997) Brain-derived neurotrophic factor is reduced in Alzheimer's disease. *Brain Res Mol Brain Res* 49: 71–81
291 Ferrer I, Marin C, Rey MJ, Ribalta T, Goutan E, Blanco R, Tolosa E, Marti E (1999) BDNF and full-length and truncated TrkB expression in Alzheimer disease. Implications in therapeutic strategies. *J Neuropathol Exp Neurol* 58: 729–739
292 Murer MG, Boissiere F, Yan Q, Hunot S, Villares J, Faucheux B, Agid Y, Hirsch E, Raisman-Vozari R (1999) An immunohistochemical study of the distribution of brain-derived neurotrophic factor in the adult human brain, with particular reference to Alzheimer's disease. *Neuroscience* 88: 1015–1032
293 Hock C, Heese K, Muller-Spahn F, Hulette C, Rosenberg C, Otten U (1998) Decreased trkA neurotrophin receptor expression in the parietal cortex of patients with Alzheimer's disease. *Neurosci Lett* 241: 151–154
294 Mufson EJ, Lavine N, Jaffar S, Kordower JH, Quirion R, Saragovi HU (1997) Reduction in p140-TrkA receptor protein within the nucleus basalis and cortex in Alzheimer's disease. *Exp Neurol* 146: 91–103
295 Boissiere F, Hunot S, Faucheux B, Hersh LB, Agid Y, Hirsch EC (1997) Trk neurotrophin receptors in cholinergic neurons of patients with Alzheimer's disease. *Dement Geriatr Cogn Disord* 8: 1–8
296 Salehi A, Verhaagen J, Dijkhuizen PA, Swaab DF (1996) Co-localization of high-affinity neurotrophin receptors in nucleus basalis of Meynert neurons and their differential reduction in Alzheimer's disease. *Neuroscience* 75: 373–387
297 Boissiere F, Lehericy S, Strada O, Agid Y, Hirsch EC (1996) Neurotrophin receptors and selective loss of cholinergic neurons in Alzheimer disease. *Mol Chem Neuropathol* 28: 219–223
298 Boissiere F, Faucheux B, Ruberg M, Agid Y, Hirsch EC (1997) Decreased TrkA gene expression in cholinergic neurons of the striatum and basal forebrain of patients with Alzheimer's disease. *Exp Neurol* 145: 245–252
299 Mufson EJ, Li JM, Sobreviela T, Kordower JH (1996) Decreased trkA gene expression within basal forebrain neurons in Alzheimer's disease. *Neuroreport* 8: 25–29
300 Connor B, Young D, Lawlor P, Gai W, Waldvogel H, Faull RL, Dragunow M (1996) Trk receptor alterations in Alzheimer's disease. *Brain Res Mol Brain Res* 42: 1–17

301 Allen SJ, Wilcock GK, Dawbarn D (1999) Profound and selective loss of catalytic TrkB immunoreactivity in Alzheimer's disease. *Biochem Biophys Res Commun* 264: 648–651
302 Garlind A, Brauner A, Hojeberg B, Basun H, Schultzberg M (1999) Soluble interleukin-1 receptor type II levels are elevated in cerebrospinal fluid in Alzheimer's disease patients. *Brain Res* 826: 112–116
303 Yasuhara O, Matsuo A, Terai K, Walker DG, Berger AE, Akiguchi I, Kimura J, McGeer PL (1997) Expression of interleukin-1 receptor antagonist protein in post-mortem human brain tissues of Alzheimer's disease and control cases. *Acta Neuropathol (Berlin)* 93: 414–420
304 Hampel H, Sunderland T, Kotter HU, Schneider C, Teipel SJ, Padberg F, Dukoff R, Levy J, Moller HJ (1998) Decreased soluble interleukin-6 receptor in cerebrospinal fluid of patients with Alzheimer's disease. *Brain Res* 780: 356–359
305 Hampel H, Teipel SJ, Padberg F, Haslinger A, Riemenschneider M, Schwarz MJ, Kotter HU, Scheloske M, Buch K, Stubner S et al (1999) Discriminant power of combined cerebrospinal fluid tau protein and of the soluble interleukin-6 receptor complex in the diagnosis of Alzheimer's disease. *Brain Res* 823: 104–112
306 Lippa CF, Flanders KC, Kim ES, Croul S (1998) TGF-beta receptors-I and -II immunoexpression in Alzheimer's disease: a comparison with aging and progressive supranuclear palsy. *Neurobiol Aging* 19: 527–533
307 de la Monte SM, Sohn YK, Wands JR (1997) Correlates of p53- and Fas (CD95)-mediated apoptosis in Alzheimer's disease. *J Neurol Sci* 152: 73–83
308 Nishimura T, Akiyama H, Yonehara S, Kondo H, Ikeda K, Kato M, Iseki E, Kosaka K (1995) Fas antigen expression in brains of patients with Alzheimer-type dementia. *Brain Res* 695: 137–145
309 Birecree E, Whetsell WOJ, Stoscheck C, King LEJ, Nanney LB (1988) Immunoreactive epidermal growth factor receptors in neuritic plaques from patients with Alzheimer's disease. *J Neuropathol Exp Neurol* 47: 549–560
310 Styren SD, Mufson EJ, Styren GC, Civin WH, Rogers J (1990) Epidermal growth factor receptor expression in demented and aged human brain. *Brain Res* 512: 347–352
311 Takami K, Matsuo A, Terai K, Walker DG, McGeer EG, McGeer PL (1998) Fibroblast growth factor receptor-1 expression in the cortex and hippocampus in Alzheimer's disease. *Brain Res* 802: 89–97
312 Ferrer I, Marti E (1998) Distribution of fibroblast growth factor receptor-1 (FGFR-1) and FGFR-3 in the hippocampus of patients with Alzheimer's disease. *Neurosci Lett* 240: 139–142
313 Xia MQ, Bacskai BJ, Knowles RB, Qin SX, Hyman BT (2000) Expression of the chemokine receptor CXCR3 on neurons and the elevated expression of its ligand IP-10 in reactive astrocytes: *in vitro* ERK1/2 activation and role in Alzheimer's disease. *J Neuroimmunol* 108: 227–235
314 Xia MQ, Qin SX, Wu LJ, Mackay CR, Hyman BT (1998) Immunohistochemical study of the beta-chemokine receptors CCR3 and CCR5 and their ligands in normal and Alzheimer's disease brains. *Am J Pathol* 153: 31–37

315 Ishizuka K, Kimura T, Igata-yi R, Katsuragi S, Takamatsu J, Miyakawa T (1997) Identification of monocyte chemoattractant protein-1 in senile plaques and reactive microglia of Alzheimer's disease. *Psychiatry Clin Neurosci* 51: 135–138
316 Horuk R, Martin AW, Wang Z, Schweitzer L, Gerassimides A, Guo H, Lu Z, Hesselgesser J, Perez HD, Kim J et al (1997) Expression of chemokine receptors by subsets of neurons in the central nervous system. *J Immunol* 158: 2882–2890
317 Xia M, Qin S, McNamara M, Mackay C, Hyman BT (1997) Interleukin-8 receptor B immunoreactivity in brain and neuritic plaques of Alzheimer's disease. *Am J Pathol* 150: 1267–1274
318 Tooyama I, Kimura H, Akiyama H, McGeer PL (1990) Reactive microglia express class I and class II major histocompatibility complex antigens in Alzheimer's disease. *Brain Res* 523: 273–280
319 McGeer PL, McGeer EG, Kawamata T, Yamada T, Akiyama H (1991) Reactions of the immune system in chronic degenerative neurological diseases. *Can J Neurol Sci* 18: 376–379
320 Frohman EM, Frohman TC, Gupta S, de Fougerolles A, van den Noort S (1991) Expression of intercellular adhesion molecule 1 (ICAM-1) in Alzheimer's disease. *J Neurol Sci* 106: 105–111
321 Itagaki S, Akiyama H, Saito H, McGeer PL (1994) Ultrastuctural localization of complment membrane attack complex (MAC)-like immunoreactivity in brains of patients with Alzheimer's disease. *Brain Res* 645: 78–84
322 Mattiace LA, Davies P, Dickson DW (1990) Detection of HLA-DR on microglia in the human brain is a function of both clinical and technical factors. *Am J Pathol* 136: 1101–1114
323 McGeer PL, Itagaki S, Tago H, McGeer EG (1987) Reactive microglia in patients with senile dementia of the Alzheimer type are positive for the histocompatibility glycoprotein HLA-DR. *Neurosci Lett* 79: 195–200
324 Styren SD, Civin WH, Rogers J (1990) Molecular, cellular, and pathologic characterization of HLA-DR immunoreactivity in normal elderly and Alzheimer's disease brain. *Exp Neurol* 110: 93–104
325 Ross BM, Moszczynska A, Erlich J, Kish SJ (1998) Phospholipid-metabolizing enzymes in Alzheimer's disease: increased lysophospholipid acyltransferase activity and decreased phospholipase A2 activity. *J Neurochem* 70: 786–793
326 Gattaz WF, Cairns NJ, Levy R, Forstl H, Braus DF, Maras A (1996) Decreased phospholipase A2 activity in the brain and in platelets of patients with Alzheimer's disease. *Eur Arch Psychiatry Clin Neurosci* 246: 129–131
327 Gattaz WF, Maras A, Cairns NJ, Levy R, Forstl H (1995) Decreased phospholipase A2 activity in Alzheimer brains. *Biol Psychiatry* 37: 13–17
328 Stephenson DT, Lemere CA, Selkoe DJ, Clemens JA (1996) Cytosolic phospholipase A2 (cPLA2) immunoreactivity is elevated in Alzheimer's disease brain. *Neurobiol Dis* 3: 51–63
329 Yasojima K, Schwab C, McGeer EG, McGeer PL (1999) Distribution of cyclooxygenase-

1 and cyclooxygenase-2 mRNAs and proteins in human brain and peripheral organs. *Brain Res* 830: 226–236

330 Yermakova AV, Rollins J, Callahan LM, Rogers J, O'Banion MK (1999) Cyclooxygenase-1 in human Alzheimer and control brain: quantitative analysis of expression by microglia and CA3 hippocampal neurons. *J Neuropathol Exp Neurol* 58: 1135–1146

331 Lukiw WJ, Bazan NG (1997) Cyclooxygenase 2 RNA message abundance, stability, and hypervariability in sporadic Alzheimer neocortex. *J Neurosci Res* 50: 937–945

332 Lukiw WJ, Bazan NG (1998) Strong nuclear factor-kappaB-DNA binding parallels cyclooxygenase-2 gene transcription in aging and in sporadic Alzheimer's disease superior temporal lobe neocortex. *J Neurosci Res* 53: 583–592

333 O'Banion MK, Chang JW, Coleman PD (1997) Decreased expression of prostaglandin G/H synthase-2 (PGHS-2) in Alzheimer's disease brain. *Adv Exp Med Biol* 407: 171–177

334 Chang JW, Coleman PD, O'Banion MK (1996) Prostaglandin G/H synthase-2 (cyclooxygenase-2) mRNA expression is decreased in Alzheimer's disease. *Neurobiol Aging* 17: 801–808

335 Wong PT, McGeer PL, McGeer EG (1992) Decreased prostaglandin synthesis in postmortem cerebral cortex from patients with Alzheimer's disease. *Neurochem Int* 21: 197–202

336 Iwamoto N, Kobayashi K, Kosaka K (1989) The formation of prostaglandins in the postmortem cerebral cortex of Alzheimer-type dementia patients. *J Neurol* 236: 80–84

337 Montine TJ, Sidell KR, Crews BC, Markesbery WR, Marnett LJ, Roberts LJ, Morrow JD (1999) Elevated CSF prostaglandin E2 levels in patients with probable AD. *Neurology* 53: 1495–1498

338 Montine TJ, Beal MF, Cudkowicz ME, O'Donnell H, Margolin RA, McFarland L, Bachrach AF, Zackert WE, Roberts LJ, Morrow JD (1999) Increased CSF F2-isoprostane concentration in probable AD. *Neurology* 52: 562–565

339 Pratico D, Lee MY, V, Trojanowski JQ, Rokach J, Fitzgerald GA (1998) Increased F2-isoprostanes in Alzheimer's disease: evidence for enhanced lipid peroxidation *in vivo*. *FASEB J* 12: 1777–1783

340 Nourooz-Zadeh J, Liu EH, Yhlen B, Anggard EE, Halliwell B (1999) F4-isoprostanes as specific marker of docosahexaenoic acid peroxidation in Alzheimer's disease. *J Neurochem* 72: 734–740

341 Berzin TM, Zipser BD, Rafii MS, Kuo-Leblanc V, Yancopoulos GD, Glass DJ, Fallon JR, Stopa EG (2000) Agrin and microvascular damage in Alzheimer's disease. *Neurobiol Aging* 21: 349–355

342 Akiyama H, Ikeda K, Kondo H, McGeer PL (1992) Thrombin accumulation in brains of patients with Alzheimer's disease. *Neurosci Lett* 146: 152–154

343 Akiyama H (1997) Thrombin deposition in brains of patients with Alzheimer's disease – activation of the coagulation system in the central nervous system. *Rinsho Byori* (Suppl) 104: 117–123

344 McGeer PL, Klegeris A, Walker DG, Yasuhara O, McGeer EG (1994) Pathological proteins in senile plaques. *Tohoku J Exp Med* 174: 269–277
345 Akiyama H (1994) Inflammatory response in Alzheimer's disease. *Tohoku J Exp Med* 174: 295–303
346 Kalaria RN, Golde T, Kroon SN, Perry G (1993) Serine protease inhibitor antithrombin III and its messenger RNA in the pathogenesis of Alzheimer's disease. *Am J Pathol* 143: 886–893
347 McComb RD, Miller KA, Carson SD (1991) Tissue factor antigen in senile plaques of Alzheimer's disease. *Am J Pathol* 139: 491–494
348 Hollister RD, Kisiel W, Hyman BT (1996) Immunohistochemical localization of tissue factor pathway inhibitor-1 (TFPI-1), a Kunitz proteinase inhibitor, in Alzheimer's disease. *Brain Res* 728: 13–19
349 Yasuhara O, Walker DG, McGeer PL (1994) Hageman factor and its binding sites are present in senile plaques of Alzheimer's disease. *Brain Res* 654: 234–240
350 Rebeck GW, Harr SD, Strickland DK, Hyman BT (1995) Multiple, diverse senile plaque-associated proteins are ligands of an apolipoprotein E receptor, the alpha 2-macroglobulin receptor/low- density-lipoprotein receptor-related protein. *Ann Neurol* 37: 211–217
351 Alonso DF, Farias EF, Famulari AL, Dominguez RO, Kohan S, de Lustig ES (1996) Excessive urokinase-type plasminogen activator activity in the euglobulin fraction of patients with Alzheimer-type dementia. *J Neurol Sci* 139: 83–88
352 Sutton R, Keohane ME, VanderBerg SR, Gonias SL (1994) Plasminogen activator inhibitor-1 in the cerebrospinal fluid as an index of neurological disease. *Blood Coagul Fibrinolysis* 5: 167–171
353 Akiyama H, Ikeda K, Kondo H, Kato M, McGeer PL (1993) Microglia express the type 2 plasminogen activator inhibitor in the brain of control subjects and patients with Alzheimer's disease. *Neurosci Lett* 164: 233–235
354 Wagner SL, Geddes JW, Cotman CW, Lau AL, Gurwitz D, Isackson PJ, Cunningham DD (1989) Protease nexin-1, an antithrombin with neurite outgrowth activity, is reduced in Alzheimer disease. *Proc Natl Acad Sci USA* 86: 8284–8288
355 Vaughan PJ, Su J, Cotman CW, Cunningham DD (1994) Protease nexin-1, a potent thrombin inhibitor, is reduced around cerebral blood vessels in Alzheimer's disease. *Brain Res* 668: 160–170
356 Choi BH, Kim RC, Vaughan PJ, Lau A, Van Nostrand WE, Cotman CW, Cunningham DD (1995) Decreases in protease nexins in Alzheimer's disease brain. *Neurobiol Aging* 16: 557–562
357 Rosenblatt DE, Geula C, Mesulam MM (1989) Protease nexin I immunostaining in Alzheimer's disease. *Ann Neurol* 26: 628–634
358 Akiyama H, Kondo H, Ikeda K, Arai T, Kato M, McGleer PL (1995) Immunohistochemical detection of coagulation factor XIIIa in postmortem human brain tissue. *Neurosci Lett* 202: 29–32
359 Verbeek MM, Otte-Holler I, Westphal JR, Wesseling P, Ruiter DJ, de Waal RM (1994)

Accumulation of intercellular adhesion molecule-1 in senile plaques in brain tissue of patients with Alzheimer's disease. *Am J Pathol* 144: 104–116
360 Gillian AM, Brion JP, Breen KC (1994) Expression of the neural cell adhesion molecule (NCAM) in Alzheimer's disease. *Neurodegeneration* 3: 283–291
361 Yew DT, Li WP, Webb SE, Lai HW, Zhang L (1999) Neurotransmitters, peptides, and neural cell adhesion molecules in the cortices of normal elderly humans and Alzheimer patients: a comparison. *Exp Gerontol* 34: 117–133
362 Akiyama H, Tooyama I, Kawamata T, Ikeda K, McGeer PL (1993) Morphological diversities of CD44 positive astrocytes in the cerebral cortex of normal subjects and patients with Alzheimer's disease. *Brain Res* 632: 249–259
363 Lawlor BA, Swanwick GR, Feighery C, Walsh JB, Coakley D (1996) Acute phase reactants in Alzheimer's disease. *Biol Psychiatry* 39: 1051–1052
364 Abraham CR, Selkoe DJ, Potter H (1988) Immunochemical identification of the serine protease inhibitor alpha 1-antichymotrypsin in the brain amyloid deposits of Alzheimer's disease. *Cell* 52: 487–501
365 Abraham CR, Shirahama T, Potter H (1990) Alpha 1-antichymotrypsin is associated solely with amyloid deposits containing the beta-protein. Amyloid and cell localization of alpha 1-antichymotrypsin. *Neurobiol Aging* 11: 123–129
366 Rozemuller JM, Stam FC, Eikelenboom P (1990) Acute phase proteins are present in amorphous plaques in the cerebral but not in the cerebellar cortex of patients with Alzheimer's disease. *Neurosci Lett* 119: 75–78
367 Rozemuller JM, Abbink JJ, Kamp AM, Stam FC, Hack CE, Eikelenboom P (1991) Distribution pattern and functional state of alpha 1-antichymotrypsin in plaques and vascular amyloid in Alzheimer's disease. A immunohistochemical study with monoclonal antibodies against native and inactivated alpha 1-antichymotrypsin. *Acta Neuropathol (Berlin)* 82: 200–207
368 Licastro F, Morini MC, Polazzi E, Davis LJ (1995) Increased serum alpha 1-antichymotrypsin in patients with probable Alzheimer's disease: an acute phase reactant without the peripheral acute phase response. *J Neuroimmunol* 57: 71–75
369 Licastro F, Parnetti L, Morini MC, Davis LJ, Cucinotta D, Gaiti A, Senin U (1995) Acute phase reactant alpha 1-antichymotrypsin is increased in cerebrospinal fluid and serum of patients with probable Alzheimer disease. *Alzheimer Dis Assoc Disord* 9: 112–118
370 Lieberman J, Schleissner L, Tachiki KH, Kling AS (1995) Serum alpha 1-antichymotrypsin level as a marker for Alzheimer-type dementia. *Neurobiol Aging* 16: 747–753
371 Van Gool D, De Strooper B, Van Leuven F, Triau E, Dom R (1993) alpha 2-Macroglobulin expression in neuritic-type plaques in patients with Alzheimer's disease. *Neurobiol Aging* 14: 233–237
372 Wetterling T, Tegtmeyer KF (1994) Serum alpha 1-antitrypsin and alpha 2-macroglobulin in Alzheimer's and Binswanger's disease. *Clin Investig* 72: 196–199
373 Liang JS, Sloane JA, Wells JM, Abraham CR, Fine RE, Sipe JD (1997) Evidence for local production of acute phase response apolipoprotein serum amyloid A in Alzheimer's disease brain. *Neurosci Lett* 225: 73–76

374 Elovaara I, Maury CP, Palo J (1986) Serum amyloid A protein, albumin and prealbumin in Alzheimer's disease and in demented patients with Down's syndrome. *Acta Neurol* Scand. 74: 245–250
375 Coria F, Castano E, Prelli F, Larrondo-Lillo M, van Duinen S, Shelanski ML, Frangione B (1988) Isolation and characterization of amyloid P component from Alzheimer's disease and other types of cerebral amyloidosis. *Lab Invest* 58: 454–458
376 Duong T, Pommier EC, Scheibel AB (1989) Immunodetection of the amyloid P component in Alzheimer's disease. *Acta Neuropathol (Berlin)* 78: 429–437
377 Akiyama H, Yamada T, Kawamata T, McGeer PL (1991) Association of amyloid P component with complement proteins in neurologically diseased brain tissue. *Brain Res* 548: 349–352
378 Iwamoto N, Nishiyama E, Ohwada J, Arai H (1994) Demonstration of CRP immunoreactivity in brains of Alzheimer's disease: immunohistochemical study using formic acid pretreatment of tissue sections. *Neurosci Lett* 177: 23–26
379 Duong T, Nikolaeva M, Acton PJ (1997) C-reactive protein-like immunoreactivity in the neurofibrillary tangles of Alzheimer's disease. *Brain Res* 749: 152–156
380 Loeffler DA, DeMaggio AJ, Juneau PL, Brickman CM, Mashour GA, Finkelman JH, Pomara N, Lewitt PA (1994) Ceruloplasmin is increased in cerebrospinal fluid in Alzheimer's disease but not Parkinson's disease. *Alzheimer Dis Assoc Disord* 8: 190–197
381 Loeffler DA, Lewitt PA, Juneau PL, Sima AA, Nguyen HU, DeMaggio AJ, Brickman CM, Brewer GJ, Dick RD, Troyer MD et al (1996) Increased regional brain concentrations of ceruloplasmin in neurodegenerative disorders. *Brain Res* 738: 265–274
382 Connor JR, Tucker P, Johnson M, Snyder B (1993) Ceruloplasmin levels in the human superior temporal gyrus in aging and Alzheimer's disease. *Neurosci Lett* 159: 88–90
383 Kawamata T, Tooyama I, Yamada T, Walker DG, McGeer PL (1993) Lactotransferrin immunocytochemistry in Alzheimer and normal human brain. *Am J Pathol* 142: 1574–1585
384 Leveugle B, Spik G, Perl DP, Bouras C, Fillit HM, Hof PR (1994) The iron-binding protein lactotransferrin is present in pathologic lesions in a variety of neurodegenerative disorders: a comparative immunohistochemical analysis. *Brain Res* 650: 20–31
385 Mecocci P, MacGarvey U, Beal MF (1994) Oxidative damage to mitochondrial DNA is increased in Alzheimer's disease. *Ann Neurol* 36: 747–751
386 Lovell MA, Gabbita SP, Markesbery WR (1999) Increased DNA oxidation and decreased levels of repair products in Alzheimer's disease ventricular CSF. *J Neurochem* 72: 771–776
387 Lovell MA, Ehmann WD, Mattson MP, Markesbery WR (1997) Elevated 4-hydroxynonenal in ventricular fluid in Alzheimer's disease. *Neurobiol Aging* 18: 457–461
388 Markesbery WR, Lovell MA (1998) Four-hydroxynonenal, a product of lipid peroxidation, is increased in the brain in Alzheimer's disease. *Neurobiol Aging* 19: 33–36
389 Lovell MA, Xie C, Markesbery WR (1998) Decreased glutathione transferase activity in brain and ventricular fluid in Alzheimer's disease. *Neurology* 51: 1562–1566
390 Van Muiswinkel FL, DeGroot C, Rozemuller-Kwakkel J, Eikelenboom P (1999)

Enhanced expression of microglial NADPH-oxidase (p22-phox) in Alzheimer's disease. In: K Iqbal, D Swaab, B Winblad, HM Wisniewski (eds): John Wiley & Sons, London, UK, 451–456

391 Samudralwar DL, Diprete CC, Ni BF, Ehmann WD, Markesbery WR (1995) Elemental imbalances in the olfactory pathway in Alzheimer's disease. *J Neurol Sci* 130: 139–145

392 Thompson CM, Markesbery WR, Ehmann WD, Mao YX, Vance DE (1988) Regional brain trace-element studies in Alzheimer's disease. *Neurotoxicology* 9: 1–7

393 Ehmann WD, Markesbery WR, Alauddin M, Hossain TI, Brubaker EH (1986) Brain trace elements in Alzheimer's disease. *Neurotoxicology* 7: 195–206

394 Good PF, Perl DP, Bierer LM, Schmeidler J (1992) Selective accumulation of aluminum and iron in the neurofibrillary tangles of Alzheimer's disease: a laser microprobe (LAMMA) study. *Ann Neurol* 31: 286–292

395 Grundke-Iqbal I, Fleming J, Tung YC, Lassmann H, Iqbal K, Joshi JG (1990) Ferritin is a component of the neuritic (senile) plaque in Alzheimer dementia. *Acta Neuropathol (Berlin)* 81: 105–110

396 Fleming J, Joshi JG (1987) Ferritin: isolation of aluminum-ferritin complex from brain. *Proc Natl Acad Sci USA* 84: 7866–7870

397 Kennard ML, Feldman H, Yamada T, Jefferies WA (1996) Serum levels of the iron binding protein p97 are elevated in Alzheimer's disease. *Nat Med* 2: 1230–1235

398 Jefferies WA, Food MR, Gabathuler R, Rothenberger S, Yamada T, Yasuhara O, McGeer PL (1996) Reactive microglia specifically associated with amyloid plaques in Alzheimer's disease brain tissue express melanotransferrin. *Brain Res* 712: 122–126

399 Lovell MA, Ehmann WD, Butler SM, Markesbery WR (1995) Elevated thiobarbituric acid-reactive substances and antioxidant enzyme activity in the brain in Alzheimer's disease. *Neurology* 45: 1594–1601

400 Subbarao KV, Richardson JS, Ang LC (1990) Autopsy samples of Alzheimer's cortex show increased peroxidation *in vitro*. *J Neurochem* 55: 342–345

401 Balazs L, Leon M (1994) Evidence of an oxidative challenge in the Alzheimer's brain. *Neurochem Res* 19: 1131–1137

402 Palmer AM, Burns MA (1994) Selective increase in lipid peroxidation in the inferior temporal cortex in Alzheimer's disease. *Brain Res* 645: 338–342

403 Lee SC, Zhao ML, Hirano A, Dickson DW (1999) Inducible nitric oxide synthase immunoreactivity in the Alzheimer disease hippocampus: association with Hirano bodies, neurofibrillary tangles, and senile plaques. *J Neuropathol Exp Neurol* 58: 1163–1169

404 Terai K, Matsuo A, McGeer PL (1996) Enhancement of immunoreactivity for NF-kappa B in the hippocampal formation and cerebral cortex of Alzheimer's disease. *Brain Res* 735: 159–168

405 Ferrer I, Marti E, Lopez E, Tortosa A (1998) NF-kB immunoreactivity is observed in association with beta A4 diffuse plaques in patients with Alzheimer's disease. *Neuropathol Appl Neurobiol* 24: 271–277

406 Kitamura Y, Shimohama S, Ota T, Matsuoka Y, Nomura Y, Taniguchi T (1997) Alter-

ation of transcription factors NF-kappaB and STAT1 in Alzheimer's disease brains. *Neurosci Lett* 237: 17–20

407 Boissiere F, Hunot S, Faucheux B, Duyckaerts C, Hauw JJ, Agid Y, Hirsch EC (1997) Nuclear translocation of NF-kappaB in cholinergic neurons of patients with Alzheimer's disease. *Neuroreport* 8: 2849–2852

408 Yamamoto-Sasaki M, Ozawa H, Saito T, Rosler M, Riederer P (1999) Impaired phosphorylation of cyclic AMP response element binding protein in the hippocampus of dementia of the Alzheimer type. *Brain Res* 824: 300–303

409 Yamada T, Yoshiyama Y, Kawaguchi N (1997) Expression of activating transcription factor-2 (ATF-2), one of the cyclic AMP response element (CRE) binding proteins, in Alzheimer disease and non-neurological brain tissues. *Brain Res* 749: 329–334

410 Lu W, Mi R, Tang H, Liu S, Fan M, Wang L (1998) Over-expression of c-fos mRNA in the hippocampal neurons in Alzheimer's disease. *Chin Med J (Engl)* 111: 35–37

411 Marcus DL, Strafaci JA, Miller DC, Masia S, Thomas CG, Rosman J, Hussain S, Freedman ML (1998) Quantitative neuronal c-fos and c-jun expression in Alzheimer's disease. *Neurobiol Aging* 19: 393–400

412 Anderson AJ, Cummings BJ, Cotman CW (1994) Increased immunoreactivity for Jun- and Fos-related proteins in Alzheimer's disease: association with pathology. *Exp Neurol* 125: 286–295

413 MacGibbon GA, Lawlor PA, Walton M, Sirimanne E, Faull RL, Synek B, Mee E, Connor B, Dragunow M (1997) Expression of Fos, Jun, and Krox family proteins in Alzheimer's disease. *Exp Neurol* 147: 316–332

414 Ferrer I, Segui J, Planas AM (1996) Amyloid deposition is associated with c-Jun expression in Alzheimer's disease and amyloid angiopathy. *Neuropathol Appl Neurobiol* 22: 521–526

415 El Khoury J, Hickman SE, Thomas CA, Loike JD, Silverstein SC (1998) Microglia, scavenger receptors, and the pathogenesis of Alzheimer's disease. *Neurobiol Aging* 19: S81–S84

416 Honda M, Akiyama H, Yamada Y, Kondo H, Kawabe Y, Takeya M, Takahashi K, Suzuki H, Doi T, Sakamoto A et al (1998) Immunohistochemical evidence for a macrophage scavenger receptor in Mato cells and reactive microglia of ischemia and Alzheimer's disease. *Biochem Biophys Res Commun* 245: 734–740

417 Christie RH, Freeman M, Hyman BT (1996) Expression of the macrophage scavenger receptor, a multifunctional lipoprotein receptor, in microglia associated with senile plaques in Alzheimer's disease. *Am J Pathol* 148: 399–403

418 Shirai H, Murakami T, Yamada Y, Doi T, Hamakubo T, Kodama T (1999) Structure and function of type I and II macrophage scavenger receptors. *Mech Ageing Dev* 111: 107–121

Clinical Research Overview

Anti-inflammatory agents as possible protective factors for Alzheimer's disease: Analysis of relevant epidemiological studies

Patrick L. McGeer[1], Michael Schulzer[2] and Edith G. McGeer[1]

Kinsmen Laboratory of Neurological Research, [1]Department of Psychiatry and [2]Departments of Medicine and Statistics, University of British Columbia, 2255 Wesbrook Mall, Vancouver, B.C., V6T 1Z3, Canada

Introduction

Alzheimer's disease (AD), an intractable disorder which primarily affects the elderly, is the cause of more than two-thirds of all dementia cases. Currently available drugs may give some symptomatic relief but are not designed to prevent the disease or arrest its progression. As reviewed elsewhere in this book, many studies have now shown the presence of a chronic inflammatory reaction in affected regions of AD brain. Particularly noteworthy is the presence of many activated microglia and greatly elevated levels of inflammatory cytokines and all the components of the classical complement cascade, including the membrane attack complex. This complex, as well as free radicals and other molecules produced in abundance by activated microglia, may damage host tissue. This has led to the hypothesis that antiinflammatory agents may slow the progress of AD or inhibit its onset [1, 2].

There are now 18 published epidemiological studies in which antiinflammatory drugs or arthritis have been included as risk factors for AD [2–19]. This chapter reviews these studies, and applies methods of statistical meta-analysis to combine the results in order to estimate the extent of risk reduction and its statistical significance.

Statistical methods

The outcome of a risk factor analysis is often expressed as an odds ratio. This is a commonly used statistic for estimation of the relative risk of developing the dis-

Neuroinflammatory Mechanisms in Alzheimer's Disease: Basic and Clinical Research,
edited by Joseph Rogers

order if there is exposure to a particular factor. It measures the odds that a person in an exposed group will develop AD, relative to the corresponding odds for a person in a control, or non-exposed group. The relative risk can be calculated directly only from cross-sectional or prospective studies. The odds ratio, however, provides comparable estimates of the association between the antecedent factor and the outcome (AD) from retrospective (case-control) studies, as well as from cross-sectional and prospective study designs [20, 21]. A negative risk, corresponding to a protective factor, yields an odds ratio less than one, while a positive risk factor is associated with an odds ratio greater than one. Estimating overall odds ratios using data from multiple reports requires that the studies be similar in design.

Accordingly, the available epidemiological studies were grouped according to their design type and the risk factor being assessed.

Six categories were identified: case control studies in which arthritis was considered as a risk factor; case control and population-based studies in which rheumatoid arthritis was considered as a risk factor; case control studies in which steroids were considered as a risk factor; and case control and population-based studies in which non-steroidal antiinflammatory drugs (NSAIDs) were considered as a risk factor.

The logarithms of the reported odds ratios for each study in a given category were combined according to the meta-analytic method of Fleiss [20]. His technique is appropriate for situations where the number of studies to be combined is small, and the within-study sample sizes are reasonably large [20, 22]. Standard errors of the logarithms of the odds ratios for the individual studies were inferred from the confidence intervals reported. When no confidence intervals were given, the standard errors were calculated from the data.

A test of statistical homogeneity was then performed to ensure that there were no inconsistent odds-ratios within the group [20, 22, 23]. This test formally evaluates the hypothesis that the individual odds ratios are estimates of a common parameter, against the alternative that they estimate different parameters. The test statistic Q is a weighted sum of squares of the estimated odds ratios about their weighted mean, and, if the hypothesis holds, Q has a chi-square distribution with k-1 degrees of freedom, where k is the number of studies in the group [23]. If the homogeneity test failed ($p(H) < 0.05$), no further calculations were performed. If the hypothesis of homogeneity was not rejected ($p(H) > 0.05$), a fixed effects model was used to obtain a point estimate of the combined odds ratio for the group, along with a 95% confidence interval and a corresponding test of significance [20–22]. Also calculated was the minimum number of studies with null results that would need to reside in "file drawers" to overturn the significance of the combined odds ratio. This is obtained by applying the method of Rosenthal [24] to judge the effect of publication bias. Publication bias represents the tendency of authors and journals to omit publication of non-significant findings [23, 25].

Results

Case control studies where arthritis was considered as a risk factor

Seven case control studies were conducted in which arthritis was included as a risk factor. They involved cohorts from the United States [3, 4, 9, 10, 11], Australia [5], China [7] and Canada [8]. In the initial study of Heyman et al. [3], a nested cohort of 40 AD cases, who had previously participated in a comprehensive, genetic and epidemiological study at Duke University Medical Center was compared with a matched community control group selected by random-digit telephone dialing. Exposure to various factors was determined by personal interview. The odds ratio for arthritis was 1.19. This was followed by the study of French et al. [4] who compared 78 clinically diagnosed male AD cases from the Veterans Administration Medical Center in Minneapolis with two different control groups, a hospital control group selected from records at the same medical center and non-hospital controls from surveys of the surrounding areas. Exposure was determined by interview with random reconfirmation in 15% of the interviews. The odds ratio was given only for the hospital control group and was 0.62. Broe et al. [5] compared a group of 178 clinically diagnosed AD cases obtained from a Sydney, Australia, catchment area and 178 controls selected from names suggested by the general practice physicians referring the AD cases to the clinic. Exposure to various risk factors was determined by personal interview, and the odds ratio for arthritis was 0.56. Breteler et al. [6] published a reanalysis of these early data, but this report was not included in the overall analysis because of the redundancy of the data presented. Li et al. [7] compared a series of 70 clinically diagnosed AD patients from several cities in China with 140 controls drawn from the registration offices of the neighborhoods of the patients. Relatives of both the patients and the controls were used as informants for risk factors which were analyzed by direct interview. The odds ratio found for arthritis was very low, 0.16. In the Canadian Health Study [8], 201 AD subjects were recruited from both communities and institutions across Canada through initial cognitive impairment screening, followed by clinical examination. They were matched against 468 cognitively normal people identified by the same screening procedure. Risk factor questionnaires were completed by proxy respondents, usually a close relative, for both cases and controls. The odds ratio for arthritis was 0.54.

The two studies of Breitner et al. [9, 10] were designed to eliminate, or at least minimize, genetic factors. In the initial study, Breitner et al. [9] identified 50 elderly twin pairs from across the United States, 26 of whom were homozygotes, where one twin developed AD three or more years before the other. Subjects suspected of having AD were examined at home by standard neuropsychological test procedures. Similar procedures were followed for unaffected twins. Exposure information was obtained by self-reporting or, where that was not possible, from surrogates. In the second study [10], sibships were selected from 45 pedigrees that had been studied at

Table 1 - Meta-analysis of homogeneous studies on arthritis or use of antiinflammatory drugs as a risk factor for Alzheimer disease (Drug or disease group/control group)

Drug or disease group	Study type	Odds ratio	P
Controls	Case controlled	1.000	
Steroids (4 studies)	Case controlled	0.656	0.049
Arthritis (7 studies)	Case controlled	0.556	< 0.0001
NSAIDs (4 studies)	Case controlled	0.475	< 0.0001
Rheumatoid arthritis (2 studies)	Population-based	0.194	< 0.0001

Duke University. They were not connected to the twin studies. For inclusion sibships met one of two criteria: presence of 2 or more cases of AD with onsets that differed in age by 3 or more years; or at least one affected individual and one or more unaffected sibs who had survived 3 or more years beyond the onset age of the index case. Telephone interviews were then conducted with subjects or collateral informants to determine exposures. The odds ratios found for arthritis in the two studies were 0.64 [9] and 0.454 [10].

In all but the final study of Breitner et al. [10], arthritis was included as one of a multitude of medical conditions and stood out as the only one consistently identified as a protective or negative risk factor. Details regarding the type of arthritis were not specified in any of these studies. Age was carefully controlled in all the studies but genetic factors were addressed only in the two studies of Breitner et al. In any event, genetic factors would only confound the results if arthritis was distributed differently in subpopulations genetically susceptible to AD than in the general population, and if these subpopulations constituted a significant proportion of the total AD cohort included. The fact that the odds ratios for the two Breitner et al. studies were in the same range as in most of the other studies, diminishes the possibility that genetic makeup was a confounding factor.

On testing the seven studies for homogeneity, the hypothesis of homogeneity was not rejected ($p(H) < 0.194$). Therefore a combined odds ratio was calculated, with a value of 0.556 (95% confidence interval 0.442–0.700) (Tab. 1). This odds ratio was highly significant ($p < 0.0001$), and it would require at least 36 null studies to overturn the significance of the odds ratio [24].

Case control studies where rheumatoid arthritis was considered as a risk factor

Rheumatoid arthritis is much less common than osteoarthritis. It is typically of earlier onset and is more severe than osteoarthritis, requiring aggressive antiinflammatory treatment. Only two case control studies considered rheumatoid arthritis as a risk factor [11, 12]. Graves et al. [11] selected 130 clinically diagnosed AD cases from two Seattle, Washington clinics. They were matched with 130 controls made up of friends, surrogates or non-blood relatives of the patients. Exposure to a variety of factors, including rheumatoid arthritis, was determined through telephone interviews with patient and control surrogates. The study of Jenkinson et al. [14] was restricted to AD and rheumatoid arthritis. They surveyed 192 consecutive inpatients coming to a London geriatric unit, four of whom were excluded from the study due to schizophrenia. The remainder included 96 AD and 92 non-AD cases. The presence or absence of rheumatoid arthritis was determined in each case by clinical examination using criteria established by the American Rheumatism Association.

The results of the two studies differed. Graves et al. [11] found 6.2% of their AD patients to be exposed compared with 3.8% of their controls. The age-adjusted odds ratio of 1.18 was not considered significant. By contrast, Jenkinson et al. [12] found only 2% of their AD cases suffering from rheumatoid arthritis compared with 13% of their controls, for a highly significant odds ratio of 0.17. The test for homogeneity of the two studies gave a p(H) value of 0.0393, i.e. <0.05, indicating that homogeneity was not acceptable. Further case control studies are necessary for reliable odds ratios to be calculated.

Population-based studies in which rheumatoid arthritis was considered as a risk factor

Three population based studies considered rheumatoid arthritis as a risk factor.

McGeer et al. [2] examined the records of 973 rheumatoid arthritics aged 65 and older who had been followed for long periods of time in established clinics in Saskatchewan and Arizona. Only 4 cases of dementia (0.41%) were identified. They also gathered statistics from the discharge records of hospitals in three Canadian provinces and Arizona. Of 7490 patients aged 65 or older with the diagnosis of rheumatoid arthritis, a concomitant diagnosis of AD was found in only 0.39% of these cases. The prevalence of AD in the 65 and older general population was conservatively estimated to be about 2.7% based on studies using comparable survey methods. This is considerably less than the 5.1% reported later by the Canadian Study of Health and Aging Working Group from their 1991–1992 survey [26]. However, that survey used detailed diagnostic methods which detected early and mild AD cases that are often missed in more general surveys.

Beard et al. [13] examined data from the Rochester, Minnesota AD incidence cohort covering the years 1950–1975. They identified 521 cases of rheumatoid arthritis, of which 23 (4.4%) subsequently developed AD. They concluded that the prevalence of AD amongst rheumatoid arthritics reported by McGeer et al. [2] was

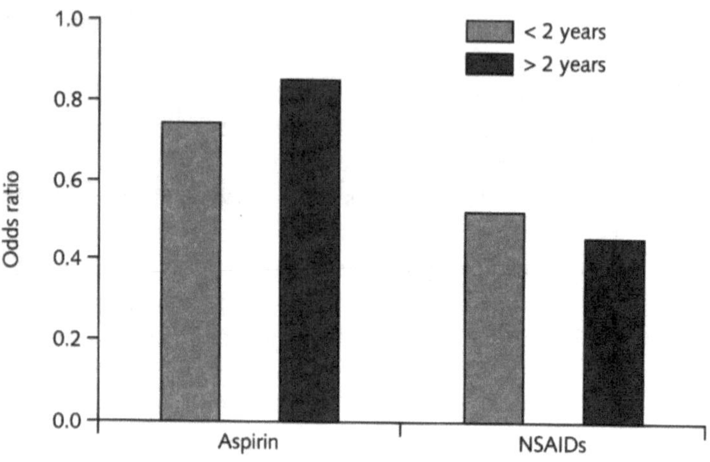

Figure 1
Odds ratios reported by Stewart et al. [18] for the use of aspirin as compared with NSAIDs as risk factors for Alzheimer disease; and effect of duration of use.

too low. Since the age specificity of their survey was not included, it cannot be determined whether this incidence was higher or lower than would be expected in an age-matched general population. Nevertheless, it is unlikely that age distribution alone could account for such a large difference. One possibility might be differing methods of treatment for rheumatoid arthritis used in the periods covered by the two surveys. The Beard et al. series was derived from records of an era when salicylates were widely used for rheumatoid arthritis. All but one of their AD cases had received such treatment. By the time of the McGeer et al. survey, salicylates had been largely replaced by the more powerful NSAIDs. Breitner et al. [10] did an orthogonal comparison of the effect of aspirin and other NSAIDs in reducing the risk of AD. Their data suggested that aspirin alone produced a similar but weaker effect compared with other NSAIDs. Stewart et al. [18] also found a very marked difference between the protective effects of aspirin and various NSAIDs (Fig. 1).

Myllykangas-Luosujarvi and Isomaki [14], using official statistics, investigated the causes of death during the year 1989 for the whole Finnish population over age 55. Only 2 rheumatoid arthritic patients died with AD, which was 0.12% of the rheumatoid arthritic subpopulation. In the general population, 227 individuals died with AD, which was 0.54% of the cohort. The odds ratio was 0.23 with a 95% confidence interval of 0.065–0.826. They concluded their data supported the suggested negative association between AD and rheumatoid arthritis.

For overall statistical analysis, the rheumatoid arthritic clinic data of McGeer et al. [2] and Myllykangas-Luosujarvi and Isomaki [14] were combined, and the hypothesis of homogeneity was not rejected ($p(H) = 0.735$). The overall odds ratio was 0.194 (95% confidence interval 0.092–0.410, $p < 0.0001$; Tab. 1). Eight null studies would be required to overturn the significance of this result. The Beard et al. study could not be included due to the lack of age specificity.

The most logical explanation for the negative associations between arthritis generally, and rheumatoid arthritis specifically, is the long term use of antiinflammatory drugs.

NSAIDs are by far the most commonly used agents for these conditions. Steroids are probably the next most commonly used class although their use is restricted to the more severely affected cases, and the administration is usually intermittent. Both classes of agents have been considered as possible protective factors in epidemiological studies of AD.

Case control studies in which steroids were considered as a risk factor

Four of the previously described case control studies included steroids as a risk factor [8–11]. Each of the four studies showed an odds ratio below 1, although only in the twin study of Breitner et al. [9] was the odds ratio (3/12 or 0.25) considered to be statistically significant ($p = 0.04$).

Interestingly, in their subsequent larger study of sibships at equal risk for AD, Breitner et al. [10] found the odds ratio to be of considerably lower significance than in the initial study, although the numbers exposed in the AD and non-AD groups combined were still small (9/151, odds ratio 0.57). The case numbers in the studies by Graves et al. [11] and the Canadian Health Study [8] were considerably larger than in the Breitner studies, with the odds ratios being very close (0.73 and 0.75, respectively). The hypothesis of homogeneity was not rejected ($p(H) = 0.538$), and the overall odds ratio was estimated. The value was 0.656 (95% confidence interval 0.431–0.999, $p = 0.0492$). Only two null studies would be required to overturn the significance of the odds ratio.

Case control studies in which NSAIDs were considered as a risk factor

Three of the four case control studies in which steroids were considered as a risk factor also included NSAIDs as a risk factor [8–10]. An additional study by Stewart et al. [18] used data collected on biennial examinations between 1980 and 1995 of 1686 participants in the Baltimore Longitudinal Study of Aging. The use of aspirin or other NSAID was based on self-reports.

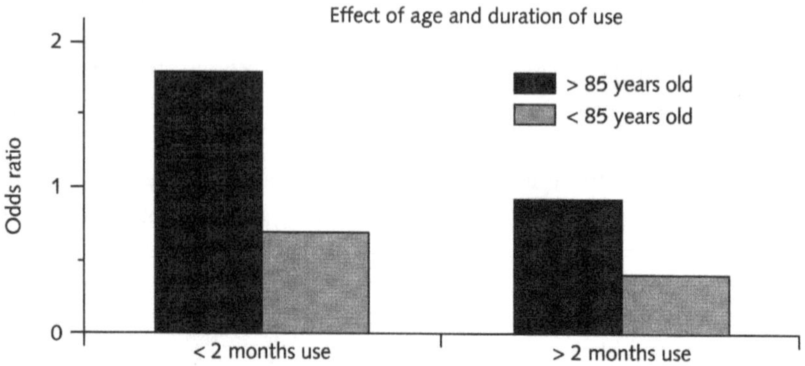

Figure 2
Effects of the duration of use of NSAIDs reported by Veld et al. [19] on the odds ratios obtained for them as risk factors for Alzheimer disease.

Veld et al. [19] used 74 AD patients and 232 age and sex-matched controls from the population-based Rotterdam study. NSAID use was abstracted from general practitioners' medical records and expressed as cumulative prescription days. This recent study could not, however, be incorporated into the meta-analysis since it differed in design from the other case controlled studies.

The odds ratios for the four NSAID case control studies used for meta-analysis [8–10, 18] did not support rejection of the hypothesis of homogeneity ($p(H) = 0.264$), and so the combined odds ratio was estimated. This was 0.475 (95% confidence interval 0.343–0.695, $p < 0.0001$). Thus, the odds ratio was smaller and the level of significance greater than for steroids.

An interesting aspect of the two most recent studies [18, 19] is that they considered the effect of length of NSAID use. As shown in Figure 1 for the Baltimore study [18] and in Figure 2 for the Rotterdam study [19], both groups found prolonged use of NSAIDs decreased the odds ratio. Another interesting aspect of the Rotterdam study is that NSAID use only appeared to be protective in persons below the age of 85 (Fig. 2).

Population-based studies in which NSAIDs were considered as a risk factor

Three population-based studies considered NSAIDs as a risk factor [15–17]. The methods in each case were completely different, so the results did not lend themselves to combined analysis. Lucca et al. [15], in their Italian study, approached the problem by considering whether AD patients used NSAIDs to a greater or lesser extent than elderly controls. They reviewed the data from two clinical trials involving 195 AD patients. They found NSAID users to be only 0.8% and 0% of the total cohorts in these trials designed to test the efficacy of other agents. They compared these NSAID use figures with data obtained from medical records in three general surveys of elderly patients: a sequential sample of the elderly from general practice and two randomized surveys of very old patients drawn from general practioner records. They found NSAID users were 22.8%, 20.3% and 18.5% of these control cohorts. They compared osteoarthritic pathology in the AD and control groups as a criterion to determine if they differed in their indication for NSAID use. They found that osteoarthritic pathology was present in 22% of the AD patients compared with 26% of the controls. They concluded that, because of the comparable osteoarthritic pathology, NSAID use was far lower than expected in the AD group. They considered that NSAID use may have reduced vulnerability to AD in the control group.

Andersen et al. [16] surveyed all eligible community-dwelling and institutionalized individuals in the Ommoord district of Rotterdam aged 55 years and over. They found only 1.4% of 365 NSAID users to be suffering from AD, compared with 2.5% in the total cohort of 5893. The odds ratio adjusted for gender, age, education and benzodiazepine use was 0.38. As a control subgroup of drug users, they chose a cohort of 365 topical medication users. The odds ratio using this control group increased to 0.54. In either case, they concluded their findings were compatible with a possible protective effect of NSAIDs on the risk of developing AD.

Rich et al. [17] reviewed the records of 210 patients in the John Hopkins Alzheimer Disease Research Center to evaluate the role of NSAIDs. Thirty-two AD NSAID users were compared with 177 AD non-NSAID users on clinical, cognitive and psychiatric measures. They found that the NSAID group had a significantly shorter duration of illness at study entry, and, over a one year longitudinal study in the clinic, a slower progression of AD. They concluded that NSAIDs may serve a protective role in AD.

These three studies, involving very different approaches in three different countries all reached the same general conclusion that NSAIDs have a protective function against the development or progression of AD.

Discussion

This review covers the eighteen epidemiological studies in which arthritis or antiinflammatory drugs have been considered as possible risk factors for AD. Negative associations were found in individual studies from eight different countries. Case control studies for arthritis, steroids and non-steroidal antiinflammatory drugs all showed significant negative associations. Population-based studies involving clinics, hospital separations and mortality statistics for rheumatoid arthritis, and medical practice records and community surveys for NSAIDs also indicated significant negative associations.

Statistical meta-analysis of groups of studies yielded firmer figures on odds ratios and at a much higher level of statistical significance than individual studies (Tab. 1). Age, which is a major positive risk factor and a potentially confounding variable, was considered in all but one of the surveys [13]. The genetic factor was tightly controlled in two of the studies [9, 10], both of which yielded results in the same range as other surveys.

These epidemiological data provide an impressive correlation for the existing evidence that AD lesions are characterized by a chronic neuroinflammatory state which may promote neuronal destruction [1]. Neuroinflammation is a silent process. It differs from peripheral inflammation in that some of the cardinal signs (tumor, dolor) do not exist, while others (rubor, calor) cannot, as yet, be evaluated. Moreover, it appears as if the inflammatory response in AD brain, which involves vigorous activation of the complement system, does not involve antibodies, indicating that the irritant action is not of the classical autoimmune variety [27].

The epidemiological studies provide general information that antiinflammatory agents may delay the onset and slow the progression of AD. However, the data are too uncertain to predict which drugs, or combination of drugs, might be useful. Moreover, only limited data exist on the relative ability of various NSAIDs to reach the brain. Such information has not heretofore been considered important. Steroids have ready access to the brain, but the long term consequences of their use, particularly in the elderly, create a problem. Steroids will damage hippocampal neurons in culture [28]. Such neurons are already among the most heavily damaged in AD. *In vivo*, steroids produce electrolyte disturbances that induce congestive heart failure, osteoporosis leading to bone fractures, vulnerability to infection and suppression of hypothalamic-pituitary function, causing endocrine and psychological dysfunction [29]. NSAIDs also have important side effects, the most dangerous of which is inducing gastrointestinal ulceration. Partial drug protection for this major side effect is available [30].

The odds ratios of 0.496 for NSAIDs and 0.656 for steroids suggest the possibility of substantial pharmacoeconomic benefits being attached to antiinflammatory therapy for AD. So far, there has been only one clinical trial testing this possibility. That was a small, double blind, placebo-controlled pilot trial of six months duration using the NSAID indomethacin [31]. The indomethacin patients appeared to hold their own while the placebo patients deteriorated at a rate comparable to that observed in other studies [32].

The patient population was very small, and the trial must be considered very preliminary.

Further, more comprehensive trials are required to verify whether these epidemiological data genuinely reflect a protective effect of antiinflammatory drugs for AD.

Acknowledgements
Supported by grants from the Alzheimer Society of British Columbia and the Jack Brown and Family A.D. Research Fund, as well as donations from individual British Columbians.

References

1 McGeer PL, Rogers J (1992) Anti-inflammatory agents as a therapeutic approach to Alzheimer's disease. *Neurology* 42: 447–449
2 McGeer PL, McGeer EG, Rogers J, Sibley J (1990) Anti-inflammatory drugs and Alzheimer disease. *Lancet* 335: 1037
3 Heyman A, Wilkinson WE, Stafford JA, Helms MJ, Sigmon AH, Weinberg T (1984) Alzheimer's disease: a study of epidemiological aspects. *Ann Neurol* 15: 335–341
4 French LR, Schuman LM, Mortimer JA, Hutton JT, Boatman RA, Christians B (1985) A case-control study of dementia of the Alzheimer's type. *Am J Epidemiol* 121: 414–421
5 Broe GA, Henderson AS, Creasey H, McCusker E, Korten AE, Jorm AF, Longley W, Anthony JC (1990) A case-control study of Alzheimer's disease in Australia. *Neurology* 40: 1698–1707
6 Breteler MMB, van Duijn CM, Andra VCI, Fratiglioni L, Graves AB, Heyman A, Jorm AF, Kokmen, E, Kondo K, Mortimer JA et al (1991) Medical history and the risk of Alzheimer's disease: a collaborative re-analysis of case-control studies. *Int J Epidemiol* 20: S36–S42
7 Li G, Shen YC, Chen CH, Zhau YW, Silverman JM (1992) A case-control study of Alzheimer's disease in China. *Neurology* 42: 1481–1482
8 Anon (1994) Canadian Study of Health and Aging: Risk factors for Alzheimer's disease in Canada. *Neurology* 44: 2073–2080
9 Breitner JCS, Gau BA, Welsh KA, Plassman BL, McDonald WM, Helms MJ, Anthony JC (1994) Inverse association of anti-inflammatory treatments and Alzheimer's disease. *Neurology* 44: 227–232
10 Breitner JCS, Welsh KA, Helms MJ, Gaskell PC, Gau BA, Roses AD, Pericak-Vance MA, Saunders AM (1995) Delayed onset of Alzheimer's disease with nonsteroidal anti-inflammatory and histamine H2 blocking drugs. *Neurobiol Aging* 16: 523–530
11 Graves AB, White E, Koepsell TD, Reifler BV, van Belle G, Larson EB, Raskind M (1990) A case-control study of Alzheimer's disease. *Ann Neurol* 28: 766–774
12 Jenkinson MI, Bliss MR, Brain AT, Scott DL (1989) Rheumatoid arthritis and senile dementia of the Alzheimer's type. *Brit J Rheumatol* 28: 86–87
13 Beard CM, Kokmen E, Kurland LT (1991) Rheumatoid arthritis and susceptibility to Alzheimer's disease. *Lancet* 337: 1426
14 Myllykangas-Luosujarvi R, Isomaki H (1994) Alzheimer's disease and rheumatoid arthritis. *Brit J Rheumatol* 33: 501–502

15 Lucca U, Tettamanti M, Forloni G, Spagnoli A (1994) Nonsteroidal antiinflammatory drug use in Alzheimer's disease. *Biol Psychiatry* 36: 854–856
16 Andersen K, Launer LJ, Ott A, Hoes AW, Breteler MMB, Hofman A (1995) Do nonsteroidal antiinflammatory drugs decrease the risk for Alzheimer's disease? *Neurology* 45: 1441–1445
17 Rich JB, Rasmusson DX, Folstein MF, Carson KA, Kawas C, Brandt J (1995) Nonsteroidal anti-inflammatory drugs in Alzheimer's disease. *Neurology* 45: 51–55
18 Stewart WF, Kawas C, Corrada M, Metter EJ (1997) Risk of Alzheimer's disease and duration of NSAID use. *Neurology* 48: 626–632
19 'T Veld BA, Launer LJ, Hoes AW, Ott A, Hofman A, Breteler MMB, Stricker BHC (1998) NSAIDs and incident Alzheimer's disease. The Rotterdam study. *Neurobiol Aging* 19: 607–611
20 Fleiss JL (1981) *Statistical methods for rates and proportions*, 2nd ed, John Wiley & Sons, New York, 160–176
21 Fleiss JL (1994) Measures of effect size for categorical data. In: H Cooper, LV Hedges (eds): *The handbook of research synthesis.* Russell Sage Foundation, New York, 245– 260
22 Shadish WR, Haddock CK (1994) Combining estimates of effect size. In: H Cooper, LV Hedges (eds): *The handbook of research synthesis.* Russell Sage Foundation, New York, 261–281
23 Hedges LV, Olkin I (1998) *Statistical methods for meta-analysis.* Academic Press, San Diego, 107–145, 189–203, 285–309
24 Rosenthal R (1979) The "file drawer" problem and tolerance for null results. *Psychol Bull* 86: 638–641
25 Begg CB (1994) Publication bias. In: H Cooper, LV Hedges (eds): *The handbook of research synthesis.* Russell Sage Foundation, New York, 399–409
26 Anon (1994) Canadian Study of Health and Aging: study methods and prevalence of dementia. *Can Med Assoc J* 150: 899–913
27 McGeer PL, McGeer EG (1995) The inflammatory response system of brain: Implications for therapy of Alzheimer and other neurodegenerative diseases. *Brain Res Rev* 21: 195–218
28 Landfield PW, Eldridge JC (1989) Increased affinity of type II corticosteroid binding in aged rat hippocampus. *Exp Neurol* 106: 110–113
29 Lewis DA, Smith RE (1983) Steroid-induced psychiatric syndromes. *J Affect Disord* 5: 319–332
30 Graham DY, Agrawal NM, Roth SH (1988) Prevention of NSAID-induced gastric ulcer with misoprostol: multicentre, double-blind, placebo-controlled trial. *Lancet* ii: 1277–1280
31 Rogers J, Kirby LC, Hempelman SR, Berry DL, McGeer PL, Kaszniak AW, Zalinski J, Cofield M, Mansukhani L, Willson P, Kogan F (1993) Clinical trial of indomethacin in Alzheimer's disease. *Neurology* 43: 1609–1611
32 Mortimer JA, Ebbitt B, Jun S-P, Finch MD (1992) Predictors of cognitive and functional progression in patients with probable Alzheimer's disease. *Neurology* 42: 1689–1696

Topics of Special Interest

Role and regulation of early complement activation products in Alzheimer's disease

Robert Veerhuis[1,2], Freek L. Van Muiswinkel[3], C. Erik Hack[4] and Piet Eikelenboom[1]

Research Institute Neurosciences Vrije Universiteit, Graduate School Neurosciences Amsterdam, [1]Department of Psychiatry, PCA Valeriuskliniek, Valeriusplein 9, 1075 BG Amsterdam, The Netherlands; [2]Department of Pathology, De Boelelaan 1117, 1081 HV Amsterdam, The Netherlands; [3]Department of Pharmacology, Van der Boechorststraat 7, 1081 BT Amsterdam, The Netherlands; [4]Department of Autoimmune Diseases, Central Laboratory of the Netherlands Red Cross Bloodtransfusion Service, Plesmanlaan 125, 1066 CX Amsterdam, The Netherlands

Introduction

Altered metabolism of the amyloid precursor protein (APP) and the progressive deposition of the amyloid β fragment (Aβ) in amyloid plaques may be crucial to the onset and progression of Alzheimer's disease (AD). How mismetabolism of APP accompanied by Aβ deposition leads to neurofibrillary changes is not completely known. A number of studies have suggested that these changes result from local inflammatory reactions ensuing in the brains of AD patients, since a variety of inflammatory mediators were found to be associated with both diffuse and neuritic Aβ deposits [1]. These mediators include complement activation products [2, 3], protease inhibitors [1, 4, 5] and interleukins [6]. These and other factors found in plaques (e.g. heparan sulfate proteoglycans (HSPG) [7, 8] and Apolipoprotein E (Apo E) [8, 9]) may be involved in the regulation of Aβ fibril formation.

Serum amyloid P (SAP) and HSPG probably are essential components required for amyloid fibril formation and persistance [10, 11] in virtually all chemical classes of amyloid in a variety of human diseases [12]. Apo E [13] and complement C1q [14] can accelerate Aβ fibrillogenesis, whereas α_1-antichymotrypsin (ACT) and clusterin (Apolipoprotein J), which are upregulated in AD plaque areas [15, 16], may be involved in the disaggregation of Aβ fibrils [17] or may prevent Aβ aggregation [18, 19], respectively. A delicate balance between factors that maintain Aβ in its soluble form and those that promote Aβ fibrillarization likely determines initial Aβ deposition and/or the transformation of diffuse into fibrillar plaques. This is illustrated by the distinct distribution patterns of a number of Aβ associated proteins found in brain regions that are differentially affected in AD (e.g. cerebral *versus* cerebellar

Neuroinflammatory Mechanisms in Alzheimer's Disease: Basic and Clinical Research,
edited by Joseph Rogers

cortex) and in brain specimens from cases with a different clinical status (demented *versus* non-demented) [8].

The co-localization of intercellular adhesion molecule-1 (ICAM-1; CD54) and activated microglia expressing lymphocyte function-associated antigen-1 (LFA-1; CD11a/CD18) and complement receptor type 3 (CR3; Mac-1; CD11b/CD18) [20–22], suggests a role for β_2-integrin cytoadhesion within Aβ plaques. The expression of ICAM-1 [22–24] by endothelial cells lining cerebral blood vessels and of other molecules involved in adhesion and migration of leucocytes, such as vascular cell adhesion molecule-1 (VCAM-1; CD106) [22], is not increased, whereas endothelial leukocyte adhesion molecule-1 (ELAM-1; E-selectin; CD62E) appears to be absent [25]. These findings, together with absence of immunoglobulins in amyloid plaques and of T cell subsets in AD brains [2, 21], support the view that in AD brains the neuritic plaque is closely associated with a locally-induced, aspecific, chronic inflammatory response without influx of leucocytes from the blood into the neuropil. The idea that the Aβ peptide itself can induce a local inflammatory response [26, 27] has received strong impetus by the finding that Aβ peptide can bind C1 and activate the classical complement pathway in an antibody-independent fashion [28–31].

Apart from their effects on Aβ fibril formation, a number of plaque-associated proteins may also affect neurons. In this respect, it is still uncertain whether complement activation that occurs in amyloid plaques may exert neurotoxic effects either directly through formation of the lytic membrane attack complex or indirectly through activation by its early activation products of phagocytes or other cells in the brain.

The complement system

The complement system consists of at least 20 different proteins, most of which are present in a non-activated state in plasma. Binding of complement C1, a Ca^{2+}-dependent complex of the recognition unit C1q and the proenzymes C1r and C1s, to an activator is the initial event in classical pathway activation. Not only antibody-antigen aggregates, but also non-immune activators such as polyanions, the pentraxins serum amyloid P (SAP) and C-reactive protein (CRP) [32] and Aβ peptides [28–30], can bind C1. Binding of C1 generates enzyme activity that starts with the conversion of C1r and C1s into serine-esterases and then leads to a cascade of sequential activation steps and to a repertoire of biological activities. Activated C1s cleaves C2 and C4, which can result in the formation of the classical pathway C3 convertase C4b2b that, after addition of a C3b molecule, changes its substrate specificity into that of C5-convertase. The cleavage fragments C3a, C4a and C5a have anaphylactic and chemotactic properties, e.g. for microglia [33]. In addition, C5a can induce cytokine synthesis [34].

The larger C4b and C3b fragments can covalently bind via an ester or amide bond to a target surface. The C5b fragment, together with C6 and C7, forms the C5b67 complex that can insert into a target membrane. Addition of C8 and several C9 molecules, leads to membrane attack complex (MAC) formation, that disturbs the cell membrane continuity and causes the influx of extracellular calcium, which, depending on the amount of C5b-9 complexes, may cause either cell activation or damage.

Complement activation products (C1q, iC3b) can opsonize invasive microorganisms, senescent cells and soluble or particulate immune complexes. Opsonization facilitates their uptake and degradation by mononuclear phagocytes through synergistic action of both Fc- and complement receptors. However, upon stimulation by, for example, fibronectin or SAP [35] macrophages can phagocytose C3-opsonized targets via their complement receptors CR1 (CD35) and CR3 (CD11b/CD18; Mac-1) alone.

Analogous to the C1q $(C1r\text{-}C1s)_2$ complex binding to its ligands, classical pathway complement activation can also result from the binding of mannan binding protein (MBP), a C1q-like molecule, to certain carbohydrate ligands. Binding of MBP activates its associated serine proteases (MASP 1 and 2), which are homologous to C1r and C1s, and in turn activate C4 and C3. Another mechanism by which the complement system can be activated is the alternative pathway, a positive feedback amplification system, which either is initiated by spontaneous hydrolysis of the internal thioester within C3, or by C3b, for example generated via classical pathway activation. "C3b-like" C3, just as C3b, can bind Factor B to form a C3 convertase analogous to the classical pathway C3 convertase, C4b2b. Except for spontaneous hydrolysis, C4b2b, plasmin and either leucocyte (elastase) or bacterial proteases may generate split C3, that, when associated with Factor B and either stabilized by properdin or stabilized on a "protective surface", may amplify complement activation.

Regulatory proteins that either prevent activation or inactivate factors once activated are needed to prevent harmful side effects of complement activation. Activation and effector functions of the complement system are regulated by a number of regulatory proteins, that can be divided into three categories: (1) Regulatory proteins in plasma that reduce the activity of complement proteases and prevent spontaneous activation of complement, such as inhibitors of C1 activation (C1-inhibitor; C1-Inh) and of C3 and C5 convertases (Factor I and its cofactors Factor H and C4-binding protein). (2) Membrane-bound regulatory proteins that attenuate activation of complement on the cell surface. These include regulators of the C3/C5 convertase CR1 (CD35), decay accelerating factor (CD55) and membrane cofactor protein (MCP; CD46), all co-factors of Factor I. (3) Regulatory proteins that protect cells from complement damage. These include the fluid phase regulators clusterin (Sp-40,40; ApoJ) and vitronectin (S-protein) and the membrane-bound proteins homologous restriction factor (HRF; C8 binding protein) and CD59 (HRF-20).

Complement C1 in AD

Complement activation can directly result from the binding of complement factor C1 to synthetic amyloid peptides under laboratory conditions. The absence of immunoglobulins, the most potent activator of complement, in plaques and the co-localization of complement activation products with amyloid deposits support the view that amyloid activates complement *in vivo*.

In AD neocortex, C1q is deposited in classical plaques consisting of a condensed amyloid core and a corona of less condensed Aβ deposits, and to a lesser extent in diffuse type amyloid plaques [27, 36]. In layers I–IV of the neocortex C1q immunostaining coincides with thioflavine-S positivity, indicative of a β-sheet conformation of Aβ. In deeper layers close to the white matter, thioflavin-negative diffuse-type plaques that clearly immunostain for Aβ and for C1q are found. Whether or not these deeper layer diffuse plaques constitute a subset of aged plaques, similar to those reported to be present in brain specimens of aged dogs [37], remains to be investigated.

In vitro studies have indicated that C1q can bind directly to Aβ [29], particularly when the Aβ is aggregated to a certain degree [30]. C1q interacts with a cluster of negatively charged N-terminal residues within Aβ [38, 39] and subsequently accelerates Aβ aggregation and fibril formation [14]. The identification of the precise binding sites on C1q for Aβ is important for the development of drugs that interfere with this binding, and hence may prevent complement activation in AD brains. Similar to Aβ peptides [29], a number of non-immune activators such as SAP [40] and CRP [41] were shown to bind C1 through a site near the N-terminus of the collagen-like region of C1q. This region within the N-terminal part of the A-chain domain of C1q contains a number of positively charged arginine and lysine residues that engage in an electrostatic interaction with a cluster of four negatively charged side chains in the $A\beta_{1-11}$ region [38, 39], as was shown in competition experiments with C1qA chain peptides [29] and in studies on the effect of ionic strength [38].

Interestingly, Aβ with isoaspartic acid substituted for the aspartic acid at position 7 does not activate C1 [39]. The increased presence of Aβ with isomerized aspartic acid, a phenomenon characteristic for aged proteins, in AD plaques [42, 43] may indicate that these are older amyloid plaques that no longer activate complement and consequently no longer attract and activate glial cells [39].

Early complement components in microglia in AD

The presence of complement activation products [2, 3, 44–46] and of clusters of activated microglial cells [1, 20, 21, 47–50] in neuritic plaques is highly suggestive of an inflammatory process. Microglia synthesizing IL-1 are present in increasing amounts in transition states from diffuse Aβ plaques to dense core neuritic plaques, suggesting that IL-1 expressing microglia are a driving force in the formation of dystrophic neurites [49]. Cytokines are involved in several steps of the amyloid plaque formation in AD [6, 26, 49, 51]. For instance, synthesis of amyloid precursor protein (APP) [52] and of proteins (e.g. ACT) that may determine the rate of Aβ aggregation in the plaques is stimulated by IL-1, possibly in concert with IL-6. In turn, Aβ can induce IL-1 production in microglia [53], providing a positive feedback reaction.

In contrast to neuritic plaques in AD, no microglia or acute phase proteins such as ACT, α_2-macroglobulin or the cytokine inducible adhesion molecule ICAM-1, indicative of a cerebral inflammatory process, can be found in cerebrovascular amyloidosis (CA) in AD brains, although the deposition of various complement activation products, including C1q, C4c, C3c and especially of the membrane attack complex (C5b-9), may be more intense in vascular amyloid than in amyloid plaques. In dyshoric angiopathy (DA), characterized by perivascular Aβ immunoreactivity around cortical vessels, immunostaining for various inflammatory factors as well as for activated microglia resembles that found in neuritic plaques in AD. These findings suggest that different pathogenic mechanisms may underlie the formation of plaques and DA on the one hand, and of CA on the other hand [54]. Further studies should address the question why in CA a full-blown complement activation apparently does not lead to the attraction and activation of microglia, whereas in neuritic plaques decorated with predominantly the early complement classical pathway factors many activated microglia expressing HLA class II antigens and complement iC3b receptors (CR3 and CR4) are found [20].

Although there is no evidence for their presence on human microglia, rat microglia were reported to express phagocytic C1q receptors [55]. Three types of C1q receptors have been described [56]. A 126 kDa C1q receptor (C1qRp), a transmembrane glycoprotein that is involved in phagocytosis and is expressed on monocyte/macrophages, neutrophils, endothelial cells, platelets and also on microglia. Another 50 to 60 kDa receptor, first thought to bind the C1q collagen stalk of C1q only (cC1qR), is expressed on a variety of cell types and later was shown to bind globular heads of C1q, MBP, pulmonary surfactant protein A (SPA) and conglutinin as well. This cC1qR, also called collectin receptor, is identical to calreticulin. Thirdly, a 33 kDa C1q binding site has been reported that can interact with the globular regions of C1q (gC1qR) and appears to be expressed intracellularly [56].

C1q interactions with the phagocytic C1q receptor facilitate the uptake and degradation of immune complexes by guinea pig macrophages [57] and human monocytes [58]. Likewise, C1q that remains bound to the activating substance (Aβ deposits) after complement activation may engage an interaction with C1q receptors expressed on microglia, and facilitate the uptake and degradation of Aβ. This can occur either directly or indirectly through stimulation of the cells, since human monocytes are capable of C3-mediated phagocytosis only when their C3b or iC3b receptors are in an activated state, e.g. after stimulation with substrate bound C1q [56, 59]. C1q can bind to a region within CR1, which shares homology with C1r or C1s [60]. Binding of C1q via this site to CR1, together with a simultaneous β_2 integrin signal, which occurs when LFA-1 or CR3 bind to ICAM-1, stimulates O_2^- release by polymorphonuclear leukocytes (PMN) [61]. Although the relevance of this for AD remains to be established, since CR1 is not expressed, nor are PMNs present in AD brains, C1q may have stimulatory effects on the induction of the release of reactive oxygen species (ROS) and possibly of also other potentially neurotoxic agents by the microglial cells.

Microglial cells secrete the superoxide anion in response to C3-opsonized zymosan *in vitro* [62]. In addition, Aβ was found to act as a priming stimulus for the phorbol-myristate-acetate (PMA)-induced respiratory burst of cultured rat microglia [63] and a human monocyte/macrophage cell line, THP-1 [64]. Moreover, human monocyte-derived macrophages could be stimulated to produce ROS after stimulation with Aβ, without further stimulus. This stimulatory effect is possibly mediated through the interaction of Aβ with a cellular recognition unit recognizing the N-terminal part of Aβ, since $A\beta_{1-16}$ abbrogates the binding and consequent cellular effects of Aβ [65].

The N-terminal residues 13–16 (HHQK) constitute the domain within Aβ that binds to microglia [66] and is responsible for the Aβ-induced respiratory burst activity [65]. HHQK possibly interacts with membrane-associated heparan sulfate, since it has a high binding affinity for heparan sulfate [66]. HHQK is, however, also the site that interacts with C1q and initiates C1 activation [39, 67]. This may explain the synergistic effect of simultaneously added $A\beta_{1-40}$ and C1q on the PMA-induced oxidative burst observed in rat microglia *in vitro* (Figs. 1, 2). Interestingly, immunohistochemical investigation in AD and Down cases has revealed that the N-terminal Aβ is present in plaques with C activation [43].

C1 activation by activators other than Aβ

Aβ peptides, especially when aggregated, bind and activate C1 *in vitro*. Whether this is a predominant pathway *in vivo* where Aβ deposits are decorated with different chaperone proteins remains to be investigated. Serum amyloid P component, which is frequently found associated with different types of amyloid throughout the body and may form a nucleus for amyloid fibril formation [12], can bind and activate C1 *in vitro* [40]. Hence, it seems possible that SAP may contribute to the activation of complement in AD plaques. A role for another pentraxin, C reactive protein, in the onset of AD has been suggested [68]. However, although CRP can bind and activate C1 *in vitro* [41, 69] and *in vivo* [69], at present there are no conclusive indications about the presence of CRP in AD plaques [70–72].

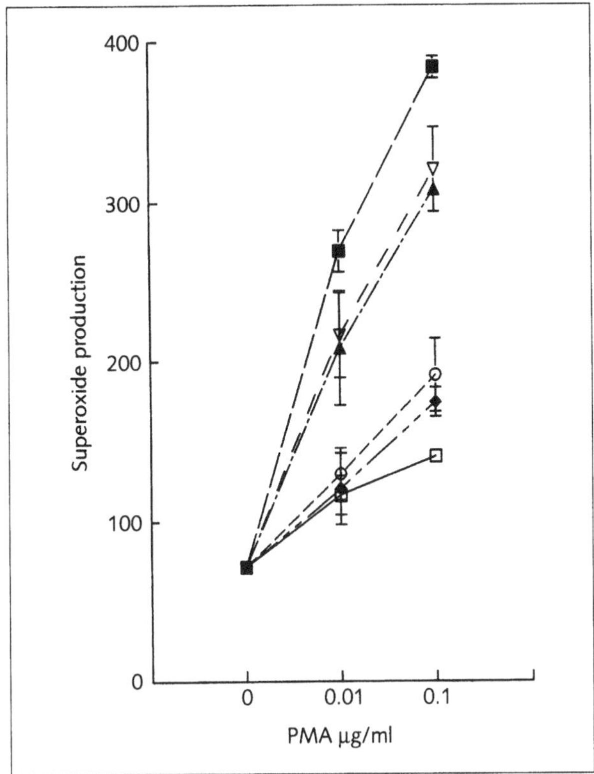

Figure 1
Phorbol 12-myristate 13-acetate (PMA)-induced superoxide production by microglial cultures isolated from cerebral cortices of 2-day-old newborn rats quantified with the INTV (iodonitrotetrazolium violet) reduction assay. Cells were treated with medium (□), 2 μM $A\beta_{1-40}$ (Bachem, Switzerland; O), 10 μM $A\beta_{1-40}$ (Δ), 2 μM $A\beta_{1-40}$ and 40 μg C1q (Quidel) (∇), 10 μM $A\beta_{1-40}$ and 40 μg C1q (■), or 40 μg C1q alone (♦) for 24 h, before the medium was replaced and the burst was triggered with 0.01 or 0.1 μg/ml PMA for 45 min. In addition, the spontaneous release by cells not treated with either Aβ, C1q or PMA Aβ and/or C1q was determined. No effects on cell viability were observed when LDH release by the cells was monitored.

Regulation of C1 activation

C1 inhibitor (C1-Inh) is a plasma glycoprotein belonging to the serine protease inhibitor (serpin) family that reacts through an exposed reactive center loop with the substrate binding site within its target protease(s) to yield stable complexes of the inactivated C1-Inh and its target protease [73, 74]. C1-Inh is the only known physiological regulator of C1 activation and a major inhibitor of the activated factors

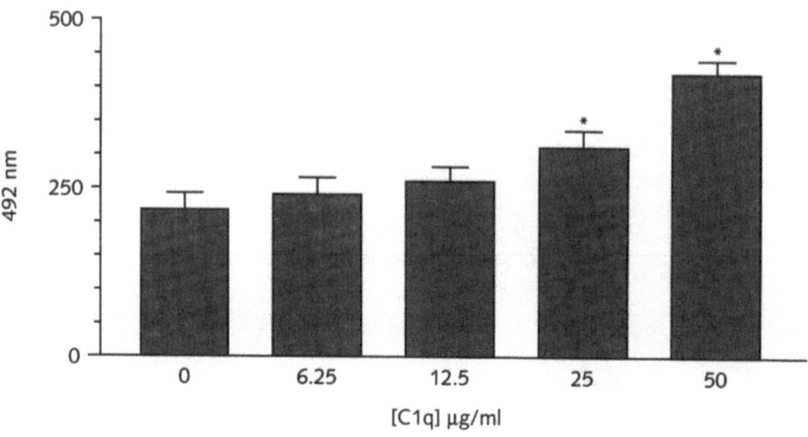

Figure 2
PMA-induced superoxide production by rat microglia after pretreatment with different doses of human C1q. Purified C1q (Quidel) was added to the cultures in medium containing 3% C1q-depleted human serum for 24 h. O_2^- release in cultures to which 0.1 µg PMA/ml was added, was determined using the INTV assay. Data are expressed as OD units and are the mean ± SD from three replicate culture wells. Significantly increased O_2^- release is seen in cells pretreated with greater than 25 µg/ml C1q ($p < 0.05$* versus *stimulated control (PMA-evoked release from untreated cultures)).*

XI, XII, and kallikrein of the contact system of coagulation. In addition, it inhibits the fibrinolytic proteases plasmin and tissue type plasminogen activator (t-PA) [73] (Fig. 3). C1-Inh forms a covalent complex with activated C1r and C1s, thereby abrogating their enzymatic activity. The complexes rapidly dissociate from the activator-bound C1q subunit [75]. Released C1r-C1-Inh and C1s-C1-Inh complexes diffuse into the interstitial fluid and may be (specifically) cleared by phagocytic cells and degraded.

Until recently no clear data were available on the regulation of complement activation at the C1 level in the brain. Native C1-Inh is not detected in amyloid plaques or vascular amyloid [3, 76], whereas inactivated C1-Inh is immunolocalized in dystrophic neurites and neuropil threads [77] and reactive astrocytes [78] in the AD neocortex. Although the very low levels of C1-Inh detected in brain homogenates with ELISA techniques and Western blotting [28, 78] were interpreted as though the C1-Inh was derived from the circulation, it is now clear that C1-Inh is produced locally [77, 78] and that in the brain C1 activation is regulated by C1-Inh.

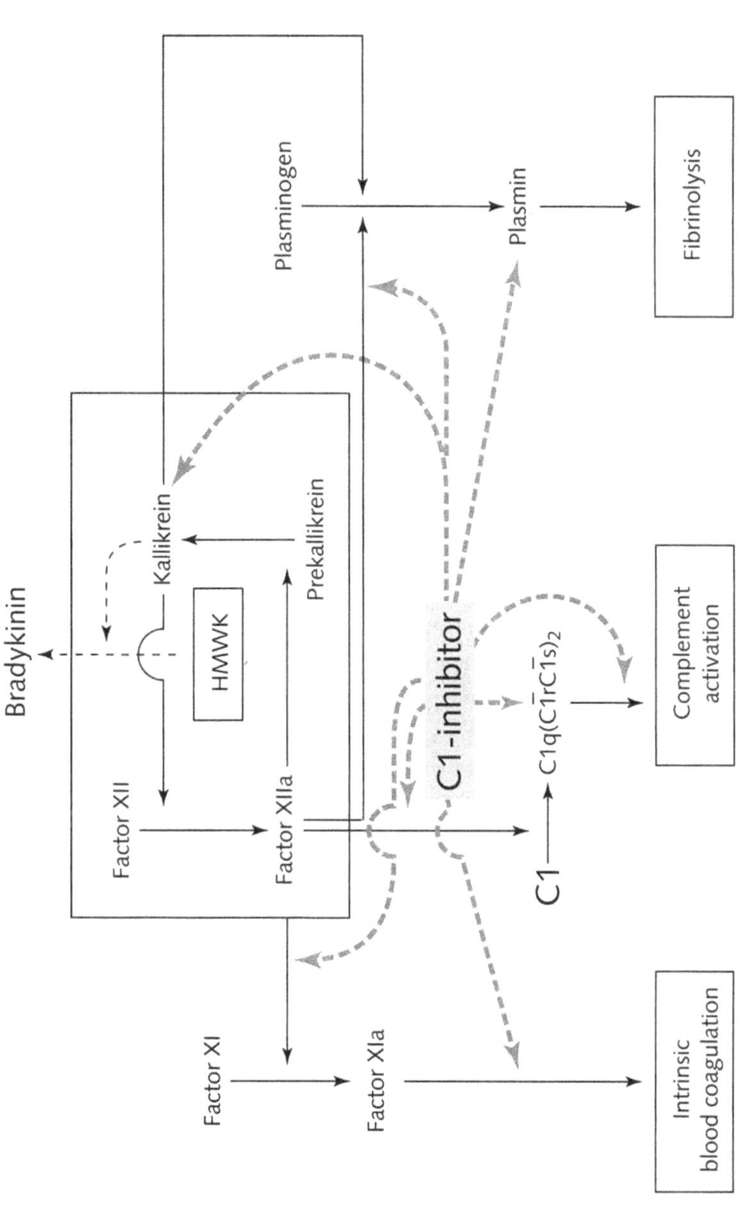

Figure 3
C1-Inhibitor is the only inhibitor of complement C1, and is the major inhibitor of factor XIIa, XIa and kallikrein and thus plays a significant role in the regulation of the complement, coagulation, fibrinolysis and kinin-forming systems.

The question remains, however, to what extent insufficient production or enhanced consumption of C1-Inh contributes to the activation of C1 in AD brains. Possibly, the ongoing C1 activation at sites of Aβ deposits accelerates when the C1/C1-Inh ratio is disturbed due to an increased production of C1 subcomponents. A 2.5-fold molar excess of C1-Inh over C1 in plasma is needed to prevent autocatalytic activation of C1. It is not known what ratio is required to inhibit C1 activation in tissue. Although C1-Inh may be less effective when cell-bound, matrix proteins in tissue may potentiate its functional activity, similar to the potentiating effect of heparin on C1s inhibition by C1-Inh [79]. Type IV collagen was shown to potentiate C1s inhibition [80] and glycosaminoglycans increase the FXIa-inhibitory potential of C1-inh [81]. Other C1 regulatory potentials of proteoglycans include the ability of dermatan sulphate proteoglycan [82] and of chondroitin sulphate proteoglycan [83] to prevent the (re)assembly of the C1 macromolecule. A similar function, i.e. binding to C1q and thereby preventing the association of C1q with C1r and C1s molecules, is suggested for secreted C1q receptor [84]. The relative contributions of these mechanisms to maintaining the balance between C1 assembly, activation and regulation *in vivo* remains to investigated.

Although C1-Inh is the only known physiological inhibitor of C1 activation in plasma, additional inhibitors may act in the brain. Protease inhibitors such as protease nexin–1 (PN-1; a potent thrombin inhibitor), plasminogen activator inhibitor-1 (PAI-1), α_2-macroglobulin, and antithrombin III can be detected in AD brain [85]. In addition, APP contains a Kunitz type protease inhibitor domain that may be involved in the regulation of activation of coagulation factors IX and XI [86]. Although the above mentioned protease inhibitors may well regulate coagulation and fibrinolysis activation and thereby prevent consumption of C1-Inh in these systems, *in vitro* studies have indicated that only PN-1 can bind activated C1s [87]. PN-1 is approximately 10-fold less potent than C1-Inh *in vitro*, but may be important as an inhibitor of C1s activation in the brain when C1-Inh is present at low levels. Indicative of the possible functional significance of PN-1 in AD is its 7-fold lower levels in AD brains compared with control brain specimens [88].

Complement synthesis by brain-derived cells

Complement factors can be synthesized by brain-derived cells [89, 90], not only by astrocytes and microglia, but also by neuroblastoma cell lines *in vitro* [91–93] (Tab. 1). RT-PCR studies have shown that, in addition to C1q, C1s and C1r are also expressed in the brain [78, 94, 95], which suggests that in the brain the C1 macromolecule can be assembled. C1q and C4 mRNA levels are known to be increased in AD brains [94, 96, 97]. In a recent study [95] comparing various brain regions of AD and non-AD brain, all classical pathway complement mRNAs were shown to be

Table 1 - Complement synthesis by brain cells

	C1q	C1r	C1s	C4	C3	C1-inh.
Constitutive						
Cell type	M	A, IMR-32 SK-N-SH	A, IMR-32 SK-N-SH		M; IMR-32	M; SK-N-SH
Effect cytokines						
Microglia	IFN, IL-1	IL-1β; TNFα	IL-1β; TNFα		IL-1β>IL-1α; TNFα>IFN	IFN
Astrocytes		IFN>IL-1α; IL-1β, IL-6 TNFα	IFN>TNFα; IL-1α IL-1β, IL-6	IFN; (IL-6)	IL-1β; TNFα (IL-1α)	IFN
neuroblastoma IMR-32		IFN; IL-1α; IL-1β	IL-1α; IL-1β	IFN	IL-1α; IL-1β>TNFα	(IFN)
neuroblastoma SK-N-SH		IL-6 (IFN; IL-1β)	TNFα	IFN	IL-1β	IFN

Human adult microglia (M), not adult astrocytes (A) or neuroblastoma cell lines (IMR-32 or SK-N-SH) constitutively secrete C1q in culture. C1r and C1s are synthesized by all three cell types. Cytokines that can be detected in AD plaques (IL-1α, IL-1β, IL6, TNFα), and in addition interferon (IFN) were tested for their effects on the production of early complement factors. Synthesis of C1r, C1s and C3 by all cell types is stimulated with cytokines that can be detected in AD plaques. C1-Inh synthesis can be stimulated by IFN only. Data adapted from [93].

expressed in the brain to various extents and to be upregulated in affected areas of AD brain, with C1q and C9 increases being most pronounced.

Not only complement factors, but also complement inhibitors are synthesized by brain derived cells [89, 90, 98]. Our recent studies show that C1-Inh is synthesized in low amounts predominantly by neuronal cells [99]. No difference in C1-Inh mRNA expression between affected and non-affected brain areas within AD brains and between AD and non-demented control cases was observed by RNA *in situ* hybridization [99]. Furthermore, these RNA *in situ* hybridization studies showed that neurons are the predominant cell type expressing C1-Inh mRNA, even in AD brain areas with neuritic plaques and activated glial cells [99]. *In vitro* adult human astrocyte cultures and neuroblastoma cell lines cannot be stimulated to secrete C1-Inh or express C1-Inh mRNA when exposed to cytokines (IL-1, IL-1β, IL-6 or tumour necrosis factor (TNF) α) [99] that are immunohistochemically detectable in activated microglia in the vicinity of neuritic plaques [6, 49, 50]. Whereas C1-Inh synthesis is refractory to stimulation by various cytokines, increased C1r and C1s synthesis by adult human brain-derived astrocytes and microglia, as well as neuroblastoma cell lines, is observed when the cells are treated with IL-1, TNFα and to a lesser extent IL-6 [93]. Even when stimulated, astrocytes or neuroblastoma cell lines do not sectrete C1q [93] or express C1qB mRNA [91]. On the other hand, rat [55] and human [93] microglia in culture express C1q intracellularly and, moreover, human microglia constitutively secrete C1q [93].

Aβ peptides can enhance the secretion of C3 by mouse microglial cells [100], suggesting that Aβ itself may be stimulatory and that activated microglial cells may produce complement in neuritic plaques. Aβ has, however, only a limited effect on C3 secretion by human microglia, and no effect on the synthesis of C1 subcomponents or C1-Inh by human microglia or astrocytes, nor by neuroblastoma cell lines, *in vitro* [93].

Taken together, these studies suggest that, in line with the reported increase in mRNA expression of these factors in AD-affected areas [95], the synthesis of the C1 subcomponents C1r and C1s by astrocytes, as well as by neurons, is increased in plaque areas where cytokines are released, whereas the production of their regulatory protein, C1-Inh, is refractory to stimulation by the aforementioned cytokines. Whether this is sufficient to cause an ongoing complement activation at sites of amyloid deposits is the subject of present investigations. In addition to a low synthesis rate of C1-Inh, its consumption in other systems such as the contact system may be crucial. Hageman factor is present in AD neuritic plaques [101], suggesting that Aβ may serve as an initiating surface for contact activation. Normally, contact activation is initiated by Factor XII autoactivation.

Conversion of prekallikrein to kallikrein by activated Factor XII can lead to the release of bradykinin that can interact with cellular bradykinin B_2 receptors, the expression of which is upregulated in AD [102]. Not only can activated factors of the contact system bind and thereby consume C1-Inh, catabolic peptides of Factor XII (FXIIa and FXIIf) can either directly (FXIIf) or via kallikrein activation (FXIIa) activate C1r and C1s *in vitro* [103]. In recent studies, Aβ aggregates were found to induce autoactivation of Factor XII *in vitro* [104]. The high levels of cleaved high molecular weight kininogen (HMWK) found in AD cerebrospinal fluid (CSF) samples, suggests that contact activation also occurs in AD brains [105]. *In vitro*, Aβ-induced FXII activation, through activation of HMWK, was shown to activate C1s and C4 independent of C1q [106]. The latter was observed with non-fibrillar Aβ and in C1q-deficient plasma, suggesting a direct effect of Aβ-induced contact activation on classical pathway complement activation *in vitro* [106]. Studies in baboons treated with a monoclonal antibody that inhibits Factor XII activation indicate that Factor XII-dependent activation of the classical pathway may also occur *in vivo* [107]. Therefore, a functional role of C1-Inh as inhibitor of Factor XII activation may be of importance. Our recent finding that C1-Inh expression remains low even in brain areas where Aβ plaque-associated inflammatory responses occur suggests more widespread effects than on complement activation only. Recent findings [103, 105, 106] suggest such an important role for C1-Inh in the regulation of contact activation in the brain. In this light the work of Akiyama [85], describing immunohistochemical evidence that coagulation and fibrinolysis systems are indeed activated in AD brains, provides a base for further research into the regulation of activation of these systems and into the interplay of these systems and the complement system in the brain.

Conclusions

Knowledge about the mechanisms of complement activation and regulation in the brain may provide new clues for therapeutic intervention to retard the onset of AD pathology. Intervention at the C1 level may prevent further activation of complement, before amplifation at the C3 level occurs with subsequent attraction and activation of glial cells. Drugs that specifically inhibit the serine protease activity of C1r and, with lesser specificity, C1s are available [108, 109] but need to be tested *in vivo*. Other possibilities for therapy include increasing the inhibitory potential of C1-Inh, either by administering genetically engineered C1-Inh that can inactivate its target proteases without being inactivated itself [110] or by administration of heparin-like substances such as low molecular weight dextran sulphate [111] that potentiate the inhibitory activity of the protease inhinbitors. Notwithstanding that heparin is most effective on AT III and C1-Inh, administration is not feasible because of the risk of bleeding. However, other ways to change the extracellular matrix proteoglycan composition in order to potentiate the inhibitors in the parenchyma may be developed.

Acknowledgements
Supported by the Netherlands Organization for Scientific Research (NWO; grant #903-51-108) and from the Internationale Stichting Alzheimer Onderzoek (ISAO; grant #95504).

References

1 Rozemuller JM, Eikelenboom P, Stam FC, Beyreuther K, Masters CL (1989) A4 protein in Alzheimer's disease: primary and secondary cellular events in extra cellulair amyloid deposition. *J Neuropathol Exp Neurol* 48: 674–691

2 Eikelenboom P, Stam FC (1982) Immunoglobulins and complement factors in senile plaques.*Acta Neuropathol (Berlin)* 57: 239–242

3 Eikelenboom P, Hack CE, Rozemuller JM, Stam FC (1989) Complement activation in amyloid plaques in Alzheimer's dementia. *Virchows Arch B (Cell Pathol)* 56: 259–262

4 Abraham CR, Selkoe DJ, Potter H (1988) Immunochemical identification of the serine protease inhibitor 1-antichymotrypsin in the brain amyloid deposits of Alzheimer's disease. *Cell* 52: 487–501

5 Rozemuller JM, Abbink J, Stam FC, Hack CE, Eikelenboom P (1991) Distribution pattern and functional state of alpha-l-antichymotrypsin in plaques and vascular amyloid in Alzheimer's disease. *Acta Neuropathol* 82: 200–207

6 Bauer J, Strauss S, Schreiter-Gasser U, Ganter U, Schlegel P, Witt I, Yolk B, Berger M (1991) Interleukin-6 and α2-macroglobulin indicate an acute-phase state in Alzheimer's disease cortices. *FEBS Lett* 285: 111–114

7 Snow AD, Sekiguchi RT, Nochlin D, Kalaria RN, Kimata K (1994) Heparan sulfate proteoglycan in diffuse plaques of hippocampus but not of cerebellum in Alzheimer's disease brain. *Am J Pathol* 144: 337–347

8 Zhan SS, Veerhuis R, Kamphorst W, Eikelenboom P (1995) Distribution of beta amyloid associated proteins in plaques in Alzheimer's disease and in the non-demented elderly. *Neurodegeneration* 4: 291–297

9 Strittmatter WJ, Saunders AM, Schmechel D, Pericak-Vance M, Enghild J, Salvesen GS, Roses AD (1993) Apolipoprotein E: High-avidity binding to β-amyloid and increased frequency of type 4 allele in late-onset familial Alzheimer disease. *Proc Natl Acad Sci USA* 90: 1977–1981

10 Emsley J, White HE, O'Hara BP, Oliva G, Srinivasan N, Tickle IJ, Blundell TL, Pepys MB, Wood SP (1994) Structure of pentameric human serum amyloid P component. *Nature* 367: 338–345

11 Snow AD, Sekiguchi R, Nochlin D, Fraser P, Kimata K, Mizutani A, Arai M, Schreier WA, Morgan DG (1994) An important role of heparan sulfate proteoglycan (Perlecan) in a model system for the deposition and persistence of fibrillar β-Amyloid in rat brain. *Neuron* 12: 219–234

12 Inoue S, Kuroiwa M, Kisilevsky R (1999) Basement membranes, microfibrils and ß amyloid fibrillogenesis in Alzheimer's disease: high resolution ultrastructural findings. *Brain Res Reviews* 29: 218–231

13 Ma J, Yee A, Brewer Jr HB, Das S, Potter H (1994) Amyloid-associated proteins 1-antichymotrypsin and apolipoprotein E promote assembly of Alzheimer β-protein into filaments. *Nature* 372: 92–94

14 Webster S, O'Barr S, Rogers J (1994) Enhanced aggregation and β structure of amyloid β peptide after coincubation with C1q. *J Neurosci Res* 39: 448–456

15 Pasternack JM, Abraham CR, Van Dyke B, Potter H, Younkin SG (1989) Astrocytes in Alzheimer's disease gray matter express α1-antichymotrypsin mRNA. *Amer J Pathol* 135: 827–834

16 May PC, Lampert-Etchells M, Johnson SA, Poirier J, Masters JM, Finch CE (1990)

Dynamics of gene expression for hippocampal glycoprotein elevated in Alzheimer's disease and in experimental lesions in rat. *Neuron* 8: 831–839
17 Eriksson S, Janciauskiene S, Lannfelt L (1995) α_1-Antichymotrypsin regulates Alzheimer β-amyloid peptide fibril formation. *Proc Natl Acad Sci USA* 92: 2313–2317
18 Ghiso J, Matsubara E, Koudinov A, Choi-Miura NH, Tomita M, Wisniewski T, Frangione B (1993) The cerebrospinal-fluid soluble form of Alzheimer's amyloid beta is complexed to SP-40,40 (apolipoprotein J), an inhibitor of the complement membrane-attack complex. *Biochem J* 293: 27–30
19 Oda T, Wals P, Osterburg HH, Johnson SA, Pasinetti GM, Morgan TE, Rozovsky I, Stine WB, Snyder SW, Holzman TF et al (1995) Clusterin (apoJ) alters the aggregation of amyloid β-peptide ($A\beta_{1-42}$) and forms slowly sedimenting Aβ complexes that cause oxidative stress. *Exp Neurol* 136: 22–31
20 Rozemuller JM, Eikelenboom P, Pals S, Stam FC (1989) Microglial cells around amyloid plaques in Alzheimer's disease express leucocyte adhesion molecules of the LFA-1 family. *Neurosci Lett* 101: 288–292
21 Eikelenboom P, Rozemuller JM, Kraal G, Stam FC, McBride PA, Bruce ME, Fraser H (1991) Cerebral amyloid plaques in Alzheimer's disease but not in scrapie-affected mice are closely associated with a local inflammatory process. *Virchows Arch* 60: 329–336
22 Eikelenboom P, Zhan S-S, Kamphorst W, van der Valk P, Rozemuller JM (1994) Cellular and substrate adhesion molecules (integrins) and their ligands in cerebral amyloid deposits in Alzheimer's disease. *Virchows Arch* 424: 421–427
23 Frohman EM, Frohman TC, Gupta S, de Fougerolles A, van de Noort S (1991) Expression of intercellular adhesion molecule 1 (ICAM-1) in Alzheimer's disease. *J Neurol Sci* 106: 105–111
24 Verbeek MM, Otte-Höller I, Wesseling P, Ruiter DJ, de Waal RMW (1996) Differential expression of intercellular adhesion molecule-1 (ICAM-1) in the Aβ-containing lesions in brains of patients with dementia of the Alzheimer type. *Acta Neuropathol* 91: 608–615
25 Blom MAA, Van Muiswinkel FL, Eikelenboom P (1996) Mechanism of inflammation in Alzheimer's disease. *Ann Psych* 6: 1–12
26 Eikelenboom P, Zhan S-S, Van Gool WA, Allsop D (1994) Inflammatory mechanisms in Alzheimer's disease. *TiPS* 15: 447–450
27 Eikelenboom P, Veerhuis R (1996) The role of complement and activated microglia in the pathogenesis of Alzheimer's disease. *Neurobiol Aging* 17: 673–680
28 Rogers J, Cooper NR, Webster S, Schultz J, McGeer PL, Styren SD, Civin WH, Brachova L, Bradt B, Ward P et al (1992) Complement activation by β-amyloid in Alzheimer's disease. *Proc Natl Acad Sci USA* 89: 10016–10020
29 Jiang H, Burdick D, Glabe CG, Cotman CW, Tenner AJ (1994) β-Amyloid activates complement by binding to a specific region of the collagen-like domain of the C1q A chain. *J Immunol* 152: 5050–5059
30 Snyder SW, Wang GT, Barrett L, Ladror US, Casuto D, Lee CM, Krafft GA, Holzman

RB, Holzman TF (1994) Complement C1q does not bind to monomeric β-amyloid. Experimental Neurol 128: 136–142

31 Bradt BM, Kolb WP, Cooper NR (1998) Complement-dependent proinflammatory properties of the Alzheimer's disease β-peptide. *J Exp Med* 188: 431–438

32 Gewurz H, Ying S-C, Jiang H, Lint TF (1993) Nonimmune activation of the classical complement pathway. *Behring Inst Mitt* 93: 138–147

33 Yao J, Harvath L, Gilbert DL, Colton CA (1990) Chemotaxis by a CNS macrophage, the microglia. *J Neurosci Res* 27: 36–42

34 Morgan EL, Sanderson S, Scholtz W, Noonan DJ, Weigle WO, Hugli TE (1992) Identification and characterization of the effector region within human C5a responsible for stimulation of Il-6 synthesis. *J Immunol* 148: 3937–3942

35 Wright SD, Craigmyle LS, Silverstein SC (1983) Fibronectin and serum amyloid P component stimulate C3b- and C3bi-mediated phagocytosis in cultured human monocytes. *J Exp Med* 158: 1338–1343

36 Afagh A, Cummings BJ, Cribbs D, Cotman CW, Tenner AJ (1996) Localization and cell association of C1q in Alzheimer's disease brain. *Exp Neurol* 138: 22–32

37 Satou T, Cummings BJ, Head E, Nielson KA, Hahn FF, Milgram NW, Velazquez P, Cribbs D, Tenner AJ, Cotman CW (1997) The progression of β-amyloid deposition in the frontal cortex of the aged canine. *Brain Res* 774: 35–43

38 Webster S, Bonnell B, Rogers J (1997) Charge-based binding of complement component C1q to the Alzheimer amyloid β-peptide. *Am J Pathol* 150: 1531–1536

39 Velazquez P, Cribbs DH, Poulos TL, Tenner AJ (1997) Aspartate residue 7 in amyloid β-protein is critical for classical complement pathway activation: Implications for Alzheimer's disease pathogenesis. *Nature Med* 3: 77–79

40 Ying S-C, Gewurz AT, Jiang H, Gewurz H (1993) Human serum amyloid P component oligomers bind and activate the classical complement pathway via residues 14–26 and 76–92 of the A chain collagen-like region of C1q. *J Immunol* 150: 169–176

41 Jiang H, Siegel JN, Gewurz H (1991) Binding and complement activation by C-reactive protein via the collagen-like region of C1q and inhibition of these reactions by monoclonal antibodies to C-reactive protein and C1q. *J Immunol* 146: 2324–2330

42 Roher A, Lowenson JD, Clarke S, Wolkow C, Wang R, Cotter RJ, Reardon IM, Zuercher-Neely HA, Heinrikson RL, Ball MJ et al (1993) Structural alterations in the peptide backbone of β-amyloid core protein may account for its deposition and stability in Alzheimer's disease. *J Biol Chem* 268: 3072–3083

43 Fonseca MI, Head E, Velazquez P, Cotman CW, Tenner AJ (1999) The presence of isoaspartic acid in β-amyloid plaques indicates plaque age. *Exp Neurol* 157: 277–288

44 Ishii T, Haga S (1984) Immuno-electron microscopic localization of complements in amyloid fibrils of senile plaques. *Acta Neuropathol* 63: 296–300

45 Pouplard A, Emile J (1985) New immunological findings in senile dementia. *Interdiscipl Topics Geront* 19: 62–71

46 McGeer PL, Akiyama H, Itagaki S, McGeer EG (1989) Immune response in Alzheimer's disease. *Canad J Neurol Sci* 16: 516–527

47 McGeer PL, Itagaki S, Tago H, McGeer EG (1987) Reactive microglia in patients with senile dementia of Alzheimer's type are positive for the histocompatibility glycoprotein HLA-DR. *Neurosci Lett* 79: 195–200
48 Rogers J, Luber-Narod J, Styren SD, Civin WH (1988) Expression of immune system-associated antigens by cells of the human central nervous system: Relationship to the pathology of Alzheimer's disease. *Neurobiol Aging* 9: 339–349
49 Griffin WST, Sheng JG, Roberts GW, Mrak RE (1995) Interleukin-1 expression in different plaque types in Alzheimer's disease: significance in plaque evolution. *J Neuropathol Exp Neurol* 54: 276–281
50 Dickson DW, Lee SC, Mattiace LA, Yen SC, Brosnan C (1993) Microglia and cytokines in neurological disease, with special reference to AIDS and Alzheimer's disease. *Glia* 7: 75–83
51 Griffin WST, Sheng JG, Royston MC, Gentleman SM, McKenzie JE, Graham DI, Roberts GW, Mrak RE (1998) Glial-neuronal interactions in Alzheimer's disease: The potential role of a 'cytokine cycle' in disease progression. *Brain Pathol* 8: 65–72
52 Vandenabeele P, Fiers W (1991) Is amyloidogenesis during Alzheimer's disease due to an Il-1/Il-6-mediated "acute phase response" in the brain? *Immunol Today* 12: 217–219
53 Araujo DM, Cotman CW (1992) Beta -amyloid stimulates glial cells *in vitro* to produce growth factors that accumulate in senile plaques in Alzheimer's disease. *Brain Res* 569: 141–145
54 Verbeek MM, Otte-Höller I, Veerhuis R, Ruiter DJ, De Waal RMW (1998) Distribution of Aβ-associated factors in cerebrovascular amyloid of Alzheimer's disease. *Acta Neuropathol* 96: 628–636
55 Korotzer AR, Watt J, Cribbs D, Tenner AJ, Burdick D, Glabe C, Cotman CW (1995) Cultured rat microglia express C1q and receptor for C1q: implications for amyloid effects on microglia. *Exp Neurol* 134: 214–221
56 Tenner AJ (1998) C1q receptors: regulating specific functions of phagocytic cells. *Immunobiol* 199: 250–264
57 Veerhuis R, Van Es LA, Daha MR (1985) Effects of soluble aggregates of Ig on the binding, uptake and degradation of the C1q subcomponent of complement by adherent guinea pig peritoneal macrophages. *Eur J Immunol* 23: 881–887
58 Guan E, Robinson SL, Goodman EB, Tenner AJ (1994) Cell-surface protein identified on phagocytic cells modulates the C1q-mediated enhancement of phagocytosis. *J Immunol* 152: 4005–4016
59 Bobak DA, Frank MM, Tenner AJ (1998) C1q acts synergistically with phorbol dibutyrate to activate CR1-mediated phagocytosis by human mononuclear phagocytes. *Eur J Immunol* 18: 2001–2007
60 Klickstein LB, Barbashov SF, Liu T, Jack RM, Nicholson-Weller A (1997) Complement receptor 1 (CR1, CD35) is a receptor for C1q. *Immunity* 7: 345–355
61 Klickstein LB, Tyagi S, Barbashov SF, Tas S, Nicholson-Weller A (1999) CR1 and β2 integrin engagement are required for C1q-triggered superoxide production in PMN. *Mol Immunol* 36: 279 (abstract)

62 Colton CA, Gilbert DL (1987) Production of superoxide anions by a CNS macrophage, the microglia. *FEBS Lett* 223: 284–288
63 Van Muiswinkel FL, Veerhuis R, Eikelenboom P (1996) Amyloid β protein (Aβ) primes cultured rat microglial cells for an enhanced phorbol-myristate-acetate induced respiratory burst activity. *J Neurochem* 66: 2468–2476
64 Klegeris A, McGeer PL (1997) β-amyloid protein enhances macrophage production of oxygen free radicals and glutamate. *J Neurosci Res* 49: 229–235
65 Van Muiswinkel FL, Raupp SFA, De Vos NM, Smits HA, Verhoef J, Eikelenboom P, Nottet HSLM (1999) The amino-terminus of the amyloid-β protein is critical for the cellular binding and consequent activation of the respiratory burst of human macrophages. *J Neuroimmunol* 96: 121–130
66 Giulian D, Haverkamp LJ, Yu J, Karshin W, Tom D, Li J, Kazanskaia A, Kirkpatrick J, Roher AE (1998) The HHQK domain of β-amyloid provides a structural basis for the immunopathology of Alzheimer's disease. *J Biol Chem* 273: 29719–29726
67 Tacnet P, Galvan M, Chevallier S, Glabe C, Tenner AJ, Arlaud GJ (1999) *In vitro* analysis of C1 activation by Aβ Alzheimer's disease-related peptides. *Mol Immunol* 36: 301 (abstract)
68 Finch CE, Marchalonis JJ (1996) Evolutionary perspectives on amyloid and inflammatory features of Alzheimer's disease. *Neurobiol Aging* 17: 809–815
69 Wolbink GJ, Brouwer MC, Buysmann S, Ten Berge IJM, Hack CE (1996) CRP-mediated activation of complement *in vivo*: assessment by measuring circulating complement-C-reactive protein complexes. *J Immunol* 157: 473–479
70 Iwamoto N, Nishiyama E, Ohwada J, Arai H (1994) Demonstration of CRP immunoreactivity in brains of Alzheimer's disease: immunohistochemical study using formic acid pretreatment of tissue sections. *Neurosci Letts* 177: 23–26
71 Duong T, Nikolaeva M, Acton PJ (1997) C-reactive protein-like immunoreactivity in the neurofibrillary tangles of Alzheimer's disease. *Brain Res* 749: 152–156
72 Kalaria RN, Harshbarger-Kelly M, Cohen DL, Premkumar RD (1996) Molecular aspects of inflammatory and immune responses in Alzheimer's disease. *Neurobiol Aging* 17: 687–693
73 Aulak KS, Donaldson VH, Coutinho M, Davis III AE (1993) C1-Inhibitor: Structure/function and biologic role. *Behring Inst Mitt* 93: 204–214
74 Patston PA, Gettins P, Beechem J, Schapira M (1991) Mechanism of serpin action: evidence that C1-inhibitor functions as a suicide substrate. *Biochemistry* 30: 8876–8882
75 Ziccardi RJ, Cooper NR (1979) Active disassembly of the first complement component, C1, by C1 inactivator. *J Immunol* 123: 788–792
76 Veerhuis R, Van der Valk P, Janssen I, Zhan S-S, Van Nostrand WE, Eikelenboom P (1995) Complement activation in amyloid plaques in Alzheimer's disease brains does not proceed further than C3. *Virchow's Archiv* 426: 603–610
77 Walker DG, Yasuhara O, Patston PA, McGeer EG, McGeer PL (1995) Complement C1 inhibitor is produced by brain tissue and is cleaved in Alzheimer disease. *Brain Res* 675: 75–82

78 Veerhuis R, Janssen I, Hack CE, Eikelenboom P (1996) Early complement components in Alzheimer's disease brains. *Acta Neuropathol* 91: 53–60
79 Sim RB, Arlaud GJ, Colomb MG (1980) Kinetics of reaction of human C1-inhibitor with the human complement system protease C1r and C1s. *Biochim Biophys Acta* 612: 433–449
80 Patston PA, Schapira M (1997) Regulation of C1-inhibitor function by binding to type IV collagen and heparin. *Biochem Biophys Res Commun* 230: 597–601
81 Wuillemin WA, Eldering E, Citarella F, de Ruig CP, ten Cate H, Hack CE (1996) Modulation of contact system proteases by glycosaminoglycans. Selective enhancement of the inhibition of factor XIa. *J Biol Chem* 271: 12913–12918
82 Krumdieck R, Hook M, Rosenberg LC, Volanakis JE (1992) The proteoglycan decorin binds C1q and inhibits the activity of the C1. *J Immunol* 149: 3695–3701
83 Kirschfink M, Blase L, Engelmann S, Schwartz-Albiez R (1997) Secreted chondroitin sulfate proteoglycan of human B cell lines binds to the complement protein C1q and inhibits complex formation of C1. *J Immunol* 158: 1324–1331
84 Van den Berg RH, Faber-Krol M, Van Es LA, Daha MR (1995) Regulation of the function of the first component of complement by human C1q receptor. *Eur J Immunol* 25: 2206–2210
85 Akiyama H (1998) Complement, coagulation and fibrinolysis pathways are involved in the pathogenesis of Alzheimer's disease. In: R Cacabelos, B Winblad, P Eikelenboom (eds): *Neurogerontology and neurogeriatrics*. Prous Science, Barcelona, vol 2, 23–34
86 Van Nostrand WE, Wagner SL, Farrow JS, Cunningham DD (1990) Immunopurification and protease inhibitory properties of protease nexin-2/ amyloid β-protein precursor. *J Biol Chem* 265: 9591–9594
87 Van Nostrand WE, McKay LD, Baker JB, Cunningham DD (1988) Functional and structural similarities between protease nexin-1 and C1 inhibitor. *J Biol Chem* 263: 3979–3983
88 Wagner SL, Geddes JW, Cotman CW, Lau AL, Gurwitz D, Isackson PJ, Cunningham DD (1989) Protease nexin-1, an antithrombin with neurite outgrowth activity, is reduced in Alzheimer's disease. *Proc Natl Acad Sci USA* 86: 8284–8288
89 Barnum SR (1995) Complement biosynthesis in the central nervous system. *Crit Rev Oral Biol Med* 6: 132–146
90 Morgan BP, Gasque P (1996) Expression of complement in the brain: role in health and disease. *Immunol Today* 17: 338–347
91 Walker DG, McGeer PL (1993) Complement gene expression in neuroblastoma and astrocytoma cell lines of human origin. *Neurosci Lett* 157: 99–102
92 Gasque P, Ischenko A, Legoedec J, Mauger C, Schouft M-T, Fontaine M (1993) Expression of the complement classical pathway by human glioma in culture. *J Biol Chem* 268: 25068–25074
93 Veerhuis R, Janssen I, De Groot CJA, Van Muiswinkel FL, Hack CE, Eikelenboom P (1999) Cytokines associated with amyloid plaques in Alzheimer's disease brain stimu-

late human glial and neuronal cell cultures to secrete early complement proteins, but not C1-inhibitor. *Exp Neurol* 160: 289–299

94 Shen Y, Li R, McGeer EG, McGeer PL (1997) Neuronal expression of mRNAs for complement proteins of the classical pathway in Alzheimer brain. *Brain Res* 769: 391–395

95 Yasojima K, Schwab C, McGeer EG, McGeer PL (1999) Up-regulated production and activation of the complement system in Alzheimer's disease brain. *Am J Pathol* 154: 927–936

96 Walker DG, McGeer PL (1992) Complement gene expression in human brain: comparison between normal and Alzheimer disease cases. *Mol Brain Res* 14: 109–116

97 Lampert-Etchells M, Pasinetti GM, Finch CE, Johnson SA (1993) Regional localization of cells containing complement C1q and C4 mRNAs in the frontal cortex during Alzheimer's disease. *Neurodegeneration* 2: 111–121

98 Gasque P, Thomas A, Fontaine M, Morgan BP (1996) Complement activation on human neuroblastoma cell lines *in vitro*: route of activation and expression of functional complement regulatory proteins. *J Neuroimmunol* 66: 29–40

99 Veerhuis R, Janssen I, Hoozemans JJM, DeGroot CJA, Hack CE, Eikelenboom P (1998) Complement C1-inhibitor expression in Alzheimer's disease. *Acta Neuropathol* 96: 287–296

100 Haga S, Ikeda K, Sato M, Ishii T (1993) Synthetic Alzheimer amyloid β/A4 peptides enhance production of complement C3 component by cultured microglial cells. *Brain Res* 601: 88–94

101 Yasuhara O, Walker DG, McGeer PL (1994) Hageman factor and its binding sites are present in senile plaques of Alzheimer brain. *Brain Res* 654: 234–240

102 Huang HM, Lin TA, Sun GY, Gibson GE (1995) Increased inositol 1,4,5-triphosphate accumulation correlates with an upregulation of bradykinin receptors in Alzheimer's disease. *J Neurochem* 64: 761–766

103 Kaplan AP, Joseph K, Shibayama Y, Reddigari S, Ghebrehiwet B, Silverberg M (1997) The intrinsic coagulation/kinin-forming cascade: assembly in plasma and cell surfaces in inflammation. *Adv Immunol* 66: 225–272

104 Shibayama Y, Joseph K, Nakazawa Y, Ghebrehiwet B, Peerschke EIB, Kaplan AP (1999) Zinc-dependent activation of the plasma kinin-forming cascade by aggregated β amyloid protein. *Clin Immunol* 90: 89–99

105 Bergamaschini L, Parnetti L, Pareyson D, Canzani S, Cugno M, Agostoni A (1998) Activation of the contact system in cerebrospinal fluid of patients with Alzheimer's β-amyloid peptides can activate the early components of complement classical pathway in a C1q-independent manner. *Alzh Dis Assoc Dis* 12: 102–108

106 Bergamaschini L, Canzani S, Bottasso B, Cugno M, Braidotti P, Agostoni A (1999) Alzheimer's β-amyloid peptides can activate the early components of complement classical pathway in a C1q-independent manner. *Clin Exp Immunol* 115: 526–533

107 Jansen PM, Pixley RA, Brouwer M, De Jong IW, Chang ACK, Hack CE, Taylor FB, Colman RW (1996) Inhibition of factor XII in septic baboons attenuates the activation of

complement and fibrinolyic systems and reduces the release of interleukin-6 and neutrophil elastase. *Blood* 87: 2337–2344

108 Spiegel K, Emmerling MR, Barnum SR (1997) Strategies for inhibition of complement activation in the treatment of neurodegenerative diseases. In: PL Wood (ed): *Neuroinflammation: mechanisms and management.* Humana Press, Totowa, NJ, 129–176

109 Hays SJ, Caprathe BW, Gilmore JL, Amin N, Emmerling MR, Nadimpalli R, Nath R, Raser KJ, Stafford D, Watson D et al (1998) 2-amino-4H-3,1-benzoxazin-4-ones as inhibitors of C1r serine protease. *J Med Chem* 41: 1060–1067

110 Eldering E, Huijbregts CM, Nuijens JH, Hack CE (1993) Recombinant C1 inhibitor P5/P3 variants display reduced susceptibility to neutrophil elastase. *J Clin Invest* 91: 1035–1043

111 Wuillemin WA, te Veldhuis H, Lubbers YT, de Ruig CP, Eldering E, Hack CE (1997) Potentiation of C1 inhibitor by glycosaminoglycans: dextran sulfate species are effective inhibitors of *in vivo* complement activation in plasma. *J Immunol* 159: 1953–1960

Complement mediator systems in Alzheimer's disease

Bonnie M. Bradt[1], Stephen A. O'Barr[2], Jack X. Yu[3] and Neil R. Cooper[3]

[1]Department of Internal Medicine, University of California Davis Medical Center, 1508 Alhambra Blvd., Sacramento, CA 95816, USA; [2]College of Pharmacy, Western University of Health Sciences, 309 E. Second St., Pomona, CA 91766-1854, USA; [3]Department of Immunology, The Scripps Research Institute, 10550 North Torrey Pines Road, La Jolla, CA 92037, USA

Introduction

The brain is "immunologically privileged" in the sense that it cannot generate primary antigen-specific humoral and cellular immune responses. This is because of the integrity of the blood brain barrier, which impedes (but does not entirely prevent) entry of naive T lymphocytes. Furthermore, brain microglia and astrocytes possess only a limited ability to process and present antigens. It is perhaps not surprising, therefore, that the brain is protected from injury due to infection, trauma, or locally damaging processes by the innate or intrinsic immune system, which includes the actions of phagocytic cells, the complement system, cytokines, chemokines, and other cell-derived soluble mediators.

Studies of Alzheimer's disease (AD) brains by Eikelenboom and Stam [1] were among the first to indicate involvement of the innate immune system in the brain in a disease process. They reported that amyloid-containing neuritic plaques (NP) in AD brains contained components of the complement system, a finding which has since been confirmed and extended by numerous investigators. It is now clear that NP and associated cells contain components of the classical complement pathway (C1q, C3 and C4) and the membrane attack pathway (C5, C7, C9), as well as complement regulatory proteins (C1 inhibitor, C4 binding protein, S-protein, CD59, clusterin) and complement receptors (CR1, CR2, CR3, CR4, C3a receptor, C5a receptor) [2–4] (Fig. 1). Since the blood brain barrier is not disrupted in AD [5], it was initially inferred, and it has been convincingly demonstrated at the mRNA and protein levels, that these inflammatory proteins are synthesized in the brain by microglia, astrocytes and, surprisingly, neurons [2, 4, 6]. Furthermore, up-regulated synthesis of various complement proteins and regulatory proteins has been demonstrated in cells from AD brains [7].

In addition to complement factors, pro-inflammatory cytokines including IL-1, IL-6 and TNFα are also present in NP and associated cells [2, 4]. Microglia, astrocytes and neurons are able to synthesize these and other cytokines, chemokines and other inflammatory mediators [2, 4].

Neuroinflammatory Mechanisms in Alzheimer's Disease: Basic and Clinical Research,
edited by Joseph Rogers

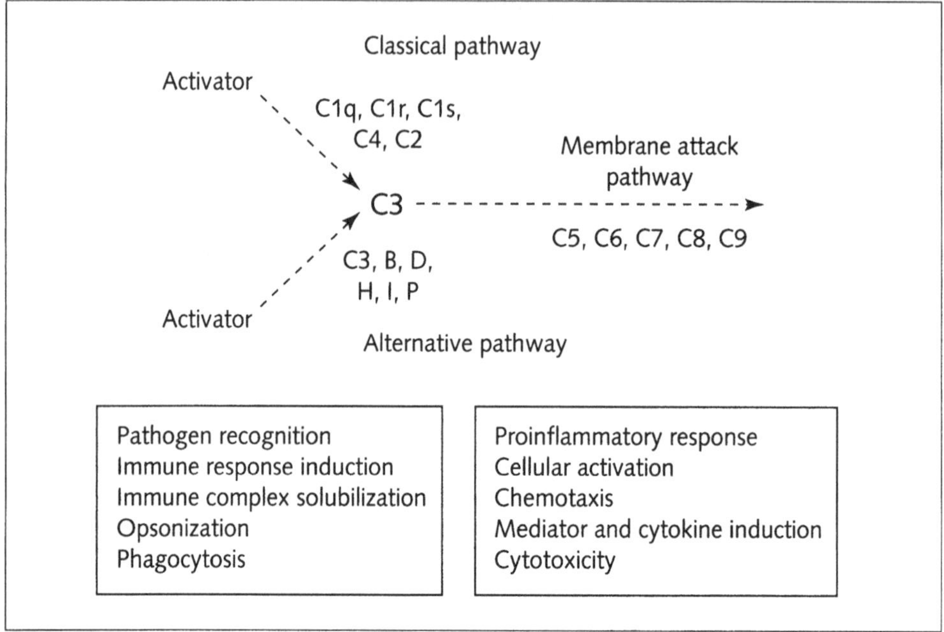

Figure 1
Pathways and biology of the complement system.

Studies of the complement system over the past 30 years have documented its many pro-inflammatory actions. Most of these derive from the multiple biological actions of C3a and C5a, which are cytokine-like cleavage products of the third and fifth complement components, respectively, and the multi-molecular C5b-9 membrane attack complex, all of which are generated during complement activation *in vitro* [8] (Fig. 1). These biological actions are sufficiently comprehensive to potentially account for the cellular changes surrounding β-amyloid deposits in NP.

A plausible scenario in AD is that complement activation in NP in the AD brain leads to the formation of covalent complexes of C3 activation fragments with the activator, since the formation of such complexes is a fundamental tenet of complement function [8]. This would account for the association of C3 with NP, since such covalent complexes not only remain bound, but they provide a nidus for chronic complement activation. Generation of the chemokine-like C5a cleavage peptide by Aβ-mediated complement activation could be responsible for the increased numbers of activated microglia and astrocytes around NP, since these cells possess C5a receptors and migrate in response to C5a [9–11]. Furthermore, C5a could trigger the release of pro-inflammatory cytokines from these glial cells, as it does from other cell types [12], leading to further cellular activation. Incoming glial cells would bind and remain adherent, via their complement receptors [6], to C3 activation fragments covalently attached to Aβ. C5b-9 insertion into cell membranes provides an explanation for the association of this complex with dystrophic neurites in NP [3]. Low-level triggering of cellular signaling pathways by the inserted complexes [13] would then be responsible for alterations in neuronal functions.

Fibrillar Aβ activates the classical and alternative complement pathways leading to covalent binding of C3 activation fragments

In vitro studies

In order for complement to play a role in AD, it must be activated, since this is a prerequisite for the system to manifest biological activity [8] (Fig. 1). In this regard, an early report that fibrillar Aβ efficiently activated the complement system in the absence of antibody [3] has been confirmed by many investigators using various experimental approaches (see [14–16] for examples). Aβ-mediated complement activation also leads to generation of the C3 activation product, C3b [3]. These findings, however, do not indicate whether the classical complement pathway (CCP) or the alternative complement pathway (ACP) is responsible for C3 activation, since both activation pathways culminate with the generation of a labile, but highly efficient enzyme able to cleave and activate large numbers of C3 molecules (Fig. 1) [8]. Various approaches demonstrated conclusively that fibrillar Aβ is an efficient activator of the CCP [3, 14]. Binding of residues 14–26 of the collagen-like portion of the A polypeptide chain of the C1q molecule has been implicated in binding to residues 1–11 of fibrillar Aβ in triggering CCP activation [14, 17, 18]. Using purified complement components and other approaches it was determined that fibrillar Aβ also independently activates the ACP [16, 19].

In order for complement activation to proceed past the C3 stage, the C3 cleaving enzymes generated by the activation pathways must be anchored to the complement activator *via* covalent ester or amide bonds involving the C4b or C3b moieties of the CCP or the ACP enzymes, respectively [8]. Various complement-based and chemical approaches have been used, together with ELISA assays (Fig. 2A) and co-localization analyses on Western blots [16, 19], to show that a significant proportion of the C3 activation fragments binding to Aβ during Aβ-mediated complement activation are covalently attached *via* ester bonds.

In vivo correlates

C3 is among the most prominent of the complement components found in NP. The demonstration of C3 in association with a known activator (Aβ) in NP (Fig. 2B) provides suggestive evidence that the complement system is activated in the context

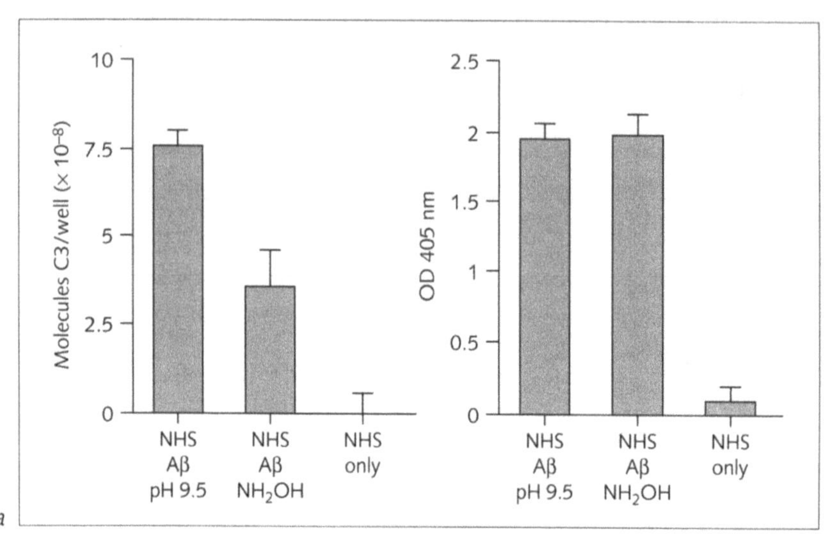

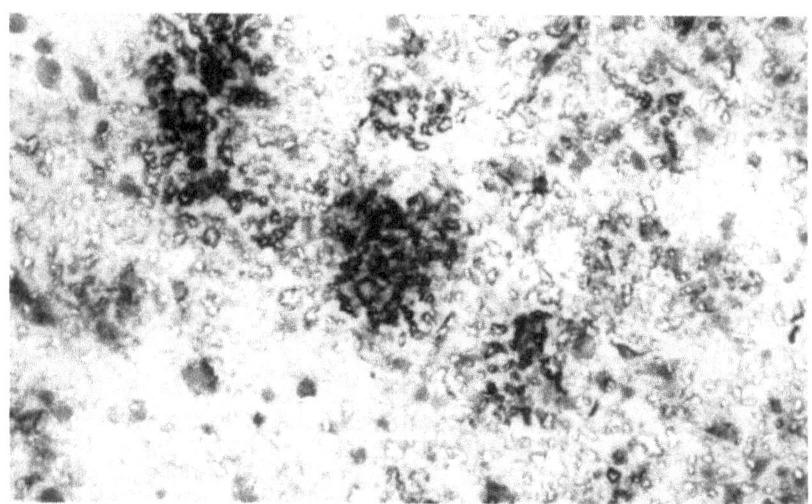

Figure 2
Involvement of C3 in complement activation by Aβ in vitro *and by NP in AD* in vivo.
(A) Formation of covalent, ester-linked complexes of Aβ with C3 activation products in vitro. *Aggregated Aβ was incubated with normal human serum (NHS) as a source of complement and captured on wells coated with antibody to Aβ. Replicate samples were treated with pH 9.5 buffer or with 1 M hydroxylamine in pH 9.5 buffer (alkaline hydroxylamine dissociates ester bonds) and remaining bound C3 quantitated by ELISA with a specific antibody (left panel) and remaining bound Aβ assessed by ELISA with an antibody to Aβ (right panel) Reprinted from [19] with permission.*
(B) Immunochemical demonstration of the presence of C3 in NP.

of NP *in vivo*. The finding that various components of an activation pathway are present (C1q, C3, C4) lends further support to this contention. Although neither finding alone proves complement activation, two additional results prove that complement is activated in NP. These are, first, the demonstration that antibodies directed against activation fragments of C4 and C3 also decorate NP [2–4], and second, evidence that the C5b-9 membrane attack complex is present on dystrophic neurites in NP, also through the use of an activation-specific antibody [2–4]. As further considered below, C5b-9 assembly only occurs after the formation of a C5 cleaving enzyme [8], which requires productive activation of the system through the C3 stage. The finding of CCP components, as just noted, together with the evidence of productive C3 activation, indicates involvement of this pathway in C3 activation. ACP complement proteins, including Factor B and properdin [2, 4], have not yet been detected in immunohistochemical studies of NP. These findings have been interpreted to indicate the lack of involvement of the ACP in NP. However, recent work has documented the ability of fibrillar Aβ to directly activate the ACP *in vitro* [19] and has demonstrated ACP activation products in the AD brain [20].

Complement activation by fibrillar Aβ generates the cytokine-like C3a and C5a biological mediators

In vitro studies

Complement activation by fibrillar Aβ generates the C3a activation cleavage fragment of C3 [16], a cytokine-like mediator with numerous pro-inflammatory actions, including regulation of the synthesis of IL-6, TNFα and other pro-inflammatory factors by macrophages, monocytes and lymphocytes [12]. These effects are initiated by binding of C3a to a 7-transmembrane domain G-protein coupled receptor (C3aR) present on numerous different cell types [12].

Aβ-triggered complement activation *in vitro* leads to generation of the potent chemokine-like C5 activation fragment, C5a [19] (Fig. 3A). In the periphery, C5a possesses the ability to induce directed migration (chemotaxis) of monocytes, neutrophils and eosinophils [12], as well as to regulate the synthesis and release of pro-inflammatory cytokines, including IL-1 and IL-6, by monocytes [12]. These effects are triggered by binding of C5a to a widely distributed G-protein coupled receptor (C5aR, CD88) which is distinct from the C3aR [12].

Numerous areas of the brain express C3aR and C5aR mRNAs [21, 22]. Furthermore, RT-PCR and Western blotting and other antibody-based approaches show that primary human astrocytes and astrocytic cell lines express a C3aR identical to the leukocyte C3aR [6, 23] which is up-regulated during CNS inflammatory conditions [21, 23]. Similar approaches demonstrate that primary human astrocytes and astrocytic cell lines also express a C5aR indistinguishable from the leuko-

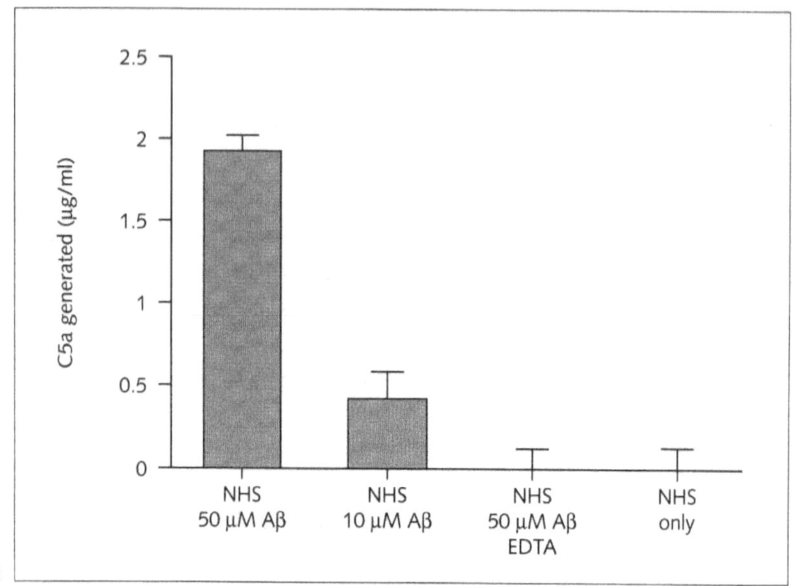

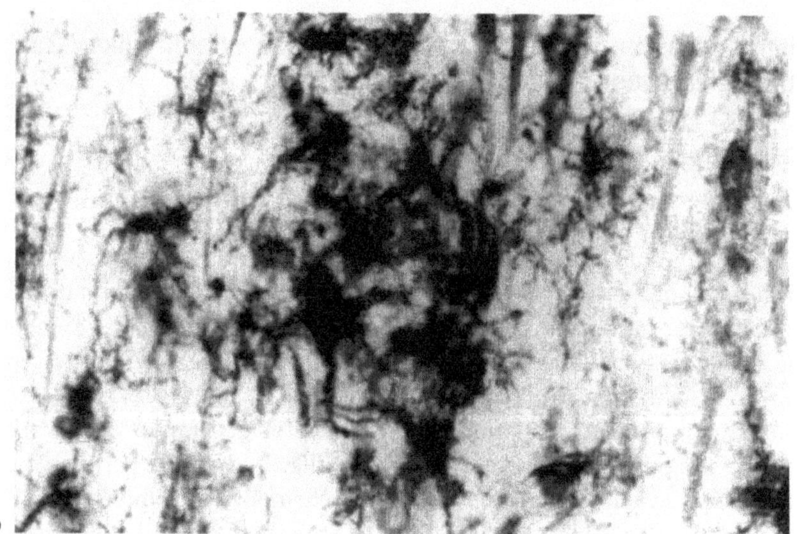

Figure 3

Generation of C5a during Aβ-mediated complement activation in vitro, *and evidence of glial cell accumulation in NP* in vivo.

(A) Aβ was incubated with a complement source and C5a generation was quantitated by radioimmunoassay. EDTA blocks complement activation and represents the negative control. Reprinted from [19] with permission.

(B) Accumulation of microglia in NP in an AD brain.

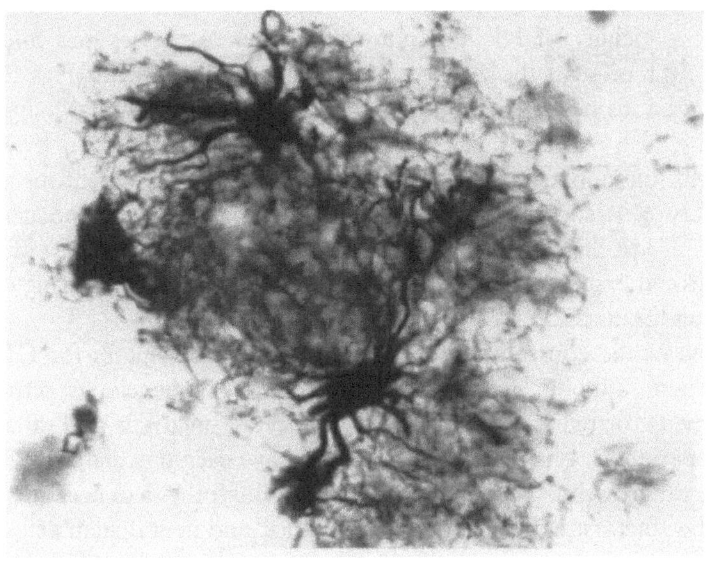

Figure 3 (continued)
(C) Accumulation of astrocytes in NP in an AD brain.

cyte receptor [6, 23] and expression is upregulated in some CNS inflammatory conditions [23]. The astrocyte receptors for C3a and C5a are functional since ligand binding triggers transient changes in intracellular calcium levels [24, 25]. Microglia also express functional C3a and C5a receptors indistinguishable from those found on inflammatory cells in the periphery [6, 23, 26], and, as with astrocytes, expression of both receptors is upregulated in certain inflammatory conditions [23, 27].

Astrocytes and microglia exhibit chemotactic behavior in response to C5a [10, 28, 29]. Human astrocytoma cells respond to C3a and C5a with increased IL-6 mRNA expression [30]. Recent results show that a differentiated human monocytic cell line, as a surrogate for microglia, synthesizes and secretes the pro-inflammatory cytokines IL-1β and IL-6 in response to C5a plus fibrillar Aβ (O'Barr and Cooper, unpublished observations).

In vivo correlates

The presence of the functional C5aR on astrocytes and microglia, the ability of C5a to induce chemotactic migration of the glial cells, and the induction of further proinflammatory changes in the cells by C5a together with Aβ are all entirely consistent with the hypothesis that complement activation by fibrillar Aβ in NP generates C5a which triggers the activation and chemotactic migration of astrocytes and microglia into the vicinity of NP. The halo of reactive astrocytes and microglia around fibrillar Aβ represents the *in vivo* manifestation of these events (Figs. 3B, C).

Surprisingly, various neuronal subpopulations, including pyramidal neurons of the hippocampus, also express C3a and C5a receptors, as determined by *in situ* hybridization and immunohistochemical approaches [22, 23, 31]. Neurons appear to be the primary cells expressing the C3aR in the normal brain, and neuronal expression of the C3aR does not significantly change during inflammation [23, 31]. In contrast, neuronal expression of the C5a receptor is up-regulated during certain inflammatory conditions [22, 23].

The functions of the constitutively expressed neuronal receptors for C3a and C5a are not known, although it is unlikely that they mediate cellular activation, migration and mediator release as they do for astrocytes, microglia and inflammatory cells in the periphery. Numerous novel actions have been postulated, including roles in dendrite outgrowth, cytoskeletal reorganization, synthesis of neurotrophins, cytokines or other factors, clearance of C3a and C5a, and neural stem cell migration [23], all of which represent topics for further investigation. Another possibility, for which there is some emerging evidence, is that binding of C5a to the neuronal C5aR is neuroprotective. The evidence is that C5-deficient mice, which cannot generate C5a, exhibit heightened hippocampal neurodegeneration in response to intraventricularly infused kainic acid, an excitotoxin, as compared to C5 sufficient mice [32], and co-infusion of C5a markedly reduces neurodegeneration [33]. C5a also protects primary neurons in C5 sufficient mice from glutamate toxicity [33]. Since C5a is generated during many and probably most inflammatory processes, a more general related hypothesis is that the binding of C5a to neuronal C5aRs protects the neurons from injury produced by reactive oxygen products and other toxic products generated in inflammatory lesions. A mechanism capable of protecting neurons in proximity to inflammatory or neurodegenerative lesions from "bystander" damage would seem to be imperative. In support of the protective effects of the C5aR, it has been shown that C5a protects differentiated human neuroblastoma cells from the neurotoxic effects of fibrillar Aβ (O'Barr and Cooper, unpublished observations). Further studies in this area are needed.

Complement activation by fibrillar Aβ generates the pro-inflammatory C5b-9 complex

In vitro studies

The ability of fibrillar Aβ to activate complement leading to the generation of C5a indicates that Aβ mediates the successful assembly of a C5 cleaving enzyme. Since the C5b-9 membrane attack complex of the complement system self-assembles after cleavage of C5, and further enzymatic action is not needed [8], it was predicted that complement activation by fibrillar Aβ *in vitro* would generate the C5b-9 complex, and this has been demonstrated [19, 34]. The C5b-9 complex formed as a consequence of Aβ-mediated complement activation is functionally competent, since it possesses the ability to insert into the membranes of neuronal precursor cells (Fig. 4A), and render their cell membranes permeable to small molecules [19]. The neuronal precursor cells are not lysed, undoubtedly due to the actions of cell membrane and plasma molecules which prevent complement-mediated damage to autologous cells [8]. Of these complement regulatory molecules, neuronal cell membranes express CD59 [35], and astrocytes and other CNS cells synthesize S protein and clusterin, two fluid phase complement regulators [6]. However, the C5b-9 complex and the earlier assembly intermediates, C5b-7 and C5b-8, possess numerous other signaling functions when inserted into the membrane of various cell types [13] (Fig. 5). These actions are likely to be cell type specific. Some of the actions, including the release of cytokines, eicosanoids and reactive oxygen species, are pro-inflammatory, while others, such as ERK kinase activation and protein kinase C activation are considered survival signals. None of these possible consequences of C5b-7, C5b-8 or C5b-9 binding to neurons has yet been evaluated.

In vivo correlates

Antibodies to the C5b-9 complex are reactive with dystrophic neurites in the vicinity of NP in AD (Fig. 4B) [2, 3], as well as with neuropil threads and the amyloid deposit itself [3, 34] in immunofluorescence studies. C5b-9 binding to neurites and neuronal membranes is also evident in electron microscopic analyses [34]. It is clear that the structures visualized in these studies represent C5b-9 complexes, since several antibodies to the complex detect comparable structures, including antibodies which detect neoantigens present only in the assembled C5b-9 complex [34]. The demonstration of C5b-9 reactivity on neuronal cell membranes associated with fibrillar Aβ-containing deposits in NP is consistent with the findings discussed above which show that the Aβ peptide efficiently activates complement *in vitro* leading to formation of the C5b-9 complex and its insertion into neuronal cell membranes. The finding of C5b-9 complexes on dystrophic membranes suggests that the complex has damaged the neurites, which would be consistent with the known cytotoxic and intracellular signaling properties of the membrane attack complex. A further indication of the functional nature of the complex deposited in NP is the finding of the C5b-9 complex on endocytosed and exocytosed vesicles or blebs on neuronal membranes [34]. Such blebbing or extrusion is a common feature of C5b-9 action on oligodendroglia and on cells in the periphery [13, 36], and strongly implies that the C5b-9 complex is functionally active. Potential signaling functions occurring in response to C5b-7, C5b-8 and C5b-9 binding to neurons *in vivo* have not been examined.

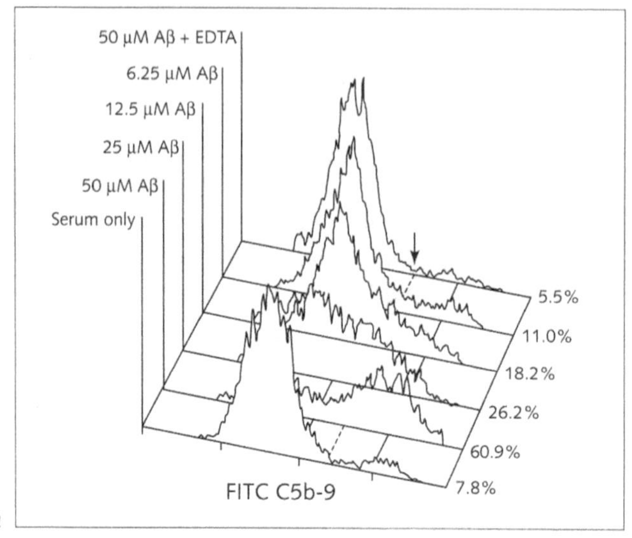

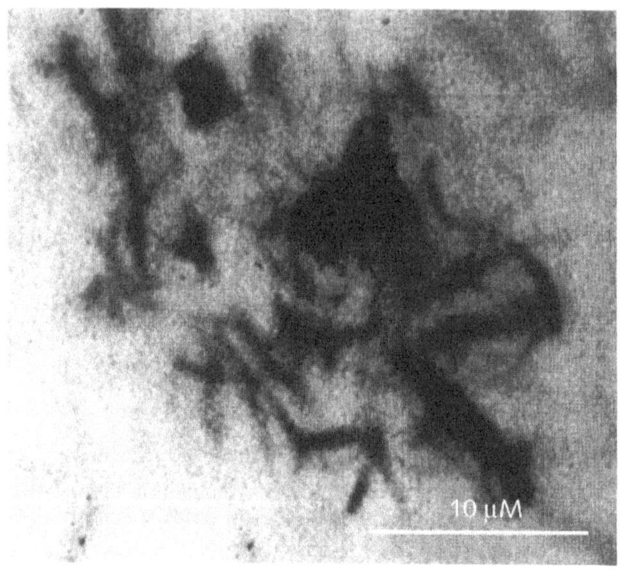

Figure 4
C5b-9 generation by Aβ-mediated complement activation in vitro, *and demonstration of the C5b-9 complex in NP* in vivo. *(A) Neuronal precursor cells were incubated with varying concentrations of Aβ and a complement source and analyzed by flow cytometry with antibody to C5b-9 neoantigens which recognize only activation-induced antigens. The numbers on the right indicate the percentage of C5b-9 positive cells, as determined by their relationship to the marker arrow in the EDTA-containing sample. Reprinted from [19] with permission. (B) Immunochemical demonstration of C5b-9 in NP. Reprinted from [34] with permission.*

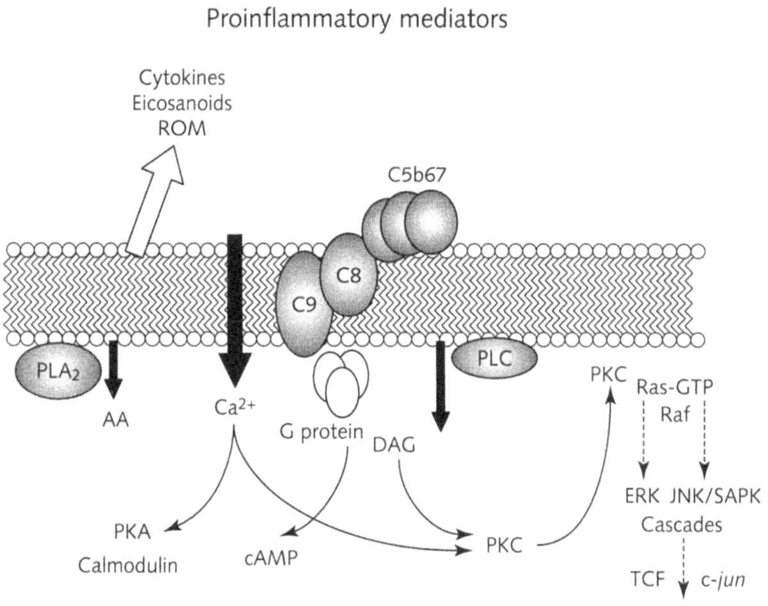

Figure 5
Induction of signaling pathways and proinflammatory mediator release by C5b-9. Modified and reprinted from [13] with permission.

Conclusions

In the periphery, acute and chronic inflammatory processes contain evidence for an initiating stimulus, and show influx of inflammatory cells, damage to tissues and augmented phagocytosis. NP also exhibit the physical and cellular hallmarks of a focal acute or chronic inflammatory reaction, since they contain a centrally located noxious substance, the fibrillar Aβ deposit, surrounded by a focal accumulation of activated microglia and astrocytes. Numerous studies in multiple systems have shown that inflammatory processes in the brain exhibit increased numbers of activated microglia and astrocytes; thus these cells function as the inflammatory cells of the CNS. Additionally, NP show evidence for damage to cell membranes, in the form of dystrophic neurites, and active phagocytic processes are implicated by studies of the interaction between Aβ and microglia [37]. Finally, NP and their associated cells contain pro-inflammatory complement components and cytokines, which are the protein mediators of the cellular changes associated with focal inflammatory reactions. Production of an inflammatory response in the CNS does not require disruption of the blood-brain barrier since neurons, microglia and astrocytes possess the ability to synthesize the complement components and pro-inflammatory cytokines necessary for the induction of an acute inflammatory response.

The complement system plays a crucial role in many inflammatory processes in the periphery. Considerable evidence suggests central involvement of the complement system in NP in AD. These include the *in vitro* demonstration that fibrillar Aβ efficiently activates both complement activation pathways leading to the formation of covalent complexes of Aβ with activation products of the third complement component, to generation of the chemokine-like C5a activation fragment, and to formation of the pro-inflammatory C5b-9 complex in functionally active form able to insert into and permeabilize the membranes of neuronal precursor cells. *In vitro* studies have also shown that C5a possesses the ability to activate both microglia and astrocytes, and to trigger their chemotactic migration.

There is no reason to doubt that these pro-inflammatory complement-dependent reactions occur in NP *in vivo*. There is, in fact, evidence for this since complement activation fragments and neoantigens specific for complement activation are found in NP, and the activation-specific pro-inflammatory C5b-9 complement membrane attack complex is readily demonstrable on damaged neuronal processes. The precise role of complement-dependent interactions in mediating the physical and cellular changes associated with fibrillar Aβ deposits in the AD brain remains to be determined.

Acknowledgments
These studies were supported in part by RO1 NS34682 and PO1 AG04342 from the NIH and SFP 1247 from the Novartis Corporation. J.X. Yu was supported by U.S.P.H.S. Training Grant T32 AG00080. This is publication 12933-IMM from The Scripps Research Institute. We thank Brian J. Cummings, Institute for Brain Aging and Dementia, University of California, Irvine, CA for permission to use his photomicrographs of astrocytes and microglia in plaques. The authors also wish to thank Catalina Hope and Joan Gausepohl for assistance with the preparation of the manuscript.

References

1 Eikelenboom P, Stam FC (1982) Immunoglobulins and complement factors in senile plaques. *Acta Neuropathol* 57: 239–242
2 McGeer PL, McGeer EG (1995) The inflammatory response system of brain: Implications for therapy of Alzheimer and other neurodegenerative diseases. *Brain Res Rev* 21: 195–218

3 Rogers J, Cooper NR, Webster S, Schultz J, McGeer PL, Styren SD, Civin WH, Brachova L, Bradt B, Ward P et al (1992) Complement activation by β-amyloid in Alzheimer disease. *Proc Natl Acad Sci USA* 89: 10016–10020

4 Rogers J, O'Barr S (1997) Inflammatory mediators in Alzheimer's disease. In: W Wasco, RE Tanzi (eds): *Molecular mechanisms of dementia.* Humana Press, Totowa, 177–198

5 Frölich L, Kornhuber J, Ihl R, Fritze J, Maurer K, Riederer P (1991) Integrity of the blood-CSF barrier in dementia of Alzheimer type: CSF/serum ratios of albumin and IgG. *Eur Arch Psy Clin Neurosci* 240: 363–366

6 Morgan BP, Gasque P (1996) Expression of complement in the brain: role in health and disease. *Immunol Today* 17: 461–466

7 Yasojima K, Schwab C, McGeer EG, McGeer PL (1999) Up-regulated production and activation of the complement system in Alzheimer's disease brain. *Am J Pathol* 154: 927–936

8 Cooper NR (1999) Biology of the complement system. In: J Gallin, R Snyderman (eds): *Inflammation: basic principles and clinical correlates.* Lippincott-Raven, Philadelphia, 281–315

9 Armstrong RC, Harvath L, Dubois-Dalcq ME (1990) Type I astrocytes and oligodendrocyte-type 2 astrocyte glial progenitors migrate toward distinct molecules. *J Neurosci Res* 27: 400–407

10 Yao J, Harvath L, Gilbert DL, Colton CA (1990) Chemotaxis by a CNS macrophage, the microglia. *J Neurosci Res* 27: 36–42

11 Lacy M, Jones J, Whittemore SR, Haviland DL, Wetsel RA, Barnum SR (1995) Expression of the receptors for the C5a anaphylatoxin, interleukin-8 and FMLP by human astrocytes and microglia. *J Neuroimmunol* 61: 71–78

12 Ember JA, Jagels MA, Hugli TE (1999) Characterization of complement anaphylatoxins and their biological responses. In: JE Volanakis, MM Frank (eds): *The human complement system in health and disease.* Marcel Dekker Inc., New York, 241–284

13 Mold C (1998) Cellular responses to the membrane attack complex. In: JE Volanakis, MM Frank (eds): *The human complement system in health and disease.* Marcel Dekker Inc., New York, 309–325

14 Jiang H, Burdick D, Glabe CG, Cotman CW, Tenner AJ (1994) β-Amyloid activates complement by binding to a specific region of the collagen-like domain of the C1q A chain. *J Immunol* 152: 5050–5059

15 Chen S, Frederickson RCA, Brunden KR (1996) Neuroglial-mediated immunoinflammatory responses in Alzheimer's disease: Complement activation and therapeutic approaches. *Neurobiol Aging* 17: 781–787

16 Watson MD, Roher AE, Kim KS, Spiegel K, Emmerling MR (1997) Complement interactions with amyloid-β 1–42: a nidus for inflammation in AD brains. *Amyloid: Int J Exp Clin Invest* 4: 147–156

17 Velazquez P, Cribbs DH, Poulos TL, Tenner AJ (1997) Aspartate residue 7 in amyloid β-protein is critical for classical complement pathway activation: Implications for Alzheimer's disease pathogenesis. *Nature Med* 3: 77–79

18 Webster S, Bonnell B, Rogers J (1997) Charge-based binding of complement component C1q to the Alzheimer amyloid β-peptide. *Am J Pathol* 150: 1531–1536
19 Bradt BM, Kolb WP, Cooper NR (1998) Complement-dependent proinflammatory properties of the Alzheimer's disease β-peptide. *J Exp Med* 188: 431–438
20 Strohmeyer R, Shen Y, Rogers J (2000). Detection of complement alternative pathway mRNA and proteins in the Alzheimer's disease brain. *Brain Res Mol Brain Res* 81 (1–2): 7–18
21 Gasque P, Singhrao SK, Neal JW, Wang P, Sayah S, Fontaine M, Morgan BP (1998) The receptor for complement anaphylatoxin C3a is expressed by myeloid cells and non-myeloid cells in inflamed human central nervous system: analysis in multiple sclerosis and bacterial meningitis. *J Immunol* 160: 3543–3554
22 Osaka H, McGinty A, Höepken UE, Lu B, Gerard C, Pasinetti GM (1999) Expression of C5a receptor in mouse brain: Role in signal transduction and neurodegeneration. *Neuroscience* 88: 1073–1082
23 Nataf S, Stahel PF, Davoust N, Barnum SR (1999) Complement anaphylatoxin receptors on neurons: new tricks for old receptors. *Trends Neurosci* 22: 397–402
24 Gasque P, Chan P, Fontaine M, Ischenko A, Lamacz M, Götze O, Morgan BP (1995) Identification and characterization of the complement C5a anaphylatoxin receptor on human astrocytes. *J Immunol* 155: 4882–4889
25 Ischenko A, Sayah S, Patte C, Andreev S, Gasque P, Schouft M-T, Vaudry H, Fontaine M (1998) Expression of a functional anaphylatoxin C3a receptor by astrocytes. *J Neurochem* 71: 2487–2496
26 Möller T, Nolte C, Burger R, Verkhratsky A, Kettenmann H (1997) Mechanisms of C5a and C3a complement fragment-induced $[Ca^{2+}]_i$ signaling in mouse microglia. *J Neurosci* 17(2): 615–624
27 Gasque P, Singhrao SK, Neal JW, Götze O, Morgan BP (1997) Expression of the receptor for complement C5a (CD88) is up-regulated on reactive astrocytes, microglia, and endothelial cells in the inflamed human central nervous system. *Am J Pathol* 150: 31–41
28 Armstrong RC, Harvath L, Dubois-Dalcq ME (1990) Type 1 astrocytes and oligodendrocyte-type 2 astrocyte glial progenitors migrate toward distinct molecules. *J Neurosci Res* 27: 400–407
29 Nolte C, Möller T, Walter T, Kettenmann H (1996) Complement 5a controls motility of murine microglial cells *in vitro via* activation of an inhibitory G-protein and the rearrangement of the actin cytoskeleton. *Neuroscience* 73: 1091–1107
30 Sayah S, Ischenko AM, Zhakhov A, Bonnard AS, Fontaine M (1999) Expression of cytokines by human astrocytomas following stimulation by C3a anaphylatoxins: specific increase in interleukin-6 mRNA expression. *J Neurochem* 72: 2426–2436
31 Davoust N, Jones J, Stahel PF, Ames RS, Barnum SR (1999) Receptor for the C3a anaphylatoxin is expressed by neurons and glial cells. *GLIA* 26: 201–211
32 Pasinetti GM, Tocco G, Sakhi S, Musleh WD, DeSimoni MG, Mascarucci P, Schreiber S, Baudry M, Finch CE (1997) Hereditary deficiencies in complement C5 are associated

with intensified neurodegenerative responses that implicate new roles for the C-system in neuronal and astrocytic functions. *Neurobiol Disease* 3: 197–204
33 Osaka H, Mukherjee P, Aisen PS, Pasinetti GM (1999) Complement-derived anaphylatoxin C5a protects against glutamate-mediated neurotoxicity. *J Cell Biochem* 73: 303–311
34 Webster S, Lue L-F, Brachova L, Tenner AJ, McGeer PL, Terai K, Walker DG, Bradt B, Cooper NR, Rogers J (1997) Molecular and cellular characterization of the membrane attack complex, C5b-9, in Alzheimer's disease. *Neurobiol Aging* 18 (4): 415–421
35 Shen Y, Halperin JA, Lee C-M (1995) Complement-mediated neurotoxicity is regulated by homologous restriction. *Brain Res* 671: 282–292
36 Scolding NJ, Morgan BP, Houston WAJ, Linington C, Campbell AK, Compston DAS (1989) Vesicular removal by oligodendrocytes of membrane attack complexes formed by activated complement. *Nature* 339: 620–622
37 Chung H, Brazil MI, Soe TT, Maxfield FR (1999) Uptake, degradation, and release of fibrillar and soluble forms of Alzheimer's amyloid β-peptide by microglial cells. *J Biol Chem* 274: 32301–32308

Amyloid β peptide interactions with the classical pathway of complement

Scott D. Webster

Department of Molecular Biology and Biochemistry, 3205 Biological Sciences II, University of California, Irvine, CA 92697, USA

Introduction

Complement is a term used to collectively refer to a group of over thirty serum proteins that is classified as part of the innate immune system. One hundred years after its original description as a factor "complementing" the ability of antibodies to lyse bacteria, complement is recognized for its crucial role as a multi-component effector system that is normally involved in host defense. However, as more studies are done on patients presenting with complement regulatory protein deficiencies [1], more is understood about complement's potential role as a source for damage of "self" tissue in circumstances involving inappropriate activation.

The complement system

The current understanding of the complement system shows the existence of three pathways, distinctive in their components and modes of activation but interrelated by their convergence at the assembly of the membrane attack complex (Fig. 1) (for recent reviews see references [2–5]). The classical pathway begins with C1, a macromolecular complex consisting of one C1q, two C1r and two C1s proteins. Activation is initiated by the binding of C1q to activating substances, and for this reason C1q is frequently referred to as the recognition subcomponent of the classical pathway. C1q binding activates C1r, which in turn cleaves and activates C1s. C1s then activates the next two proteins of the classical pathway, C4 and C2. C4 is cleaved to generate fragments C4a and C4b, the latter of which binds back to the activating substance and acts as an anchor for C2. Cleavage of C2 into C2a and C2b by C1s results in the formation of a C4b2a complex called C3 convertase, so named for its ability to cleave C3. One of the products of C3 cleavage, C3b, also binds back to the activating substance and thereby generates C4b2a3b, otherwise known as C5 convertase due to its ability to cleave C5. The C5b fragment that results from this cleavage initiates addition of the terminal complement components, C6, C7, C8 and

Neuroinflammatory Mechanisms in Alzheimer's Disease: Basic and Clinical Research,
edited by Joseph Rogers

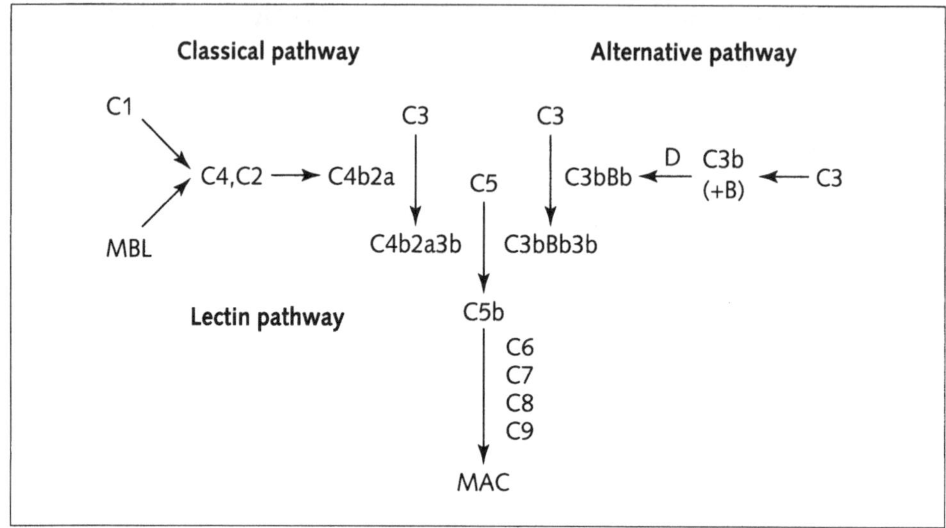

Figure 1
Pathways of complement activation. There are currently three known mechanisms for activation of complement: The classical pathway, the mannose binding lectin (MBL) pathway and the alternative pathway. Note that, although there is in vitro *evidence that MBL can interact with C1r and C1s, it appears that it is MASP-1 and MASP-2 that interact with MBL and lead to complement activation* in vivo *[84, 85].*

multiple C9 molecules to form C5b-9, the membrane attack complex (MAC). This macromolecular assembly forms a ring-like structure on membranous surfaces, and the ensuing transmembrane channel establishes a continuum between the cytoplasm and the extracellular space. As a result, ions and small molecules are able to diffuse into and out of the cell according to their concentration gradients, a circumstance that results in effects that range from disruptions in cellular homeostasis to cell lysis if a sufficient number of MAC complexes have assembled.

A second mechanism for activation of complement is the mannose binding lectin (MBL) pathway. Following interaction with complex carbohydrate constituents of bacterial surfaces, MBL acquires the capacity to interact with two proteases referred to as MASP's (for MBL-associated serine proteases). MASP-1 and MASP-2 share approximately 40% identity with C1r and C1s, and activated MASP-2 is capable of activating complement at the level of C4/C2 in a manner similar to that exhibited by C1s.

The third arm of complement is the alternative pathway. Central to this mechanism is a slow rate of spontaneous activation of C3. This active form of C3 is capable of cleaving other C3 molecules, thereby generating C3b, which will bind to substances such as bacterial cell wall polysaccharides if available. Under such circumstances, C3b is capable of binding factor B, which will in turn be cleaved into Ba and Bb fragments by another alternative pathway complement protein, factor D. The resulting C3bBb complex behaves much like the classical pathway C3 convertase (C4b2a) in that it cleaves C3 and results in the formation of a C5 convertase, C3bBb3b. As described for the classical pathway, generation of C5b by C5 convertase initiates the formation of the MAC.

There are numerous points at which complement displays cytopathic potential in Alzheimer's disease (AD). In addition to MAC formation [6], many complement subcomponents and activation fragments have pathological relevance. The anaphylatoxins C3a and C5a, the opsonins C4b and C3b, and subcomponent C1q provide chemotactic and activating signals to inflammatory cells, and microglia and/or astrocytes express receptors for numerous complement proteins/activation fragments, including $C1qR_P$, CR1, CR3, CR4, C3aR and C5aR [7–12]. An important mechanism whereby the complement system becomes integrated into AD pathology is *via* activation by the amyloid β peptide (Aβ), and this chapter will focus on interactions that are unique to the classical pathway. However, as discussed elsewhere in this volume, Aβ exhibits the capacity to activate the alternative pathway [13, 14].

Endogenous sources of complement

Components of the classical complement pathway were among the first inflammatory mediators implicated in the pathogenesis of AD [15]. Every component from C1 through C9 is synthesized in the human CNS [16], and every component has been shown to be upregulated in the AD brain at both the mRNA and protein levels [17–20]. Several cell types in the brain appear capable of synthesizing complement. Although microglia and astrocytes have been shown to produce complement proteins [21–26], studies suggest that neurons appear to be a major source of complement in the AD brain [18, 19, 27, 28].

Mechanism of Aβ activation

Charged residues mediate Aβ/C1q binding

Activation of the classical complement pathway by Aβ was first described in the seminal work of Rogers and colleagues [29], who demonstrated that activation derived from the binding of C1q to the amino terminal region of Aβ. Subsequent studies by Rogers and others have revealed much of the details of Aβ-mediated classical pathway activation, and of Aβ/C1q binding in particular. Tenner and colleagues [30] demonstrated that it was the collagen-like region (CLR) of C1q that mediated the binding of C1q to Aβ and the ensuing activation of the classical complement pathway, a finding that is in line with the mechanism of action of other antibody-independent activators of the classical pathway such as DNA, fibronectin, serum amyloid P, bacterial lipopolysaccharide and C-reactive protein (reviewed in [31]).

The most notable feature of the Aβ-binding region described by Tenner [30] (residues 14–26 of the C1q A chain polypeptide) is that, unlike much of the C1q CLR, it is highly cationic in composition. Five of the thirteen residues contained in this region (Arg16, Arg19, Arg20, Arg22 and Lys26) exhibit positive charge at physiological pH, suggestive of a mechanism based on ionic interaction, and indeed, binding of C1q to Aβ has been found to be highly dependent on ionic strength [32]. This charge-based hypothesis is also supported by the observations of Chen et al. [33] who investigated the abilities of a series of synthetic peptides corresponding to the C1qA14–26 sequence to inhibit Aβ-mediated classical complement activation. They found that peptides with truncations or substitutions resulting in the loss of Arg16, Arg19 or Arg20 exhibited substantially reduced capacities as inhibitors of Aβ-mediated complement activation.

If cationic side chains contained in C1qA14-26 mediate Aβ/C1q binding, it follows that anionic residues in Aβ must be available for interaction with C1q. The initial report of Rogers et al. [29] suggested that the N-terminal region of Aβ mediates C1q binding and activation of complement, and subsequent studies using peptide fragments narrowed this to the 1–11 region [32] and ultimately the 4–11 region [34] of Aβ, which contains two negatively charged side chains, Asp7 and Glu11, that are capable of interacting with C1qA14–26.

Modeling and ultrastructural studies of Aβ and C1q

Structural correlates of the Aβ/C1q interaction can be discussed at several levels. First, modeling studies show that Arg16, Arg19 and Arg20 are found at the exterior of the collagen-like triple helix of C1q [34] and that Asp7 and Glu11 are exposed at the surface of aggregated Aβ [35, 36], suggesting that these side chains are available for interaction. Furthermore, the model presented by Velazquez et al. [34] demonstrates that, when Aβ is constrained to the β-sheet configuration, the negatively charged Asp7 and Glu11 are appropriately spaced to interact with either the Arg16/Arg19 or Arg19/Arg20 positive charge pairs, consistent with a role for these arginines in binding [33]. Therefore, the currently understood structures of both molecules are entirely consistent with an interaction based on attraction between negative charges in the Aβ amino terminus and positive charges in the C1q CLR.

Electron micrographs reveal C1q as a large, multimeric molecule composed of six identical subunits, the structure of which has been likened to a bouquet of six tulips, with the carboxy-terminal globular heads representing the blossoms and the amino-terminal collagen-like regions the bundled stalks (Fig. 2A) (reviewed in [37]).

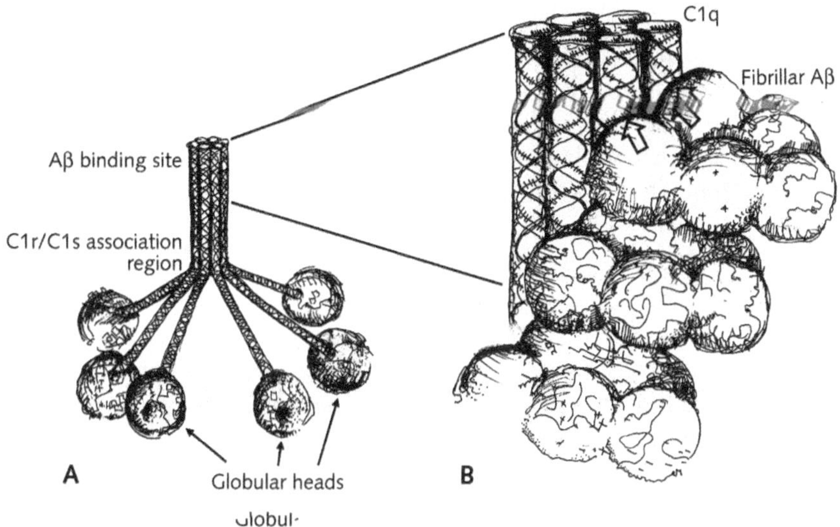

Figure 2
Model of the Aβ/C1q interaction.
(A) Representation of the complex C1q structure. In this depiction the bundled "stems" (the collagen-like region) are oriented upward. Indicated are the globular heads (site of immunoglobulin binding), the region where C1r and C1s interact with C1q and the non-immunoglobulin activation site to which Aβ binds.
(B) The spacing among A chain binding sites on C1q (one per "stem") is closely matched to the repeating structure that characterizes Aβ fibrils in vivo *(arrows) [39, 40]. Although the precise nature of the repeating globular subunits which characterize Aβ fibrils is not clear, their size is consistent with Aβ dimers [86]. Illustration courtesy of C.A. Cotman.*

Each subunit is composed of three polypeptides (designated A,B and C) intertwined in a collagen-like triple helix, and the A chain binding site is therefore replicated at regular intervals six times around the collagen-like region of each C1q molecule. Based on the known dimensions of C1q, the distance between these binding sites is predicted to be 2–3 nm [38]. Electron microscopic analysis of platinum replicas of fibrillar Aβ in AD and Down's brain show a helical arrangement of globular structures which are approximately 3–5 nm in diameter, and in reality are likely somewhat smaller if the thickness of the platinum layer is taken into account [39, 40]. These considerations suggest that the spatial arrangements of A chain binding sites in C1q and Aβ moieties in amyloid fibrils are ideally situated for multimeric binding (Fig. 2B).

Activation by Aβ derives from multimeric interaction

The tendency of Aβ to form fibrils has been rigorously examined in recent years, and the assembly state of Aβ appears to regulate its ability to activate complement. Jiang et al. [30] observed that Aβ preparations exhibiting greater proportions of sedimentable peptide both bound C1q and activated the classical pathway of complement more effectively than did less sedimentable preparations. These observations have been confirmed and extended to conclude that, beyond simple sedimentability, the ability of Aβ to initiate the classical complement pathway through activation of C1 correlates with thioflavine- and Congo red-positivity [41], the presence of fibrils as assessed by electron microscopy [34, 41, 42] and the presence of β sheet structure as judged by circular dichroism measurement [34, 42], although conflicting data exists [33]. This requirement for assembled peptide correlates with the known biological properties of C1, as an integral step in the activation of C1 by immunoglobulin is the induction of a conformational shift among the six subunits of C1q by the binding of C1q globular heads to immune complexes containing multiple IgG molecules or pentavalent IgM (reviewed in [43]). Such a mechanism based on multimeric interaction between C1q and activating molecules likely extends to the collagen-like region as well, since a common structural feature of non-immunoglobulin activators of C1 is a polymeric or oligomeric structure such that binding sites for C1q are presented in a regular, repeating array [44–51]. Aβ would clearly be a member of this group when in an assembled state. The concept of C1q interacting with assembled peptide is also consistent with the work of Snyder et al. [52] who showed that C1q does not bind to monomeric Aβ.

Bergamaschini et al. [53] recently demonstrated that $A\beta_{1-42}$ was capable of inducing C1s and C4 activation under conditions that inhibited formation of the C1 complex. This study is interesting in that plasma was used instead of serum, and therefore the clotting and contact systems were still intact. The authors showed that factor XII appears to have the capacity to mediate Aβ-induced cleavage of C4. This finding awaits confirmation, but does raise the possibility of an additional point of interaction of Aβ with the complement system.

Factors that modify Aβ-mediated activation

In addition to the action of numerous complement regulatory proteins [1], other molecules can affect the extent of complement activation. McGeer et al. [54] demonstrated that the E4 isoform of apolipoprotein E produced an approximately 20–25% enhancement of Aβ-mediated activation of the classical complement pathway *in vitro*. Although the mechanism of Apo E4 enhancement *in vitro* has not been established and a link between Apo E4 and enhanced complement activation has yet to be proved in the AD brain, this finding is interesting in light of the ability of Apo E to bind Aβ [55] and the well documented association of the E4 isoform with AD (for reviews see [56–58]).

Modification of complement activation may represent a therapeutic target in AD. A true prospective clinical trial [59] and numerous retrospective clinical studies (reviewed in [60]) have demonstrated that antiinflammatory paradigms have efficacy with regard to delaying the onset and/or slowing the progression of AD. The significant incidence of adverse side effects associated with traditional antiinflammatory medications has prompted efforts to discover agents with a more focused mechanism of action. Complement offers an attractive target for therapeutic intervention in AD, since successful inhibition would ameliorate both MAC deposition onto neuronal surfaces and the generation of microglia-activating C3, C4 and C5 cleavage products. Inhibition of the Aβ/C1q interaction has been proposed as a possible mechanism for inhibiting classical pathway activation in the AD brain [34, 61], and would have the added benefit of eliminating the enhancing effect of C1q on Aβ aggregation (see next section), but other sites for intervention may also exist. Hays et al. [62] presented data demonstrating that a class of organic molecules known as benzoxazinones can inhibit C1r, and the vaccinia virus complement control protein has been shown to diminish Aβ-mediated activation of both the classical and alternative pathways of complement [63].

Influences of C1q on Aβ aggregation

Repeating structure is exhibited not only by fibrillar Aβ, as described above, but also by oligomeric Aβ. Interestingly, oligomers that contain some minimum moiety of the repeating structure that characterizes mature fibrils are a critical intermediate in the mechanism of nucleation-dependent polymerization that characterizes Aβ fibrillogenesis [64, 65]. C1q enhances the fibrillar aggregation of Aβ in a fashion that suggests a promotion of the nucleation phase; by stabilizing already-formed oligomers of Aβ, C1q appears to nucleate the formation of mature Aβ fibrils [38, 66]. If the appearance of neuritic, Aβ fibril-containing plaques is a critical event in the pathogenesis of AD, then the ability of C1q to enhance fibrillar Aβ aggregation is likely to be an important contributory factor for disease progression.

The requirement of some level of assembly within Aβ for C1q binding/complement activation and for the ability of C1q to accelerate fibril formation suggests that C1q would be found preferentially in fibrillar plaques in the AD brain. However, a consensus on this issue has yet to be reached. Using plaque morphology as a basis for distinguishing subtypes, McGeer et al. [67] reported that C1q was absent from diffuse plaques, whereas Zhan et al. [68] found that C1q was present in both neuritic and diffuse plaques. Results have also varied when the tinctorial properties of

Aβ deposits were employed. Eikelenboom et al. [69] reported a colocalization of C1q with Congo Red positive (and therefore fibril-containing) plaques and Afagh et al. [70] found a similar colocalization of C1q to thioflavine positive plaques, whereas Rozemuller et al. [71] found C1q in both congophilic and non-congophilic plaques. Furthermore, reports of the existence of clusters of fibrils in diffuse plaques blur the distinction between plaque types [72–74].

A likely scenario may be that C1 binds with the formation of the first fibrillar/oligomeric Aβ structure in the region of a developing plaque, resulting in a low level of activation. However, following activation, C1 dissociates leaving subcomponent C1q in contact with the nascent plaque. Because of the hexameric structure of C1q, some of the A chain binding sites would be expected to remain accessible, allowing C1q to bind and stabilize oligomers of Aβ and thereby promote further generation of fibrils, which would in turn foster binding of additional C1 and therefore further complement activation. This hypothesis may help explain the variable results seen for immunodetection of complement components in diffuse plaques but their consistent detection in neuritic plaques.

Transgenic models

In recent years several models of AD have been generated in the form of transgenic mice that express mutant forms of the human amyloid precursor protein (APP) alone or in conjunction with another protein relevant to AD such as one of the human presenilin mutants. These mice are valuable tools in the study of AD, yet some of the hallmarks of the disease are not expressed. For example, the existence of neurofibrillary tangles has not been reported, and neuronal loss is modest at best. Furthermore, such loss is only observed after deposition of Aβ at levels far exceeding those generally observed in severe AD cases [75, 76]. One possible explanation for this phenomenon is that the mice are deficient in some fashion that is critical for the development of the full range of AD pathology.

Interestingly, the mouse C1q A chain sequence contains two significant differences in the 14–26 region compared to the human, specifically Arg16→Asn and Arg20→Pro. Inasmuch as the Tenner model of Aβ/C1q binding [34] suggests that Asp7 and Glu11 of Aβ interact with either the Arg16/Arg19 pair or the Arg19/Arg20 pair in the C1qA14–26 region, the fact that mouse C1q contains only one of these three (Arg19) infers that it will bind Aβ less avidly than will human C1q. This would be predicted to lead to a diminished ability of mouse C1 to be activated by the human Aβ peptide in comparison to human C1, a hypothesis which was confirmed in a recent report showing that activation of mouse C1 by fibrillar Aβ was significantly lower than activation of human C1 [77].

In addition to this decrease in the ability of mouse C1 to respond to human Aβ due to the loss of Arg16 and Arg20 in the C1q A chain, the mouse exhibits deficiencies in other components of complement such as C4 [78], and possesses an acute phase response that is quite different from that found in humans [79, 80]. This suggests the existence of a diminished Aβ-driven cycle of complement activation and associated inflammatory events in the CNS of transgenic mice, and may in turn explain the limited neurodegeneration seen in the currently available mouse transgenic models of AD when compared to human AD brain pathology.

Preliminary reports of complement proteins associated with amyloid plaques in transgenic mice that overexpress mutant human APP genes [81, 82] are consistent with the observation that mouse C1 does respond to human Aβ, albeit with a lower efficiency than does human C1 [77]. It will be critical to assess the extent to which complement deposition in these animals compares to that seen in the AD brain in order to determine whether additional modifications to the mouse genome are necessary to effectively mimic the Aβ-driven cycle of complement activation, inflammatory events, and neurodegeneration seen in AD. For example, in a recent study Schenk and colleagues [83] found that inoculation of human APP transgenic mice slowed the development of AD-like amyloid plaques in the brains of those mice. This work suggested that recruitment of the immune system by immunization with Aβ can counteract deposition of the peptide. This is an intriguing concept; however, as noted above, laboratory mice can be deficient or significantly different in components of the inflammatory response when compared to humans. Therefore, human clinical trials of Aβ immunization should be constructed with this factor in mind, as the possibility exists that inoculation with the peptide could induce significant inflammatory damage that was not foreseen based on the animal studies.

Acknowledgments

This work was supported in part by NIH grant AG-17289. The author wishes to thank Cheryl A. Cotman for her original illustration (Fig. 2).

References

1 Morgan BP, Harris CL (1999) *Complement regulatory proteins*. Academic Press, San Diego

2 Reid KBM, Colomb MG, Loos M (1998) Complement component C1 and the collectins: parallels between routes of acquired and innate immunity. Immunol Today 19: 56–59

3 Rother K, Till GO, Hansch GM (eds) (1998) *The complement system*. Springer-Verlag, New York

4 Turner MW (1998) Mannose-binding lectin (MBL) in health and disease. *Immunobiology* 199: 327–339

5 Volanakis JE, Frank MM (eds) (1998) *The human complement system in health and disease.* Marcel Dekker Inc., New York
6 Webster S, Lue L-F, Brachova L, Tenner AJ, McGeer PL, Terai K, Walker DG, Bradt B, Cooper NR, Rogers J (1997) Molecular and cellular characterization of the membrane attack complex, C5b-9, in Alzheimer's disease. *Neurobiol Aging* 18: 415–421
7 Ulvestad E, Williams K, Bjerkvig R, Tiekotter K, Antel J, Matre R (1994) Human microglial cells have phenotypic and functional characteristics in common with both macrophages and dendritic antigen-presenting cells. *J Leukoc Biol* 56: 732–740
8 Lacy M, Jones J, Whittemore SR, Haviland DL, Wetsel RA, Barnum SR (1995) Expression of the receptors for the C5a anaphylatoxin, interleukin-8 and FMLP by human astrocytes and microglia. *J Neuroimmunol* 61: 71–78
9 Gasque P, Singhrao SK, Neal JW, Gotze O, Morgan BP (1997) Expression of the receptor for complement C5a (CD88) is up-regulated on reactive astrocytes, microglia, and endothelial cells in the inflamed human central nervous system. *Am J Pathol* 150: 31–41
10 Gasque P, Singhrao SK, Neal JW, Wang P, Sayah S, Fontaine M, Morgan BP (1998) The receptor for complement anaphylatoxin C3a is expressed by myeloid cells and non-myeloid cells in inflamed human central nervous system: analysis in multiple sclerosis and bacterial meningitis. *J Immunol* 160: 3543–3554
11 Gasque P, Tenner A, Morgan BP (1998) Expression of the C1q/MBL/SPA receptor involved in phagocytosis and innate immune defense on human glia. *Molec Immunol* 35: 379
12 Webster S, Park M, Fonseca MI and Tenner AJ (2000) Structural and functional evidence for a microglial C1q receptor that enhances phagocytosis. *J Leukoc Biol* 67: 109–116
13 Watson, MD, Roher AE, Kim KS, Spiegel K, Emmerling MR (1997) Complement interactions with amyloid-β 1–42: a nidus for inflammation in AD brains. *Amyloid* 4: 147–156
14 Bradt BM, Kolb WP, Cooper NR (1998) Complement-dependent proinflammatory properties of the Alzheimer's disease beta-peptide. *J Exp Med* 188: 431–438
15 Eikelenboom P, Stam FC (1982) Immunoglobulins and complement factors in senile plaques. An immunoperoxidase study. *Acta Neuropathol* 57: 239–242
16 Barnum SR (1995) Complement biosynthesis in the central nervous system. *Crit Rev Oral Biol Med* 6: 132–146
17 Johnson SA, Lampert-Etchells M, Pasinetti GM, Rozovsky I, Finch CE (1992) Complement mRNA in the mammalian brain: responses to Alzheimer's disease and experimental brain lesioning. *Neurobiol Aging* 13: 641–648
18 Shen Y, Li R, McGeer EG, McGeer PL (1997) Neuronal expression of mRNAs for complement proteins of the classical pathway in Alzheimer brain. *Brain Res* 769: 391–395
19 Terai K, Walker DG, McGeer EG, McGeer PL (1997) Neurons express proteins of the classical complement pathway in Alzheimer disease. *Brain Res* 769: 385–390
20 Yasojima K, Schwab C, McGeer EG, McGeer PL (1999) Up-regulated production and

activation of the complement system in Alzheimer's disease brain. *Am J Pathol* 154: 927–936

21 Levi-Strauss M, Mallat M (1987) Primary cultures of murine astrocytes produce C3 and factor B, two components of the alternative pathway of complement activation. *J Immunol* 139: 2361–2366

22 Gasque P, Ischenko A, Legoedec J, Mauger C, Schouft MT, Fontaine M (1993) Expression of the complement classical pathway by human glioma in culture. A model for complement expression by nerve cells. *J Biol Chem* 268: 25068–25074

23 Gasque P, Fontaine M, Morgan BP (1995) Complement expression in human brain. Biosynthesis of terminal pathway components and regulators in human glial cells and cell lines. *J Immunol* 154: 4726–4733

24 Walker DG, Kim SU, McGeer PL (1995) Complement and cytokine gene expression in cultured microglial derived from postmortem human brains. *J Neurosci Res* 40: 478–493

25 Haga S, Aizawa T, Ishii T, Ikeda K (1996) Complement gene expression in mouse microglia and astrocytes in culture: comparisons with mouse peritoneal macrophages. *Neurosci Lett* 216: 191–194

26 Walker DG, Kim SU, McGeer PL (1998) Expression of complement C4 and C9 genes by human astrocytes. *Brain Res* 809: 31–38

27 Lampert-Etchells M, Pasinetti GM, Finch CE, Johnson SA (1993) Regional localization of cells containing complement C1q and C4 mRNAs in the frontal cortex during Alzheimer's disease. *Neurodegeneration* 2: 111–121

28 Fischer B, Schmoll H, Riederer P, Bauer J, Platt D, Popa-Wagner A (1995) Complement C1q and C3 mRNA expression in the frontal cortex of Alzheimer's patients. *J Mol Med* 73: 465–471

29 Rogers J, Cooper NR, Webster S, Schultz J, McGeer PL, Styren SD, Civin WH, Brachova L, Bradt B, Ward P et al (1992) Complement activation by beta-amyloid in Alzheimer disease. *Proc Natl Acad Sci USA* 89: 10016–10020

30 Jiang H, Burdick D, Glabe CG, Cotman CW, Tenner AJ (1994) β-Amyloid activates complement by binding to a specific region of the collagen-like domain of the C1q A chain. *J Immunol* 152: 5050–5059

31 Trinder PK, Maeurer MJ, Kaul M, Petry E, Loos M (1993) Functional domains of the human C1q A-chain. *Behring Inst Mitt* 93: 180–188

32 Webster S, Bonnell B, Rogers J (1997) Charge based binding of complement component C1q to the Alzheimer amyloid β-peptide. *Am J Pathol* 150: 1531–1536

33 Chen S, Frederickson RC, Brunden KR (1996) Neuroglial-mediated immunoinflammatory responses in Alzheimer's disease: complement activation and therapeutic approaches. *Neurobiol Aging* 17: 781–787

34 Velazquez P, Cribbs DH, Poulos TL, Tenner AJ (1997) Aspartate residue 7 in amyloid beta-protein is critical for classical complement pathway activation: implications for Alzheimer's disease pathogenesis. *Nat Med* 3: 77–79

35 Soreghan B, Kosmoski J, Glabe C (1994) Surfactant properties of Alzheimer's A beta peptides and the mechanism of amyloid aggregation. *J Biol Chem* 269: 28551–28554
36 Chaney MO, Webster SD, Kuo YM, Roher AE (1998) Molecular modeling of the Abeta1–42 peptide from Alzheimer's disease. *Protein Eng* 11: 761–767
37 Cooper NR (1985) The classical complement pathway: activation and regulation of the first complement component. *Adv Immunol* 37: 151–216
38 Webster S, Glabe C, Rogers J (1995) Multivalent binding of complement protein C1q to the amyloid beta-peptide (A beta) promotes the nucleation phase of A beta aggregation. *Biochem Biophys Res Commun* 217: 869–875
39 Miyakawa T, Katsuragi S, Watanabe K, Shimoji A, Ikeuchi Y (1986) Ultrastructural studies of amyloid fibrils and senile plaques in human brain. *Acta Neuropathol* 70: 202–208
40 Miyakawa T, Watanabe K, Katsuragi S (1986) Ultrastructure of amyloid fibrils in Alzheimer's disease and Down's syndrome. *Virch Archiv* 52: 99–106
41 Webster S, Bradt B, Rogers J, Cooper N (1997) Aggregation state-dependent activation of the classical complement pathway by the amyloid beta peptide. *J Neurochem* 69: 388–398
42 Cribbs DH, Velazquez P, Soreghan B, Glabe CG, Tenner AJ (1997) Complement activation by cross-linked truncated and chimeric full-length beta-amyloid. *Neuroreport* 8: 3457–3462
43 Heinz HP (1989) Biological functions of C1q expressed by conformational changes. *Behring Inst Mitt* 84: 20–31
44 Rosenberg AM, Prokopchuk PA, Lee JS (1988) The binding of native DNA to the collagen-like segment of Clq. *J Rheumatol* 15: 1091–1096
45 Hicks PS, Saunero-Nava L, Du Clos TW, Mold C (1992) Serum amyloid P component binds to histones and activates the classical complement pathway. *J Immunol* 149: 3689–3694
46 Jiang H, Cooper B, Robey FA, Gewurz H (1992) DNA binds and activates complement via residues 14–26 of the human C1q A chain. *J Biol Chem* 267: 25597–25601
47 Jiang H, Robey FA, Gewurz H (1992) Localization of sites through which C-reactive protein binds and activates complement to residues 14–26 and 76–92 of the human C1q A chain. *J Exp Med* 175: 1373–1379
48 Krumdieck R, Hook M, Rosenberg LC, Volanakis JE (1992) The proteoglycan decorin binds C1q and inhibits the activity of the C1 complex. *J Immunol* 149: 3695–3701
49 Bunse R, Heinz HP (1993) Interaction of the capsular polysaccharide of Haemophilus influenzae type B with C1q. *Behring Inst Mitt* 93: 148–164
50 Gewurz H, Ying SC, Jiang H, Lint TF (1993) Nonimmune activation of the classical complement pathway. *Behring Inst Mitt* 93: 138–147
51 Ying SC, Gewurz AT, Jiang H, Gewurz H (1993) Human serum amyloid P component oligomers bind and activate the classical complement pathway via residues 14–26 and 76–92 of the A chain collagen-like region of C1q. *J Immunol* 150: 169–176
52 Snyder SW, Wang GT, Barrett L, Ladror US, Casuto D, Lee CM, Krafft GA, Holzman

RB, Holzman TF (1994) Complement C1q does not bind monomeric beta-amyloid. *Exp Neurol* 128: 136–142

53 Bergamaschini L, Canziani S, Bottasso B, Cugno M, Braidotti P, Agostoni A (1999) Alzheimer's beta-amyloid peptides can activate the early components of complement classical pathway in a C1q-independent manner. *Clin Exp Immunol* 115: 526–533

54 McGeer PL, Walker DG, Pitas RE, Mahley RW, McGeer EG (1997) Apolipoprotein E4 (ApoE4) but not ApoE3 or ApoE2 potentiates beta-amyloid protein activation of complement *in vitro*. *Brain Res* 749: 135–138

55 Naslund J, Thyberg J, Tjernberg LO, Wernstedt C, Karlstrom AR, Bogdanovic N, Gandy SE, Lannfelt L, Terenius L, Nordstedt C (1995) Characterization of stable complexes involving apolipoprotein E and the amyloid beta peptide in Alzheimer's disease brain. *Neuron* 15: 219–228

56 Mayeux R (1998) Gene-environment interaction in late-onset Alzheimer disease: the role of apolipoprotein-epsilon 4. *Alzh Dis Assoc Disord* 12 (Suppl 3): S10–S15

57 Roses AD (1998) Apolipoprotein E and Alzheimer's disease. The tip of the susceptibility iceberg. *Ann NY Acad Sci* 855: 738–743

58 Swartz RH, Black SE, St George-Hyslop P (1999) Apolipoprotein E and Alzheimer's disease: a genetic, molecular and neuroimaging review. *Can J Neurol Sci* 26: 77–88

59 Rogers J, Kirby LC, Hempelman SR, Berry DL, McGeer PL, Kaszniak AW, Zalinski J, Cofield M, Mansukhani L, Willson P et al (1993) Clinical trial of indomethacin in Alzheimer's disease. *Neurology* 43: 1609–1611

60 McGeer PL, Schulzer M, McGeer EG (1996) Arthritis and anti-inflammatory agents as possible protective factors for Alzheimer's disease: a review of 17 epidemiologic studies. *Neurology* 47: 425–432

61 Rogers J, Webster S, Lue L-F, Brachova L, Civin WH, Emmerling M, Shivers B, Walker D, McGeer P (1996) Inflammation and Alzheimer's disease pathogenesis. *Neurobiol Aging* 17: 681–686

62 Hays SJ, Caprathe BW, Gilmore JL, Amin N, Emmerling MR, Michael W, Nadimpalli R, Nath R, Raser KJ, Stafford D et al (1998) 2-Amino-4H-3,1-benzoxazin-4-ones as inhibitors of C1r serine protease. J Med Chem 41: 1060–1067

63 Daly J, Kotwal GJ (1998) Pro-inflammatory complement activation by the A beta peptide of Alzheimer's disease is biologically significant and can be blocked by vaccinia virus complement control protein. *Neurobiol Aging* 19: 619–627

64 Jarrett JT, Berger EP, Lansbury PT (1993) The C-terminus of the beta protein is critical in amyloidogenesis. *Ann NY Acad Sci* 695: 144–148

65 Harper JD, Lansbury PT (1997) Models of amyloid seeding in Alzheimer's disease and scrapie: mechanistic truths and physiological consequences of the time-dependent solubility of amyloid proteins. *Ann Rev Biochem* 66: 385–407

66 Webster S, O'Barr S, Rogers J (1994) Enhanced aggregation and beta structure of amyloid beta peptide after coincubation with C1q. *J Neurosci Res* 39: 448–456

67 McGeer PL, Akiyama H, Itagaki S, McGeer EG (1989) Immune system response in Alzheimer's disease. *Can J Neurol Sci* 16: 516–527

68 Zhan SS, Veerhuis R, Kamphorst W, Eikelenboom P (1995) Distribution of beta amyloid associated proteins in plaques in Alzheimer's disease and in the non-demented elderly. *Neurodegeneration* 4: 291–297
69 Eikelenboom P, Hack CE, Rozemuller JM, Stam FC (1989) Complement activation in amyloid plaques in Alzheimer's dementia. *Virch Arch* 56: 259–262
70 Afagh A, Cummings BJ, Cribbs DH, Cotman CW, Tenner AJ (1996) Localization and cell association of C1q in Alzheimer's disease brain. *Exp Neurol* 138: 22–32
71 Rozemuller JM, Eikelenboom P, Stam FC, Beyreuther K, Masters CL (1989) A4 protein in Alzheimer's disease: primary and secondary cellular events in extracellular amyloid deposition. *J Neuropathol Exp Neurol* 48: 674–691
72 Yamaguchi H, Nakazato Y, Shoji M, Takatama M, Hirai S (1991) Ultrastructure of diffuse plaques in senile dementia of the Alzheimer type: comparison with primitive plaques. *Acta Neuropathol* 82: 13–20
73 Yamazaki T, Yamaguchi H, Okamoto K, Hirai S (1991) Ultrastructural localization of argyrophilic substances in diffuse plaques of Alzheimer-type dementia demonstrated by methenamine silver staining. *Acta Neuropathol* 81: 540–545
74 Davies CA, Mann DM (1993) Is the "preamyloid" of diffuse plaques in Alzheimer's disease really nonfibrillar? *Am J Pathol* 143: 1594–1605
75 Games D, Adams D, Alessandrini R, Barbour R, Berthelette P, Blackwell C, Carr T, Clemes J, Donaldson T, Gillespie F et al (1995) Alzheimer-type neuropathology in transgenic mice overexpressing V717F beta-amyloid precursor protein. *Nature* 373: 523–527
76 Hsiao K, Chapman P, Nilsen S, Eckman C, Harigaya Y, Younkin S, Yang F, Cole G (1996) Correlative memory deficits, Aβ elevation, and amyloid plaques in transgenic mice. *Science* 274: 99–102
77 Webster S, Tenner AJ, Poulos TL and Cribbs DH (1999) The mouse C1q A chain sequence alters beta amyloid induced complement activation. *Neurobiol Aging* 20: 297–304
78 Ebanks RO, Isenman DE (1996) Mouse complement component C4 is devoid of classical pathway C5 convertase subunit activity. *Mol Immunol* 33: 297–309
79 Zahedi K, Whitehead AS (1993) Regulation of mouse serum amyloid P gene expression by cytokines *in vitro*. *Biochim Biophys Acta* 1176: 162–168
80 Szalai AJ, Briles DE, Volanakis JE (1995) Human C-reactive protein is protective against fatal Streptococcus pneumoniae infection in transgenic mice. *J Immunol* 155: 2557–63
81 Yu JX, Bradt BM, Hsiao K, Cooper NR (1998) The third complement component is associated with amyloid plaques in human APP695SWE transgenic mice. *Soc Neurosci Abst* 28: 730
82 Lemere CA, Maron R, Spooner E, Grenfell TJ, Mori C, Weiner HL, Selkoe DJ (1999) Mucosal administration of Aβ peptide decreases cerebral amyloid burden in PD-APP transgenic mice. *Soc Neurosci Abst* 29: 519.6
83 Schenk D, Barbour R, Dunn W, Gordon G, Grajeda H, Guido T, Hu K, Huang J, Johnson-Wood K, Khan K et al (1999) Immunization with amyloid-beta attenuates Alzheimer-disease-like pathology in the PDAPP mouse. *Nature* 400: 173–177

84 Sim RB, Dodds AW (1997) The complement system: an introduction. In: RB Sim, AW Dodds (eds): *Complement, a practical approach*. IRL Press at Oxford University Press, Oxford, 1–17
85 Matsushita M, Endo Y, Fujita T (1998) MASP1 (MBL-associated serine protease 1). *Immunobiology* 199: 340–347
86 Roher AE, Chaney MO, Kuo Y-M, Webster SD, Stine WB, Haverkamp LJ, Woods AS, Cotter RJ, Tuohy JM, Krafft GA et al (1996) Morphology and toxicity of Aβ1–42 dimer derived from neuritic and vascular amyloid deposits of Alzheimer disease. *J Biol Chem* 271: 20631–20635

Physiology and biochemistry of the interleukin-6 receptor complex: Implications for CNS disorders and Alzheimer's disease

Harald Hampel, Michael Scheloske and Andreas Haslinger

Dementia Research Section, Department of Psychiatry, Ludwig-Maximilian University, Nussbaumstr. 7, 80336 Munich, Germany

Introduction

Functional pleiotropy and redundancy are characteristic features of cytokines, including interleukins, interferons, colony-stimulating factors and growth factors. These molecules exert their biological functions through specific receptors expressed on the surface of target cells. Originally it was thought that each cytokine exerts a specific effect on its particular target cell, but in fact, most cytokines exhibit a wide range of biological effects on various tissues and cells. One receptor may interfere with different signal transduction systems and multiple receptors can couple to the same signaling pathway *via* common effectors. Therefore signaling pathways within a cell form a network with multiple interactions between different cytokine pathways. Interleukin-6 (IL-6) is an example of such a multifunctional cytokine [1] and exerts multiple effects on the immune, hematopoietic and nervous system in a finely regulated interaction with its two receptors: interleukin-6 receptor (IL-6R) and glycoprotein 130 (gp130), the component critical for signal transduction.

Interleukin-6

In 1980, interleukin-6 (IL-6) was first described as interferon-2 (IFN-2), a sub-product of interferon-β-producing fibroblasts [2]. Different terms were subsequently introduced in the literature for the same protein, each referring to the original report. In 1988, the name IL-6 was proposed in order to resolve the confusion in terminology [3] after molecular cloning studies revealed that IL-6 [4], IFN-2 [2, 5], B-cell stimulatory factor 2 (BSF 2) [6, 7], hybridoma growth factor (HGF) [3, 8], plasmacytoma growth factor (PGF) [9], hepatocyte stimulating factor (HSF) [10], T-cell replacing (TRF)-like factor [11], and 26 kDa-protein [12, 13] were identical proteins.

Neuroinflammatory Mechanisms in Alzheimer's Disease: Basic and Clinical Research,
edited by Joseph Rogers

The molecular structure of interleukin-6

In 1986, the single human IL-6 (*hIL-6*) gene was assigned to chromosome 7p21 [14]. It is approximately 5 kb in length and consists of five exons and four introns [4, 15]. The deduced amino acid sequence for *hIL-6* contains an open reading frame of 212 amino acids, including a 28 amino acid hydrophobic leader sequence with two intramolecular disulphide bonds that is suspected to undergo extensive post-translational modification including phosphorylation and both N-linked and O-linked glycosylation.

The N-terminal 28 amino acids can be deleted without loss of biological activity [16]. Deletion of more than these amino acids, however, results in functional inactivation of IL-6 [16, 17]. The C-terminal domain of IL-6 plays a dominant role in receptor recognition [18–20]. Truncation of as few as three or four C-terminal residues drastically reduces or abolishes the biological activity of IL-6 [18]. The interactions between residues of the N- and C-terminal regions of *hIL-6* are important for establishing an α-helical conformation and are critical for the ability to bind to hIL-6R [21].

Mature IL-6 is secreted as 183–185 amino acid polypeptides with different N-termini. These polypeptides are, in turn, subjected to differential N- and O-glycosylation and serine phosphorylation in a cell-type-specific manner leading to the secretion of proteins of molecular mass 19–30 kDa from different cell types [22, 23].

Somers and colleagues (1997) were able to obtain a crystal structure from a recombinant 185 amino acid IL-6-polypeptide expressed in *Escherichia coli* [17] and described the IL-6 structure as one that consisted of four anti-parallel α-helices linked by up-and-down loops [24], as previously predicted. This structure-type is known for a group of proteins including leukemia inhibitory factor (LIF), oncostatin M (OSM), ciliary neurotrophic factor (CNTF), growth hormone (GRH), prolactine and granulocyte colony-stimulating factor (G-CSF) [25, 26]. The structural results for IL-6 were confirmed by Xu and colleagues (1997) using nuclear magnetic resonance (NMR)-spectroscopy [27].

The expression of interleukin-6

IL-6 is a pleiotropic cytokine expressed by a variety of cells, e.g. endothelial cells, fibroblasts, keratinocytes, mesangium cells, stroma cells, activated T and B cells, monocytes or macrophages and several tumor cells [28].

In the CNS, the expression of IL-6 has not yet been entirely explored. Relatively scarce information is available on IL-6 CNS protein signals. However, a variety of studies reported IL-6 mRNA expression levels in different cell types, such as microglia, astroglia, neurons and endothelial cells [29, 30, 31]. Other sources of IL-6 are pituitary [32, 33] and hypothalamic cells [34, 35]. Oligodendrocytes show IL-6 mRNA expression only *in vitro*, after infection with the measles virus [36].

In rat brain, IL-6 mRNA is expressed in most brain regions at low concentration levels. High expression was observed in the cerebellum, cortex and hippocampus. Furthermore, IL-6 mRNA expression could also be traced in striatum, hypothalamus, neocortex, and brain stem. *In situ* hybridization revealed that IL-6 mRNA is predominantly expressed by neuronal cells in the CNS [37, 38]. At the cellular level a colocalization of IL-6 mRNA with the mRNA of its receptor, the interleukin-6 receptor (IL-6R), has been shown in several neuronal types throughout the CNS, including pyramidal and granular neurons of the hippocampus, neurons of the habenular nucleus, dorsomedial, cerebellar granular neurons and pyramidal neurons of the cerebral cortex [39, 40].

The exact mechanisms responsible for the regulation of IL-6 expression are still unclear. It could be demonstrated that Janus kinase-2 (JAK2) [41], protein kinase C (PKC) and cyclic adenosine monophosphate (cAMP)-dependent signal transduction pathways can trigger IL-6 gene expression [42, 43].

Physiological actions of interleukin-6

IL-6 participates in a variety of biological processes, such as immune responses, acute phase reactions and hematopoiesis, inducing growth and differentiation of cells of the immune and hematopoietic system. IL-6 also plays an important role in host defense mechanisms [28, 44–46].

Recently, IL-6 has been reported to serve as a relevant mediator of neuroregulatory and inflammatory processes in the CNS. In particular, IL-6 may play a role in controlling neuroimmune responses and protection of neurons, as well as in neuronal differentiation, growth, survival mechanisms [47, 48], differentiation [49] and modulation of neurotrophin production [29].

Multiple proinflammatory properties of IL-6 have been characterized [45, 46]. For example, in transgenic mice with astrocyte-targeted IL-6 expression, complement activation was demonstrated in brain tissue [50]. In contrast, IL-6 has also anti-inflammatory properties. Recent data suggest that IL-6 and IL-6-regulated acute phase proteins are anti-inflammatory and immunosuppressive, and may negatively regulate the acute phase response [51]. IL-6 might contribute to the resolution of acute and chronic inflammatory processes by the direct suppression of interleukin-1 (IL-1) and tumor necrosis factor (TNF), the induction of glucocorticoid release and the induction of natural antagonists of IL-1 and TNF.

IL-6 exerts its biological activity after formation of the interleukin-6 receptor complex (IL-6RC). The IL-6 RC consists of IL-6, interleukin-6 receptor (IL-6R, gp80 or α-chain) and glycoprotein 130 (gp130 or β-chain).

The interleukin-6 receptor

The human interleukin-6 receptor (hIL-6R) could be detected in two different forms, a soluble (sIL-6R) and a membrane-bound form. IL-6R is expressed on lymphoid and non-lymphoid cells in accordance with the multifunctional properties of IL-6 [52]. The molecular weight of the membrane-bound and of the soluble form is 80 kDa and 55 kDa, respectively [24]. The sIL-6R is produced either by alternative splicing of IL-6R mRNA [53] or by shedding *via* limited proteolytic cleavage [54, 55]. It was demonstrated that genetically engineered sIL-6R and plasma sIL-6R retained their capability to bind IL-6 and that the formed IL-6/sIL-6R-complexes were able to activate the gp130 transducer chain [56, 57].

The mRNA which encodes the soluble form is expressed in leukocytes, in transformed B-cell lines and in myeloma cells [58]. In rat brain IL-6R mRNA expression could be colocalized with IL-6 mRNA expression at the cellular level (see IL-6 and expression). In the nervous system the IL-6R is expressed by neurons [59].

Molecular cloning of the human IL-6R gene demonstrated that the precursor protein consists of 468 amino acids with a signal peptide of 19 amino acids. The mature protein consists of 449 amino acids including an extracellular domain of 342 amino acids, a transmembrane domain of 28 amino acids and a cytoplasmic domain of 82 amino acids [60]. The short intracytoplasmic region can be deleted without affecting IL-6 signal transduction [61], which indicates that possibly other proteins are involved in signal transduction.

Physiological actions of the interleukin-6 receptor

Recent publications have reported that soluble forms of the IL-6R induce marked effects on IL-6. The soluble IL-6R retains its ligand binding capacity [56, 61] and in the presence of IL-6 can even associate with the soluble form of gp130 [62]. In contrast to most other soluble cytokine receptors, the sIL-6R together with IL-6 acts agonistically on cells that express gp130. By this mechanism the sIL-6R might render cells IL-6 responsive which themselves cannot bind IL-6 [63]. sIL-6R together with IL-6 can activate target cells that express only gp130 on their cell surface but lack membrane-bound IL-6R [64, 65]. SIL-6R enhances IL-6 effects by making the ligand accessible to the membrane-bound signal-transducing β-subunit gp130 [61], however, it has also been shown to augment the action of sgp130 [66], which neutralizes IL-6 signals [66-68]. In heart muscle cells it was shown that the cells only respond to IL-6 in the presence of sIL-6R [69].

The glycoprotein 130

Glycoprotein 130 (gp130) was detected and described as the signal-transducing partner of the IL-6 RC. It is the structural common element of all proteins belonging to the family of IL-6-type cytokines, including IL-6, CNTF, LIF, OSM, interleukin 11 (IL-11) and cardiotrophin-1 (CT-1) [56, 61]. All members of the IL-6 family commonly use gp130 for signaling.

Gp130 is a 130 kDa membrane-bound protein, which is ubiquitously expressed within the CNS. Molecular cloning experiments revealed that gp130 consists of 918 amino acids with a single transmembrane domain [61]. In the cytoplasmic domain of 277 amino acids a region of about 60 amino acids proximal to the transmembrane domain seems to be essential for signal transduction [70].

Gp130 exists in a 100 kDa soluble form (sgp130) in human serum [66].

Physiological actions of glycoprotein 130

Gp130 cannot bind IL-6 directly, but is crucial for signal transduction of the IL-6RC and even for generating a high-affinity binding site for IL-6 in IL-6R [61]. A stimulation of target cells with the IL-6/sIL-6R-complex or other cytokines of the IL-6-family triggers homo- or heterodimerization of gp130 and the tyrosine-specific phosphorylation of gp130 [56]. sgp130 is able to bind efficiently to the IL-6/sIL-6R-complex [64] and recombinant sgp130 inhibits the growth-inhibitory activity of the IL-6/sIL-6-R-complex on some melanoma cell lines [68]. sgp130 is also a potent IL-6 antagonist on various cell types and its antagonistic activity is markedly enhanced by sIL-6R [66]. In human serum sgp130 can associate in an sIL-6R-dependent manner with IL-6 [66–68].

Monoclonal antibodies directed against gp130 have been shown to inhibit IL-6-mediated functions. Some of the antibodies inhibit the IL-6-induced association of sgp130 and sIL-6R and other were shown to inhibit IL-6-mediated biological responses such as Ig production in a human B-cell line [71, 72].

The interleukin-6 receptor complex and its formation

The human interleukin-6 receptor complex (IL-6RC) consists of IL-6, IL-6R and the signal transducer unit gp130 (Fig. 1). For the functional activity of the IL-6RC it is not necessary to have a membrane-bound IL-6R as its cytoplasmic region is not involved in signal transduction [56, 20].

Currently two different models of the IL-6RC structure, responsible for signaling, exist. One group favors a hexameric model [24, 73–75], whereas another group discusses a tetrameric model [76]. Both models were generated by molecular mod-

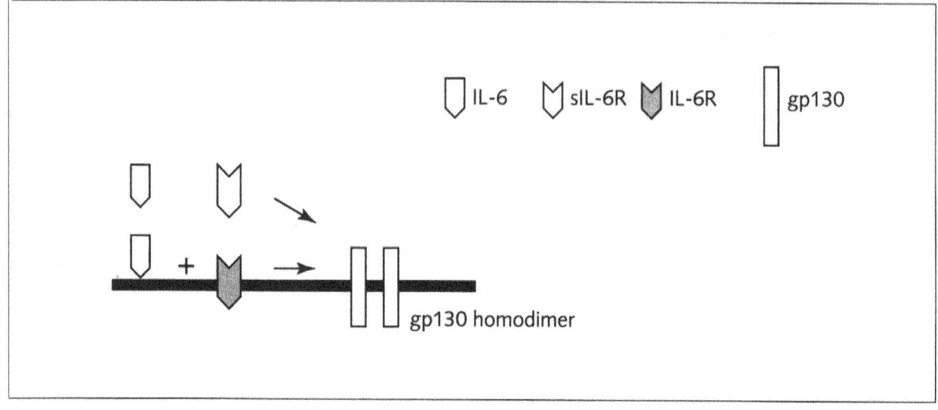

Figure 1
The interleukin-6 receptor complex (IL-6RC).

eling calculations of the protein structures for IL-6, IL-6R and gp130, deduced from existing structural information and by experimental data.

The general mechanism of the two models is that IL-6, like IL-11 or CNTF, binds to a specific α-subunit (IL-6R, IL-11R, CNTFR) which is not involved in the intracellular signal-transduction cascade. After ligand binding, the complex of cytokine and α-receptor, the IL-6/IL-6R heterodimer, is able to recruit the corresponding signal transducing receptor components, gp130. Moreover, the membrane-bound α-receptors can be functionally replaced by their soluble forms, which lack transmembrane and cytoplasmic regions [56, 77, 78].

The hexameric model for the IL-6 receptor complex

In assays with the soluble IL-6RC components (IL-6, sIL-6R and sgp130) a final structure of IL-6RC with the stoichiometry 2:2:2 (IL-6:sIL-6R:sgp130) could be detected, named hexameric complex [24, 73–75]. First, an IL-6/IL-6R heterodimer is formed, which reacts with gp130 to form a heterotrimer. Following this step different possible mechanisms are described. Somers and colleagues favor a reaction between two heterotrimers, forced by different interaction sites between the two heterotrimers forming the final hexameric complex [24], whereas Ward and colleagues favor a strong influence of IL-6 dimerization to combine the two heterotrimers [73, 79]. The resulting hexamer differs as well. Somers reports a IL-6 interaction, whereas Ward shows a direct gp130 interaction [79]. Finally, homodimerization of gp130 occurs and signal transduction is initiated after phosphorylation of gp130 and of bound JAK kinases (Figs. 2 and 3) [24, 73, 79].

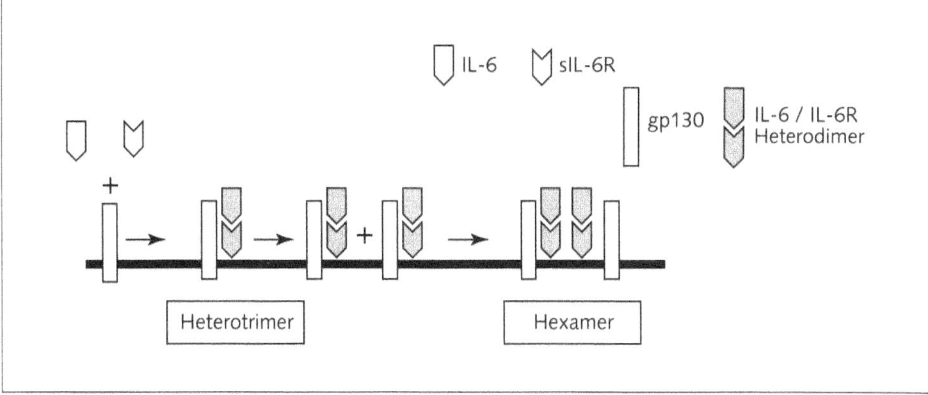

Figure 2
Hexameric model (modified after Somers [24]).

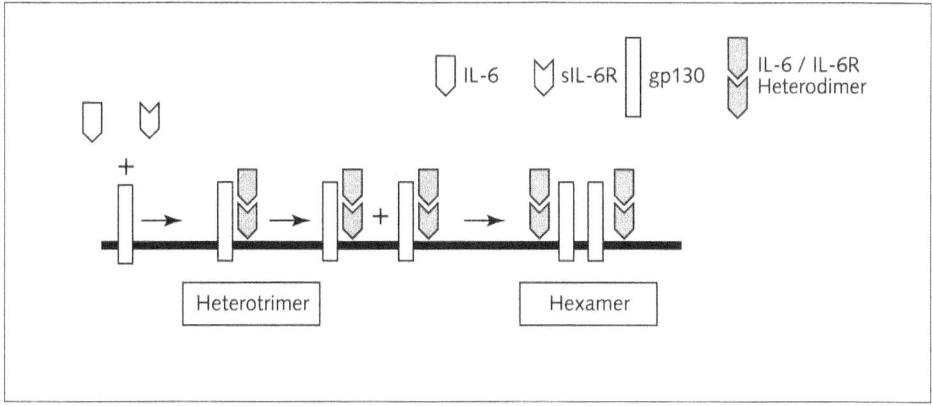

Figure 3
Hexameric model (modified after Ward [73, 79]).

The tetrameric model for the IL-6RC complex

Grötzinger and colleagues [76] predict that after forming the IL-6/IL-6R heterodimer and the reaction with gp130, only another gp130 has enough space to be associated with the heterotrimer. Their results are underlined by IL-6RC structure model calculations validated by published mutagenesis data [80-82]. Thus, the resulting stoichiometry for the signaling complex is 1:1:2 (IL-6:IL-6R:gp130). Solu-

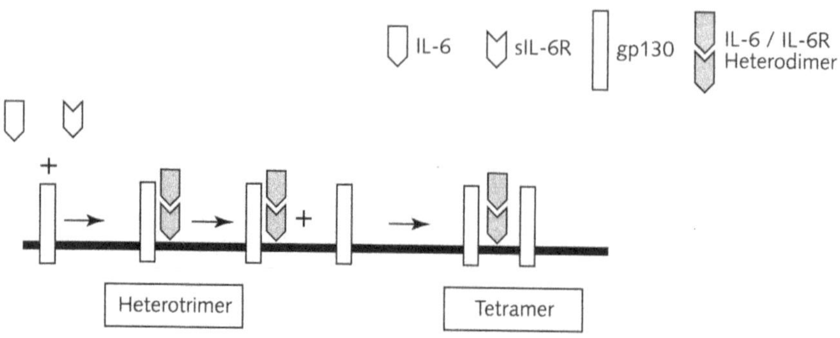

Figure 4
Tetrameric model (modified after Grötzinger [76]).

ble hexameric complexes possibly exist in solution but are not necessarily representative of the membrane situation. The hexameric structure is only formed at high protein concentrations and cannot transduce a signal (Fig. 4) [76].

Signal transduction

Studies on signal transduction mechanisms of interferons (IFNs) have shown that novel tyrosine kinases, Janus kinases (JAKs) and transcriptional factors, signal transducers and activators of transcription (STATs), play a major role in signal transduction triggered by receptors of various cytokines and hormones. It has also been shown that the JAK-STAT pathway is involved in signal transduction through gp130 [83, 84].

Normally, the cytoplasmic domain plays an important role in signal transduction for almost all receptors, but Taga and colleagues (1989) could show that the cytoplasmic domain of IL-6R is not required for signal transduction [56, 20].

Signal transduction is initiated by activation of different members of a family of cytoplasmic tyrosine kinases, known as the JAK/TYK kinases, which are associated with the cytoplasmic domain of gp130 in an inactive state. They are activated following homo- or heterodimerization of gp130 through phosphorylation of gp130 (Fig. 5) [85].

At least three JAK/TYK kinases (JAK1, JAK2 and TYK2) are activated by these cytokines, but distinct patterns of activation occur in different cell lines [87–90]. This is significant since it might give us the initial clue as to the mechanisms by

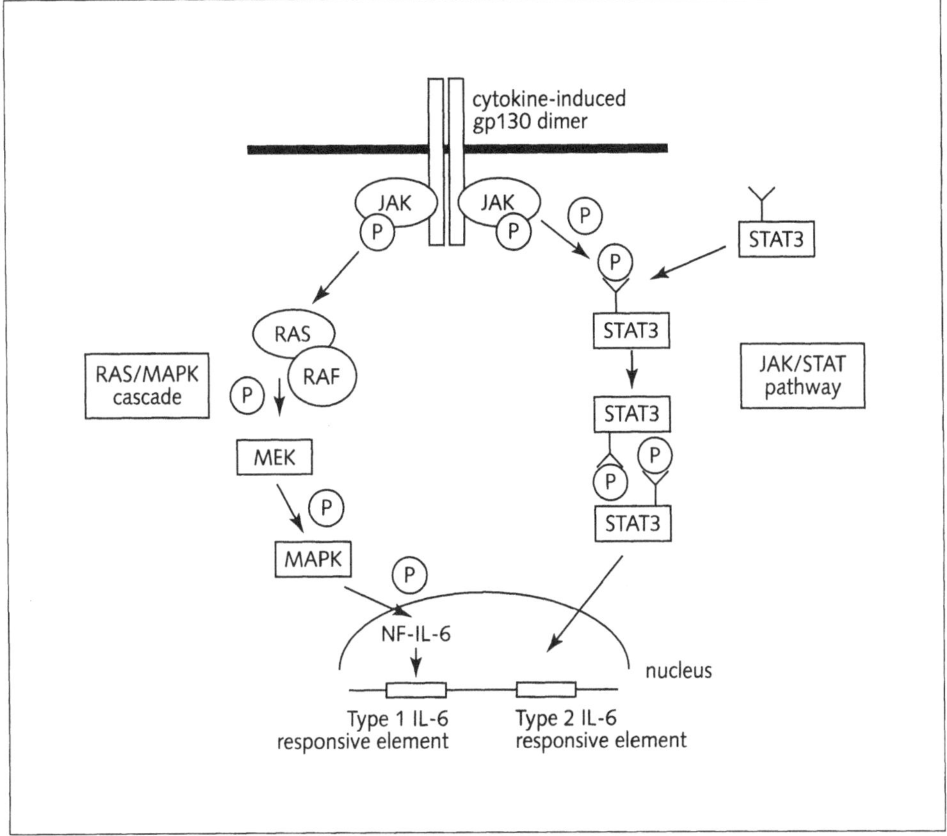

Figure 5
Signal transduction pathways.

which different cell types respond in different ways to one single factor. The JAK/TYK kinases, in turn, activate a variety of intracellular signaling molecules, such as members of the STAT family, a group of DNA-binding transcriptional activators. [91]. Six major STATs (STAT1 to STAT6) are identified and strict specificity is often observed between cytokine stimulation and gp130-mediated STAT activation. For cytokines utilizing gp130 receptor complexes, STAT3 is the most potently activated [92, 93]. STATS also become phosphorylated, form dimers and translocate to the nucleus where they regulate transcription of target genes.

Another signaling pathway which might be used is the RAS-dependent MAPK (mitogen-activated protein kinase) cascade, a pathway that is highly conserved in evolution and plays central roles in signal transduction in all eukaryotic cells. RAS is a small GTP-binding protein, which activates RAF kinase, thus phosphorylating MAPK *via* the MEK kinase. The RAS/MAPK signaling pathway is activated after stimulation of gp130 through many different kinases. The precise mechanism and which parts of gp130 are required for the activation are still unknown. Downstream of gp130, nuclear factor interleukin-6 (NF-IL-6) is phosphorylated by MAP kinases and thus transcriptionally activated. This transcription factor binds to the promotor region of the acute phase protein genes. Two types of IL-6-responsive elements exist in the promotor region, type 1 and type 2. NF-IL-6 recognizes type 1 and STAT3 binds to type 2 [86, 94, 95].

The interleukin-6 receptor complex in the CNS

Different methodological approaches have been made to gain insight into the significance of the IL-6 complex in the CNS. Information can be generated by investigating human material, such as measurements of body fluids, analysis of post-mortem brain sections or by using model systems, such as cell culture supernatants or transgenic mice.

A role for IL-6 in the pathology of neurological disorders, such as acquired immunodeficiency syndrome (AIDS) dementia [96], virus encephalopathy [96, 97], Alzheimer's disease [98, 99], multiple sclerosis [100], CNS trauma [101] and viral [102] and bacterial meningitis [103] has been hypothesized by several authors. This hypothesis is further supported by studies with transgenic mice where over-expression of IL-6 results in significant neuroanatomical and neurophysiological alterations of the CNS, similar to those observed in patients suffering from various neurological diseases [104, 105]. In IL-6-deficient mice, a resistance to a demyelinating type of experimental autoimmune encephalomyelitis (EAE), which is regarded as an animal model of multiple sclerosis (MS), was reported [106]. This resistance is not found in normal control mice and was overruled by exogeneous IL-6 administration in IL-6-deficient mice [107].

Studies of IL-6 CSF levels in various neuropathological diseases revealed altered IL-6 concentrations in the CSF of patients with HIV infection [97], systemic lupus erythematosus [108], MS [109, 110], schizophrenia [111], major depression (MD) [112] and Alzheimer's disease [98, 113, 114].

At present, few data regarding other components of the sIL-6RC, e.g. sIL-6R and sgp130, in neuropathological conditions are available. Statistically significant decreased CSF concentrations of the IL-6 and sIL-6R of MD patients compared to age-matched controls were found, whereas sgp130 showed no significant difference between patients and controls [112]. sIL-6R and sgp130 levels are significantly increased in serum of MS patients and correlate with disease severity, while IL-6 concentrations are unchanged. In CSF sgp130-levels were decreased in MS, indicating an altered IL-6 regulation in the CSF [110].

The question as to how CSF-levels of the sIL-6RC mirror neuroregulatory, neurodegenerative or inflammatory processes within the CNS cannot be answered at the present time [115]. This difficulty is due to the complex regulation of IL-6 actions by its soluble receptors and of the pleiotropic function of IL-6 itself. Moreover, the cellular source of CSF proteins and the mechanisms which influence the CSF-levels of specific proteins have to be an issue of future studies.

The interleukin-6 receptor complex in Alzheimer's disease

IL-6 has been reported to play a role in the pathogenesis of Alzheimer's disease (AD) [98, 116–118], however, the significance and mechanisms of IL-6 action in the CNS of both healthy-aging and AD patients are not yet fully understood. A putative correlation between neuropathological hallmarks of AD, such as amyloid plaques, has been hypothesized as important since IL-6, along with IL-1, seems to modulate amyloid precursor protein synthesis *via* augmented synthesis of α1-antichymotrypsin and amyloid precursor protein [99]. An enhancement of beta-amyloid precursor protein transcription and expression by the IL-6/sIL-6R-complex was reported *in vitro* [119]. In contrast, elevated IL-6 mRNA levels were shown in cultured rat cortical glial cells after stimulation with the carboxy-terminal 105 amino acids of the amyloid precursor protein [120]. Transgenic mice, chronically expressing IL-6 in astrocytes, exhibited dose- and age-related deficits in learning which closely corresponded to specific neuropathological changes [105].

Further evidence for a role of IL-6 in the pathophysiology of AD is derived from immunohistochemical studies of AD brain tissue. IL-6 has been consistently detected in the frontal-, parietal- and occipital-cortex and hippocampus of AD patients but not of non-demented elderly subjects [98, 121]. More recently, IL-6 expression has been demonstrated for diffuse early plaques without neuritic pathology in neocortical (frontal- temporal- and parietal-cortex) and hippocampal brain samples of AD patients. IL-6 immunoreactivity was rare in classical plaques and absent in compact or burned-out plaques [116, 122]. Therefore, it has been suggested that IL-6 may appear before neuritic changes rather than following neuritic degeneration. The IL-6 positive plaques also showed increased levels of α2-macroglobulin (α2-M), an acute-phase protein [123].

These observations add to previous findings indicating an inflammatory pathology of AD [118]. However, the actions of IL-6 are influenced by its receptors (IL-6R and gp130) in a complex manner. The question as to how the IL-6RC is involved is being investigated by various groups.

In a study launched to investigate the expression of all members of the IL-6RC in human brain tissue, IL-6, IL-6R and gp130 could be individually detected in astroglia across investigated rapid-brain autopsy brain samples of AD patients and controls of frontal-, temporal-, parietal- and occipital-cortex. In addition, gp130 and IL-6 expression could be shown in neurons across all investigated AD-patients and healthy subjects [124].

In brain homogenate supernatants of AD patients and healthy controls, elevated IL-6 levels were reported in temporal cortex of AD patients in combination with increased levels of α2-M and C reactive protein [117].

In AD tissue homogenate supernatants from hippocampus and area 22, expression of the sIL-6RC (IL-6, sIL-6R, sgp130) could be shown. In the corresponding pellets the membrane-bound IL-6RC (IL-6R, gp130) was detectable. Expression of the membrane-bound IL-6R and gp130 did not significantly differ in area 22 and hippocampus of AD-patients [125]. These results are in line with the elevated IL-6 mRNA expression results, described in hippocampus and area 22 AD brain tissue homogenates in comparison to non-AD cases [126].

sIL-6RC has also be investigated in serum and CSF. Only one study has addressed serum levels of AD patients. IL-6-levels were unchanged, but sIL-6R-levels from AD patients were significantly decreased compared to healthy control subjects [127]. In AD-CSF, März and colleagues (1997) found no alteration in sIL-6RC (IL-6, sIL-6R and sgp130) concentrations compared with medicated patients with major depression [128]. Hampel and colleagues reported statistically significant decreased sIL-6RC CSF concentrations in the presence of unchanged IL-6 levels in patients with AD compared to healthy age-matched control subjects [114, 129, 130]. Furthermore, it has been shown that the application of a multivariate discriminant analysis, using combined CSF τ protein and sIL-6RC components, may add more certainty to the clinical diagnosis of AD (sensitivity and specificity > 90%) [130]. The reported method, however, is still preliminary and will need to be extended to an independent group of patients, comparisons and control subjects to assess the true applicability.

In conclusion, there is increasing evidence that IL-6 and its receptors are involved in the pathophysiology of AD. How and to what extend the IL-6RC contributes to the pathophysiological processes in AD is a focus of current research.

Conclusion

Basic studies show that IL-6 exerts its biological actions only by complex interactions with specific soluble or membrane bound receptors [49, 56, 61, 131, 132], forming the biologically active IL-6 receptor complex (IL-6RC). The involved proteins, in addition to IL-6, are two membrane glycoproteins, a protein referred to as the ligand-binding α-subunit (IL-6R, gp80 or CD126) and a protein referred to as the non-ligand binding, affinity converting and signal transducing β-receptor (gp130 or CD130) [61, 133].

All members of the IL-6 cytokine family (IL-6, IL-11, oncostatin M (OSM), leukemia inhibitory factor (LIF), ciliary neurotrophic factor (CNTF), and cardiotrophin-1 (CT-1)) share gp130 as a component critical for signal transduction [61, 94, 119, 134–136].

In the nervous system IL-6 can be secreted by microglia, astroglia, neurons and endothelial cells [29, 31], IL-6R by neurons [59, 119, 137] and gp130 by all cell types [61, 138]. gp130 neuropil immunoreactivity was observed in telencephalic structures including the hippocampus, cerebral cortex and caudate-putamen [138]. Activation of membrane-bound gp130 by IL-6 and the soluble IL-6R was reported to generate a neuronal differentiation signal [139].

Soluble forms of the two receptors (sIL-6R, sgp130) arise by limited proteolysis (shedding) [140] or differential splicing [58, 54, 62, 119, 141] and it has been reported that the complex formed by soluble components (sIL-6RC) has a hexameric structure, consisting of the three different proteins with a 2:2:2 stoichiometry [24, 73, 74, 79, 141].

There is a complex regulatory interaction between all sIL-6RC components. SIL-6R enhances IL-6 effects by making the ligand accessible to the membrane-bound signal-transducing β-subunit [61], however, it has also been shown to augment the action of sgp130 [66], which neutralizes IL-6 signals [66–68].

Evidence derived from clinical and basic research suggests that IL-6 plays an important role in the pathology of neurodegenerative disorders, such as AD, and an enlargement of the research field to encompass its two receptors seems to be more than necessary in order to understand IL-6 interactions.

Optimized genetic mouse models, comprising transgenic and knockout animals, should help to further specify the physiological and pathophysiological role of IL-6 in the nervous system. Further elucidation of the specific function of the functionally-interacting IL-6 receptor system, the development of selective IL-6 agonists and antagonists, as well as the usage of soluble IL-6 receptors offers fascinating new therapeutic opportunities for neurodegenerative disorders.

References

1 Kishimoto T, Akira S, Taga T (1992) Interleukin-6 and its receptor: a paradigm for cytokines. *Science* 258: 593–597

2 Weissenbach J, Chernajovsky Y, Zeevi M, Shulman L, Soreq H, Nir U, Wallach D, Perricaudet M, Tiolleis P, Revel M (1980) Two interferon mRNAs in human fibroblasts: *in vitro* translation and *Escherichia coli* cloning studies. *Proc Natl Acad Sci USA* 77: 7152–7156

3 Van Damme J, Opdenakker G, Simpson RJ, Rubira MR, Cayphas S, Vink A, Billiau A, Van Snick J (1987) Identification of the human 26-kD protein, interferon beta 2 (IFN-beta 2), as a B cell hybridoma/plasmacytoma growth factor induced by interleukin 1 and tumor necrosis factor. *J Exp Med* 165: 914–919

4 Yasukawa K, Hirano T, Wanatabe Y, Muratani K, Matsuda T, Nakai S, Kishimoto T (1987) Structure and expression of human B cell stimulary factor 2 (BSF-2/IL-6) gene. *EMBO J* 6(10): 2939–2945

5 Zilberstein A, Ruggieri R, Horn JH, Revel M (1986) Structure and expression of cDNA and genes for human interferon-beta-2, a distinct species inducible by growth-stimulatory cytokines. *EMBO J* 5: 2529–2537
6 Hirano T, Taga T, Nakano N, Yasukawa K, Kashiwamura S, Shimizu K, Nakajima K, Pyun KH, Kishimoto T (1985) Purification to homogeneity and characterization of human B-cell differentiation factor (BCDF or BSFp2). *Proc Natl Acad Sci USA* 82(16): 5490–5494
7 Hirano T, Yasukawa K, Harda H, Taga T, Wanatabe Y, Matsuda T, Kashiwamura SI, Nakajima K, Koyama K, Iwamatsu A et al (1986) Complementary DNA for a novel human interleukin (BSF-2) that induces B lymphocytes to produce immunoglobulin. *Nature* 324 (6092): 73–76
8 Van Snick J, Cayphas S, Vink A, Uyttenhove C, Coulie PG, Rubira MR, Simpson RJ (1986) Purification and NH2-terminal amino acid sequence of a T-cell derived lymphokine with growth factor activity for B cell hybridomas. *Proc Natl Acad Sci USA* 83: 9679–9683
9 Nordan RP, Pumphrey JG, Rudikoff S (1987) Purification and NH2-terminal sequence of a plasmacytoma growth factor derived from the murine macrophage cell line P388D1. *J Immunol* 139: 813–817
10 Gauldie J, Richards C, Harnish D, Lansdorp P, Bauman H (1987) Interferon beta 2/B-cell stimulatory factor type 2 shares identity with monocyte-derived hepatocyte-stimulating factor and regulates the major acute phase protein response in liver cells. *Proc Natl Acad Sci USA* 84: 7251–7255
11 Teranishi T, Hirano T, Arima N, Onoue K (1982) Hhuman helper T cell factor(s) (ThF). II. Induction of IgG production in B lymphoblastoid cell lines and identification of T cell-replacing factor- (TRF) like factor(s). *J Immunol* 128(4): 1903–1908
12 Content J, De Wit L, Pierard D, Derynck R, De Clercq E, Fiers W (1982) Secretory proteins induced in human fibroblasts under conditions used for the production of interferon beta. *Proc Natl Acad Sci USA* 79: 2768–2772
13 Haegeman G, Content J, Volckaert G, Derynck R, Tavernier J, Fiers W (1986) Structural analysis of the sequence coding for an inducible 26kDa protein in human fibroblasts. Eur J Biochem 159(3): 625–632
14 Sehgal PB, Zilberstein A, Ruggieri RM, May LT, Ferguson-Smith A, Slate DL, Revel M, Ruddle FH (1986) Human chromosome 7 carries the beta-2interferone gene. *Proc Natl Acad Sci USA* 83: 5216–5222
15 Tanabe O, Akira S, Kamiya T, Wong G, Hirano T, Kishimoto T (1988) Genomic structure of the Murine IL-6 gene. High degree conservation of potential regulatory sequences between mouse and human. *J Immunol* 141(11): 3875–3881
16 Brakenhoff JP, Hart M, Aarden LA (1989) Analysis of human IL-6 mutants expressed in *Escherichia coli*. Biologic activities are not affected by deletion of amino acids 1–28. *J Immunol* 143(4): 1175–1182
17 Arcone R, Pucci P, Zappacosta F, Fontaine V, Malorni A, Marino G, Ciliberto G (1991) Single-step purification and structural characterization of human interleukin-6 produced

in *Escherichia coli* from a T7 RNA polymerase expression vector. *Eur J Biochem* 198: 541–547
18 Krüttgen A, Rose-John S, Möller C, Wroblowski B, Wollmer A, Müllberg J, Hirano T, Kishimoto T, Heinrich PC (1990) The three carboxy-terminal amino acids of human interleukin-6 are essential for its biological activity. *FEBS Lett* 273: 95–98
19 Leebeck FW, Kariya K, Schwabe M, Fowlkes DM (1992) Identification of a receptor binding site in the carboxyl terminus of human interleukin-6. *J Biol Chem* 267: 14832–14838
20 Fiorillo MT, Toniatti C, van Snick J, Ciliberto G (1992) Analysis of human/mouse interleukin-6-hybrid proteins: both amino and carboxy termini of human interleukin-6 are required for *in vitro* receptor binding. *Eur J Immunol* 22: 2609–2615
21 Hammacher A, Ward LD, Weinstock J, Treutlein H, Yasukawa K, Simpson RJ (1994) Structure-function analysis of human Il-6: identification of two distinct regions that are important for receptor binding. *Protein Sci* 3(12): 2280–2293
22 May LT, Santhanam U, Tatter SB, Bhardwaj N, Ghrayeb J, Seghal PB (1988) Phosphorylation of secreted forms of human β2-interferon/hepatocyte stimulating factor/interleukin-6. *Biochem Biophys Res Commun* 152: 1144–1150
23 May LT, Shaw JE, Khanna AK, Zabriskie JB, Sehgal PB (1991) Marked cell-type-specific differences in glycosylation of human interleukin-6. Cytokine 3: 204–211
24 Somers W, Stahl M, Seehra JS (1997) 1.9 Å crystal structure of interleukin 6: implications for a novel mode of receptor dimerization and signaling. *EMBO J* 16: 989–997
25 Bazan JF (1990) Haemopoietic receptors and helical cytokines. *Immunology Today* 11: 350–354
26 Bazan JF (1991) Neuropoietic cytokines in the hematopoietic fold. *Neuron* 7: 197–208
27 Xu G-Y, Yu H-A, Stahl M, McDonagh T, Kay LE, Cumming DA (1997) Solution structure of recombinant human interleukin-6. *J Mol Biol* 368: 468–481
28 Hirano T, Shizuo A, Taga T, Kishimoto T (1990) Biological and clinical aspects of interleukin 6. *Immunology Today* 11: 443–449
29 Frei K, Malipiero UV, Leist TP, Zinkernagel RM, Schwab ME, Fontana A (1989) On the cellular source and function of interleukin-6 produced in the central nervous system in viral diseases. *Eur J Immunol* 19: 689–694
30 Fabry Z, Fitzsimmons KM, Herlein JA, Moninger TO, Dobbs BM, Hart MN (1993) Production of the cytokines interleukin 1 and 6 by murine brain microvessel endothelium and smooth muscle pericytes. *J Neuroimmunol* 47: 23–34
31 März P, Cheng JG, Gadient RA, Patterson PH, Stoyan T, Otten U, Rose-John S (1998) Sympathetic neurons can produce and respond to interleukin-6. *Proc Natl Acad Sci USA* 95(6): 3251–3256
32 Vankelecom H, Carmeliet P, Van Damme J, Billau A Denef C (1989) Production of interleukin-6 by folliculo-stellate cells of the anterior pituitary gland in a histotypic cell aggregate culture system. *Neuroendocrinol* 49: 102–106
33 Spangelo BL, MacLeod RM, Isakson PC (1990) Production of interleukin-6 by anterior pituitary cells *in vitro*. *Endocrinology* 126: 582–586

34 Spangelo BL, Judd AM, MacLeod RM, Goodman DW, Isakson PC (1990) Endotoxin-induced release of interleukin-6 from rat medial basal hypothalami. *Endocrinology* 127: 1779–1783

35 Yamaguchi M, Yoshimoto Y, Komura H, Koike K, Matsuzaki N, Hirota K, Miyake A, Tanizawa O (1990) Interleukin 1 beta and tumor necrosis factor alpha stimulate the release of gonadotroin-releasing hormone and interleukin 6 by primary cultured rat hypothalamic cells. *Acta Endocrinol* 123: 476–480

36 Yamabe T, Dhir G, Cowan EP, Wolf AL, Bergey GK, Krumholz A, Barry E, Hoffmann PM, Dhib-Jalbut S (1994) cytokine-gene expression in measles-infected adult human glial cells. *J Neuroimmunol* 49: 171–179

37 Gadient RA, Otten U (1994) Identification of interleukin-6 (IL-6)-expressing neurons in the cerebellum and hippocampus of normal adult rats. *Neurosci Lett* 182: 243–246

38 Gadient RA, Otten U (1995) Interleukin-6 and interleukin-6 receptor mRNA expression in rat central nervous system. *Ann NY Acad Sci* 762: 403–406

39 Schöbitz B, Voorhuis DAM, De Kloet ER (1992) Localization of interleukin-6 mRNA and interleukin-6 recpetor mRNA in rat brain. *Neurosci Lett* 136: 189–192

40 Schöbitz B, De Kloet ER, Sutano W, Holsboer F (1993) Cellular localization of interleukin-6 mRNA and interleukin-6 receptor mRNA in rat brain. *Eur J Neurosci* 5: 1426–1435

41 Schaper F, Gendo C, Eck M, Schmitz J, Grimm C, Anhuf D, Kerr IM, Heinrich PC (1998) Activation of the protein tyrosine phosphatase SHP2 *via* the interleukin-6 signal transducing receptor protein gp130 requires tyrosine kinase Jak1 and limits acute-phase protein expression. *Biochem J* 335 (Pt 3): 557–565

42 Sehgal PB, Walther Z, Tamm I (1987) rapid enhancement of beta 2-interferon/B-cell differentiation factor BSF-2 gene expression in human fibroblasts by diacylglycerols and the calcium ionophore A23187. *Proc Natl Acad Sci USA* 84: 3663–3667

43 Zhang Y, Lin J-X, Vilcek J (1988) Synthesis of interleukin 6 (Interferon beta 2/B cell stimulatory factor 2) in human fibroblasts is triggered by an in crease in intracellular cyclic AMP. *J Biol Chem* 263: 6177–6182

44 Heinrich PC, Castell J, Andus T (1990) Interleukin-6 and the acute phase response. *Biochem J* 265: 621–636

45 Akira S, Taga T, Kishimoto T (1993) Interleukin-6 in biology and medicine. *Adv Immunol* 54: 1–78

46 Van Snick J (1990) Interleukin-6: an overview. *Annu Rev Immuno* 8: 253–278

47 Hama T, Miyamoto M, Tsukui H, Nishio C, Hatanaka H (1989) Interleukin-6 as a neurotrophic factor for promoting the survival of cultured basal forebrain cholinergic neurons from postnatal rats. *Neurosci Lett* 104: 340–344

48 Hama T, Kushima Y, Miyamoto M, Kubota M, Takei N, Hatanaka H (1991) Interleukin-6 improves the survival of mesencephalic catecholaminergic and septal cholinergic neurons from postnatal, two-week-old rats in cultures. *Neuroscience* 40: 445–452

49 Satoh T, Nakamura S, Taga T, Matsuda T, Hirano T, Kishimoto T, Kaziro Y (1988)

Induction of neuronal differentiation in PC12 cells by B-cell stimulatory factor 2/interleukin 6. *Mol Cell Biol* 8 (8): 3546–3549
50 Barnum SR, Jones JL, Muller-Ladner U, Samimi A, Campbell IL (1996) Chronic complement C3 gene expression in the CNS of transgenic mice with astrocyte-targeted interleukin-6 expression. *Glia* 18 (2): 107–117
51 Tilg H, Dinarello CA, Mier JW (1997) IL-6 and APPs: anti-inflammatory and immunosuppressive mediators. *Immunology Today* 18: 428–432
52 Taga T, Kawanishi Y, Hardy R, Hirano T, Kishimoto T (1987) Receptors for B cell stimulatory factor 2. Quantitation, specificity, distribution, and regulation of their expression. *J Exp Med* 166 (4): 967–981
53 Horiuchi S, Koyanagi Y, Zhou Y, Miyamoto H, Tanaka Y, Waki M, Matsumoto A, Yamamoto M, Yamamoto N (1994) Soluble interlukin-6 receptors released from T cell or granylocyte/macrophage cell lines and human peripheral blood mononuclear cells are generated through an alternative spicing mechanism. *Eur J Immunol* 24 (8): 1945–1948
54 Müllberg J, Schoolinkt H, Stoyan T, Heinrich PC, Rose-John S (1992) Protein kinase C activity is rate limiting for shedding of the interleukin-6 receptor. *Biochem Biophys Res Commun* 189: 794–800
55 Ehlers MRW, Riordan JF (1991) Membrane proteins with soluble counterparts: role of proteolysis in the release of transmembrane proteins. *Biochemistry* 30: 10065–10074
56 Taga T, Hibi M, Hirata Y, Yamasaki KY, Yasukawa K, Matsuda T, Hirano T, Kishimoto T (1989) Interleukin-6 triggers the association of its receptor with a possible signal transducer, gp130. *Cell* 58 (3): 573–581
57 Gaillard JP, Bataille R, Brailly H, Zuber C, Yasukawa K, Attal M, Maruo N, Taga T, Kishimoto T, Klein B (1993) Increased and highly stable levels of functional soluble interleukin-6 receptor in sera of patients with monoclonal gammopathy. *Eur J Immunol* 23: 820–824
58 Lust JA, Donovan KA, Kline MP, Greipp PR, Kyle RA, Maihle NJ (1992) Isolation of an mRNA encoding a soluble form of the human interleukin-6 receptor. *Cytokine* 4: 96–100
59 März P, Gadient RA, Otten U (1996) Expression of interleukin-6 receptor (IL-6R) and gp130 mRNA in PC12 cells and sympathetic neurons: modulation by tumor necrosis factor alpha (TNF-alpha). *Brain Res* 706 (1): 71–79
60 Yamasaki K, Taga T, Hirata Y, Yawata H, Kawanishi Y, Seed B, Taniguchi T, Hirano T, Kishimoto T (1988) Cloning and expression of the human Interleukin-6 (BSF-2/IFNb2) Receptor. *Science* 241: 825–828
61 Hibi M, Murakami M, Saito M, Hirano T, Taga T, Kishimoto T (1990) Molecular cloning and Expression of an IL-6 Signal Transducer, gp130. *Cell* 63: 1149–1157
62 Müllberg J, Dittrich E, Graeve L, Gerhartz L, Yasukawa K, Taga T, Kishimoto T, Heinrich PC, Rose-John S (1993) Differential shedding of the two subunits of the interleukin-6 receptor. *FEBS Lett* 332(1-2): 174–178
63 Müllberg J, Oberthür W, Lottspeich F, Mehl E, Dittrich E, Graeve L, Heinrich PC, Rose-

John S (1994) The soluble human IL-6 receptor, Multinational characterization of the proteolytic cleavage site. *J Immunol* 152: 4958–4968

64 Rose-John S, Heinrich PC (1994) Soluble receptors for cytokines and growth factors: generation and biological functions. *Biochem J* 300: 281–290

65 Mackiewicz A, Wiznierowicz M, Roeb E, Karczewska A, Nowak J, Heinrich PC, Rose-John S (1995) Soluble interleukin-6 receptor is biologically active *in vivo*. *Cytokine* 7: 142–149

66 Müller-Newen G, Küster A, Hemmann U, Keul R, Horsten U, Martens A, Graeve L, Wijdenes J, Heinrich PC (1998) Soluble IL-6 receptor potentates the antagonistic activity of soluble gp130 on IL-6 responses. *J Immunol* 161(11): 6347–6355

67 Narazaki M, Yasukawa K, Saito T, Ohsugi Y, Fukui H, Koishihara Y, Yancopulos GD, Taga T, Kishimoto T (1993) Soluble forms of the Interleukin-6 signal transducing receptor component gp130 in human serum possessing a potential to inhibit signals through membrane-anchored gp130. *Blood* 82: 1120–1126

68 Montero-Julian FA, Brailly H, Sautes C, Joyeux I, Dorval T, Mosseri V, Yasukawa K, Wijdenes J, Adler A, Gorin I et al (1997) Characterization of soluble gp130 released by melanoma cell lines: a polyvalent antagonist of cytokines from the interleukin-6 family. *Clin Canc Res* 3 (8): 1443–1451

69 Hirota H, Yoshida K, Kishimoto T, Taga T (1995) Continuos activation of gp130, a signal-transducing receptor component for interleukin 6-related cytokines, causes myocardial hypertophy in mice. *Proc Natl Acad Sci USA* 92 (11): 4862–4866

70 Murakami M, Narazaki M, Hibi M, Yawata H, Yasukawa K, Hamaguchi M, Taga T, Kishimoto T (1991) Critical cytoplasmic region of the interleukin 6 signal transducer gp130 is conserved in the cytokine receptor family. *Proc Natl Acad Sci USA* 88 (24): 11349–11353

71 Taga T, Narazaki M, Yasukawa K, Saito T, Miki D, Hamaguchi M Davis S, Shoyab M, Yancopoulos GD, Kishimoto T (1992) Functional inhibition of hematopoietic and neurotrophic cytokines by blocking the interleukin 6 signal transducer gp130. *Proc Natl Acad Sci USA* 89 (22): 10998–11001

72 Saito T, Taga T, Miki D, Futatsugi K, Yawata H, Kishimoto T, Yasukawa K (1993) Preparation of monoclonal antibodies against the IL-6 signal transducer, gp130, that can inhibit IL-6-mediated functions. *J Immunol* Methods 163 (2): 217–223

73 Ward LD, Howlett GJ, Disciolo G, Yasukawa K, Hammacher A, Moritz RL, Simpson R (1994) High affinity interleukin-6 receptor is a hexameric complex consisting of two molecules each of interleukin-6, interleukin-6 receptor and gp130. *J Biol Chem* 269: 23286–23289

74 Paonessa G, Graziani R, DeSerio A, Savino R, Ciapponi L, Lahm A, Salvati AL, Toniatti C, Ciliberto G (1995) Two distinct and independent sites on IL-6 trigger gp130 dimer formation and signalling. *EMBO J* 14: 1942–1951

75 DeSerio A, Graziani R, Laufer R, Ciliberto G, Paonessa G (1995) *In vitro* binding of ciliary neurotrophic factor to its receptors: Evidence for the formation of an IL-6type hexameric complex. *J Mol Biol* 254: 795–800

76 Grötzinger J, Kurapkat G, Wollmer A, Kalai M, Rose-John S (1997) The family of the IL-6-Type cytokines: specificity and promiscuity of the receptor complexes. *Proteins* 27: 96–109
77 Mackiewicz A, Rose-John S, Schooltink H, Laciak M, Gorny A, Heinrich PC (1992) Soluble human interleukin-6 receptor modulates interleukin-6-dependent N-glycosylation of alpha 1-protease inhibitor secreted by HepG2 cells. *FEBS Lett* 306: 257–261
78 Karow J, Hudson KR, Hall MA, Vernallis AB, Taylor JA, Gossler A, Heath JK (1996) Mediation of interleukin-11-dependent biological responses by a soluble form of the interleukin-11 receptor. *Biochem J* 318 (Pt2): 489–495
79 Ward LD, Hammacher A, Howlett GJ, Matthews JM, Fabri L, Moritz RL, Nice EC, Weinstock J, Simpson RJ (1996) Influence of Interleukin-6 (IL-6) Dimerization on formation of the high affinity hexameric IL-6 Receptor Complex. *J Biol Chem* 271(33): 20138–20144
80 Yawata H, Yasukawa K, Natsuka S, Murakami M, Yamasaki K, Hibi M, Taga T, Kishimoto T (1993) Structure-function analysis of human IL-6 receptor: Dissociation of amino acid residues required for IL-6 binding and for IL-6 signal transduction through gp130. *EMBO J* 12:1705–1712
81 Ehlers M, Grötzinger J, de Hon FD, Müllberg J, Brakenhoff JPJ, Liu JW, Wollmer A, Rose-John S (1994) Identification of two novel regions of hIL-6 responsible for receptor binding and signal transduction. *J Immunol* 153: 1744–1753
82 Ehlers M, de Hon FD, Bos KH, Horsten U, Kurapkat G, Schmitz van De Leurs H, Grötzinger J, Wollmer A, Brakenhoff JPJ, Rose-John S (1995) Combining two mutations of human interleukin-6 that affect gp130 activation results in a potent interleukin-6 receptor antagonist on human myeloma cells. *J Biol Chem* 270: 8158–8163
83 Ihle JN, Witthuhn BA, Quelle FW, Yamamoto K, Thierfelder WE, Kreider B, Silvennoinen O (1994) Signaling by the cytokine receptor superfamily: JAKs and STATs. *Trends Biochem Sci* 19: 222–227
84 Darnell JE Jr., Kerr IM, Stark GM (1994) Jak-STAT pathways and transcriptional activation in response to IFNs and other extracellular signaling proteins. *Science* 264: 1415–1421
85 Murakami M, Hibi M, Nakagawa N, Nakagawa T, Yasukawa K, Yamanishi K, Taga T, Kishimoto T (1993) IL-6 induced Homodimerization of gp130 and associated activation of a Tyrosine kinase. *Science* 260: 1808–1810
86 Taga T, Kishimoto T (1997) gp130 and the interleukin-6 family of cytokines. *Annu Rev Immunol* 15: 797–819
87 Lütticken C, Wegenka UM, Yuan J, Buschmann J, Schindler C, Ziemiecki A, Harpur AG, Wilks AF, Yasukawa K, Taga Tet al (1994) Association of transcription factor APRF and protein kinase JAK1 with the interleukin-6 signal transducer gp130. *Science* 263: 89–92
88 Stahl N, Boulton TG, Farruggella T, Ip NY, Davis S, Witthuhn BA, Quelle FW, Silvennoinen O, Barbieri G, Pellegrini S et al (1994) Association and activation of Jak-Tyk kinases by CNTF-LIF-OSM-IL-6 beta receptor components. *Science* 263: 92–95

89 Stahl N, Farruggella TJ, Boulton TG, Zhong Z, Darnell JE, Yancopoulos GD (1995) Choice of STATs and other substrates specified by modular tyrosine-based motifs in cytokine receptors. *Science* 267: 1349–1353
90 Narazaki M, Witthuhn BA, Yoshida K, Silvennoinen O, Yasukawa K, Ihle JN, Kishimoto T, Taga T (1994) Activation of JAK2 kinase mediated by the interleukin 6 signal transducer gp130. *Proc Natl Acad Sci USA* 91 (6): 2285–2289
91 Segal RA, Greenberg ME (1996) Intracellular signaling pathways activated by neurotrophic factors. *Ann Rev Neurosci* 19: 463–489
92 Akira S, Nishio Y, Inoue M, Wang XJ, Wei S, Matsusaka T, Yoshida K, Sudo T, Naruto M, Kishimoto T (1994) Molecular cloning of APRF, a novel IFN-stimulated gene factor 3 p91-related transcription factor involved in the gp130-mediated signaling pathway. *Cell* 77: 63–71
93 Zhong Z, Wen Z, Darnell JE Jr (1994) STAT3: a STAT family member activated by tyrosine phosphorylation in response to epidermal growth factor and interleukin-6. *Science* 264: 95–98
94 Hibi M, Nakajima K, Hirano T (1996) IL-6 cytokine family and signal transduction: a model of the cytokine system. *J Mol Med* 74: 1–12
95 Cooper GM (ed) (1997) The cell, a molecular approach. ASM press, Washington D.C.; 544–550
96 Gallo P, Frei K, Rordorf C, Lazdins J, Tavolato B, Fontana A (1989) Human immunodeficiency virus type 1 (HIV-1) infection of the central nervous system: an evaluation of cytokines in cerebrospinal fluid. *J Neuroimmunol* 23: 109–116
97 Laurenzi MA, Siden A, Persson MA, Norkkrans G, Hagberg L, Chiodi F (1990) Cerebrospinal fluid interleukin-6 activity in HIV infection and inflammatory and noninflammatory diseases of the nervous system. *Clin Immunol Immunopathol* 57: 233–241
98 Bauer J, Strauss S, Schreiter-Gasser U, Ganter U, Schlegel P, Witt I, Volk B, Berger M (1991) Interleukin-6 and α-2-macroglobulin indicate an acute phase state in Alzheimer's disease cortices. *FEBS* 285: 111–114
99 Vandenabeele P, Fiers W (1991) Is amyloidogenisis during Alzheimer's disease due to an IL-1-/IL-6-mediated 'acute phase response' in the brain? *Immunol Today* 12: 217–219
100 Hofman FM, Hinton DR, Johnson K, Merrill JE (1989) tumor necrosis factor identified in multiple sclerosis brain. *J Exp Med* 170: 607–612
101 Woodroofe MN, Sarna GS, Wadhwa M, Hayes GM, Loughlin AJ, Tinker A, Cuzner ML (1991) Detection of interleukin-1 and interleukin-6 in adult rat brain, following mechanical injury, by *in vivo* microdialysis: evidence of a role for microglia in cytokine production. *J Neuroimmunol* 33: 227–236
102 Frei K, Leist TP, Meager A, Gallo P, Leppert D, Zinkernagel RM, Fontana A (1988) Production of B cell stimulatory factor-2 and interferon gamma in the central nervous system during viral meningitis and encephalitis. Evaluation in a murine model infection and in patients. *J Exp Med* 168: 449–453
103 Houssiau FA, Bukasa K, Sindic CJ, Van Damme J, Van Snick J (1988) Elevated levels of the 26K human hybridoma growth factor (interleukin-6) in cerebrospinal fluid of

patients with acute infection of the cerebral nervous system. *Clin Exp Immunol* 71(2): 320–323

104 Campell IL, Abraham CR, Masliah E, Kemper P, Inglis JD, Oldstone MBA, Mucke L (1993) Neurologic disease induced in transgenic mice by cerebral overexpression of interleukin-6. *Proc Natl Acad Sci USA* 90 (21): 10061–10065

105 Heyser CJ, Masaliah E, Samimi A, Campbell IL, Gold LH (1997) Progressive decline in avoidance learning paralleled by inflammatory neurodegeneration in transgenic mice expressing interleukin-6 in the brain. *Proc Natl Acad Sci USA* 94 (4): 1500–1505

106 Samoilova EB, Horton JL, Hilliard B, Liu TS, Chen Y (1998) Il-6 deficient mice are resistant to experimental autoimmune encephalomyelitis: roles of IL-6 in the activation and differentiation of autoreactive T-cells. *J Immunol* 161 (12): 6480–6486

107 Mendel I, Katz A, Kozak N, Ben-Nun A, Revel M (1998) Interleukin-6 functions in autoimmune encephalomyelitis: a study in gene-targeted mice. *Eur J Immunol* 28: 1727–1737

108 Hirohata S, Miyamoto T (1990) Elevated levels of interleukin-6 in cerebrospinal fluid from patients with systemic lupus erythematosus and central nervous system involvement. *Arithris Rheum* 22: 644–649

109 Maimone D, Gregory S, Arnason BG, Reder AT (1991) Cytokine levels in the cerebrospinal fluid and serum of patients with multiple sclerosis. *J Neuroimmunol* 32 (1): 67–74

110 Padberg F, Feneberg W, Schmidt S, Schwarz MJ, Körschenhausen D, Greenberg BD, Nolde T, Müller N, Trapmann H, König N et al (1999) CSF and serum levels of soluble interleukin-6 receptors (sIL-6R and sgp130), but not of interleukin-6 are altered in multiple sclerosis. *J Neuroimmunol* 99 (2): 218–223

111 Naudin J, Menge JL, Azorin JM, Dassa D (1996) Elevated circulation levels of IL-6 in schizophrenia. *Schizophr Res* 20 (3): 269–273

112 Stübner S, Schön T, Padberg F, Teipel SJ, Schwarz MJ, Haslinger A, Buch K, Dukoff R, Lasser R, Müller N, Sunderland T et al (1999) Interleukin-6 and the soluble IL-6 receptor are decreased in cerebrospinal fluid of geriatric patients with major depression: no alteration of soluble gp130. *Neuroscience Lett* 259: 145–148

113 Yamada K, Kono K, Umegaki H, Yamada K, Iguchi A, Fukatsu T, Nakashima N, Nishiwaki H, Shimada Y, Sugita Y et al (1995) decreased interleukin-6 level in the cerebrospinal fluid of patients with Alzheimer type dementia. *Neurosci Lett* 186: 219–221

114 Hampel H, Schoen D, Schwarz MJ, Kötter HU, Schneider C, Sunderland T, Dukoff R, Ley J, Padberg F, Stübner S et al (1997) Interleukin-6 is not altered in cerebrospinal fluid of first-degree relatives and patients with Alzheimer's Disease. *Neurosci Lett* 228: 143–146

115 Cserr HF, Knopf PM (1992) Cervical lymphatics, the blood-brain-barrier and the immunoreactivity of the brain: a new view. *Immunology Today* 13 (12): 507–512

116 Hüll M, Strauss S, Volk B, Berger M, Bauer J (1995) Interleukin-6 is present in early stage of plaque formation and is restricted to the brains of Alzheimer's disease patients. *Acta Neuropathol* 89: 544–551

117 Wood JA, Wood PL, Ryan R, Graff-Radford NR, Pilapil C, Robtaille Y, Quirion R (1993) Cytokine indices in Alzheimer's temporal cortex: no changes in mature IL-1β or IL-1RA but increases in the associated acute phase proteins IL-6, α2-macroglobulin and C-reactive protein. *Brain Res* 629: 245–252
118 Rogers J, Webster S, Lue LF, Brachova L, Civin WH, Emmerling M, Shivers B, Walker D, McGeer P (1996) Inflammation and Alzheimer's disease pathogenesis. *Neurobiol Aging* 17 (5): 681–686
119 Ringheim GE, Szczepanik AM, Petko W, Burgher KL, Zhu SZ, Chao CC (1998) Enhancement of β-amyloid precursor protein transcription and expression by the soluble interleukin 6 receptor/interleukin-6 complex. *Brain Res Mol Res* 55: 35–44
120 Chong Y (1997) Effect of a carboxy-terminal fragment of the Alzheimer's amyloid precursor protein on expression of proinflammatory cytokines in rat glial cells. Life-Sci 61(23): 2323–2333
121 Strauss S, Bauer J, Ganter U, Jonas U, Berger M, Volk B (1992) Detection of Interleukin-6 and α2-macroglobulin immunoreactivity in Cortex and Hippocampus of Alzheimer's Disease patients. Lab Invest 66(2): 223–230
122 Hüll M, Strauss S, Berger M, Volk B, Bauer J (1996) Inflammatory mechanisms in Alzheimer's Disease. Eur Arch Psychiatry Clin Neurosci 246: 124–128
123 Ganter U, Strauss S, Jonas U, Weidemann A, Beyreuther K, Volk B, Berger M, Bauer J (1991) Alpha 2-macroglobulin synthesis in interleukin-6-stimulated human neuronal (SH-SY5Y neuroblastoma) cells. FEBS 282: 127–131
124 Scheloske M, Haslinger A, Unger J, Fischer P, Hulette C, Oshita R, Padberg F, Pongratz D, Möller H-J, Hampel H (1999) Expression of the Interleukin-6 receptor complex (IL-6 RC) in human rapid brain autopsy tissue. *Soc Neurosci Abstr* 25 (2): 1536
125 Haslinger A, Zarow C, Stein L, Bidlingmaier M, Teipel SJ, Scheloske M, Stein M, Padberg F, Freihöfer S, Schweiger R et al (1999) Measurement of the soluble and the membrane bound IL-6 receptor complex in human post-mortem brain homogenates of Alzheimer demented patients. *Soc Neurosci Abstr* 25 (2): 1537
126 Zarow C, Schlueter KE, Zhang Q (1996) Interleukin-6 mRNA is elevated in Alzheimer disease brain. *Soc Neurosci Abstr* Vol 22 Part 1: 214
127 Angelis P, Scharf S, Mander A, Vajda F, Christophidis N (1998) Serum interleukin-6 and interleukin-6 soluble receptor in Alzheimer's disease. *Neurosci Lett* 244: 106–108
128 März P, Heese K, Hock C, Golombowski S, Müller-Spahn F, Rose-John S, Otten U (1997) Interleukin-6 (IL-6) and soluble forms of IL-6 receptors are not altered in cerebrospinal fluid of Alzheimer's disease. *Neurosci Lett* 239: 29–32
129 Hampel H, Sunderland T, Kötter HU, Schneider C, Teipel SJ, Padberg F, Dukoff R, Ley J, Möller H-J (1998) Decreased soluble interleukin-6 receptor in cerebrospinal fluid of patients with Alzheimer's disease. *Brain Res* 780: 356–359
130 Hampel H, Teipel SJ, Padberg F, Haslinger A, Riemenschneider M, Schwarz MJ, Kötter HU, Scheloske M, Buch K, Stübner S et al (1999) Discriminant power of combined cerebrospinal fluid τ protein and of the soluble interleukin-6 receptor complex in the diagnosis of Alzheimer's disease. *Brain Res* 823 (1–2): 104–112

131 Ohara J, Paul WE (1987) Receptors for B-cell stimulatory factor-1 expressed on cells of hematopoietic lineage. *Nature* 325 (6104): 537–540

132 Saito T, Yasukawa H, Suzuki H, Futatsugi K, Fukunaga T, , Yokomizo C, Koishihara Y, Fukui H, Ohsugi Y, Yawata H et al (1991) Preparation of soluble murine IL-6 receptor and anti-murine IL-6 receptor antibodies, *J Immunol* 147: 168–173

133 Yasukawa K, Saito T, Fukunaga Y, Sekimori Y, Kishihara Y, Fukui H, Osugi Y, Mastuda T, Yawata H, Hirano T, Taga T, Kishimoto T (1990) Purification and characterization of soluble human IL-6 receptor expressed in CHO cells. *J Biochem* 108: 673–676

134 Ip NY, Nye SH, Boulton TG, Davis S Taga T, Li Y, Birren SJ, Yasukawa K, Kishimoto T, Anderson DJ (1992) CNTF and LIF act on neuronal cells *via* shared signaling pathways that involve the IL-6 signal transducing receptor component gp130. *Cell* 69 (7): 1121–1132

135 Kishimoto T, Akira S, Narazaki M, Taga T (1995) Interleukin-6 family of cytokines and gp130. *Blood* 86: 1243–1254

136 Pennica D, Wood WI, Chien KR (1996) Cardiotrophin-1: a multifunctional cytokine that signals *via* LIF receptor-gp130 dependent pathways. *Cytokine Growth Factor Rev* 7: 81–91

137 Ikeda K, Kinosita M, Tagaya N, Shiojima T, Taga T, Suzuki H, Okano A (1996) Coadministration of interleukin-6 (IL-6) and soluble IL-6 receptor delays progression of wobbler mouse motor neuron disease. *Brain Res* 726: 91–97

138 Watanabe D, Yoshimura R, Khalil M, Yoshida K, Kishimoto T, Taga T, Kiyama H (1996) Characteristic localization of gp130 (the signal-transducing receptor component used in common for IL-6/IL-11/CNTF/OSM) in the rat brain. *Eur J Neurosci* 8 (8): 1630–1640

139 März P, Herget T, Lang E, Otten U, Rose-John S (1997) Activation of gp130 by IL-6/soluble IL-6 receptor induces neuronal differentiation. *Eur J Neurosci* 9 (12): 2765–2763

140 Müllberg J, Schooltink H, Stoyan T, Günther M, Graeve L, Buse G, Mackiewicz A, Heinrich PC, Rose-John S (1993) The soluble interleukin-6 is generated by shedding. *Eur J Immunol* 23: 473–480

141 Zhang JG, Owczarek CM, Ward LD, Howlett GJ, Fabri LJ, Roberts BA, Nicola NA (1997) Evidence for the formation of a heterotrimeric complex of leukemia inhibitory factor with its subunits in solution. *Biochem J* 325: 693–700

Interactions of α2-macroglobulin and amyloid β peptide

Ikuo Tooyama

Molecular Neuroscience Research Center, Shiga University of Medical Science, Otsu 520-2192, Japan

Introduction

The pathological hallmarks of Alzheimer's disease (AD) are senile plaques and neurofibrillary tangles. A major component of senile plaque is β-amyloid peptide (Aβ) [1, 2]. Several lines of evidence suggest that a progressive deposition of aggregated Aβ is an early and necessary event in AD [3–5]. Several forms of the hydrophobic Aβ, consisting of 39–43 amino acids, are generated from the amyloid precursor protein (APP) [3–5]. Synthetic Aβ spontaneously aggregates and forms amyloid-like fibril [6, 7]. The aggregated Aβ is neurotoxic [8, 9].

The aggregation, deposition and neurotoxicity of Aβ are influenced by many local substances including immunoinflammatory factors. Among these factors α2-macroglobulin (α2-MAC) and its receptor (α2-macroglobulin receptor/low density lipoprotein receptor-related protein; α2MR/LRP) appear to be important because both proteins have been detected in senile plaques of AD patients [10–12], and genes on chromosome 12 that code for these proteins are candidate susceptibility genes for AD [13–16].

Structure and function of α2-MAC and α2MR/LRP

α2-MAC, a panproteinase inhibitor, is a member of a superfamily characterized by homologous subunit structures having a unique internal cyclic thiol ester bond [17–19]. The family of peptides includes α2-MAC, pregnancy zone protein, and the third, fourth and fifth complement proteins (C3, C4, C5). The human α2-MAC is a 720 kDa glycoprotein consisting of four identical 180 kDa subunits [18–20]. Each subunit has a bait region that acts as a substrate for virtually all proteinases. When an α2-MAC and proteinase complex is formed, cleavage of the internal thiol ester in the bait region occurs. The cleavage causes a conformational change of α2-MAC and exposure of the receptor binding site comprising the COOH-terminal 138 amino acids (activated α2-MAC). When the receptor-binding domain is exposed,

Neuroinflammatory Mechanisms in Alzheimer's Disease: Basic and Clinical Research, edited by Joseph Rogers the complex is removed by binding to its receptor, α2MR/LRP, and subsequently endocytosed [18–20].

α2-MAC binds not only proteinases but also many other proteins and peptides [20–22]. These include insulin, IL-1β, IL-6, NGF, TGFβ, PDGF, EGF, TNFα and FGF. As described later, recent studies have revealed that α2-MAC binds Aβ [23, 24]. These characteristics suggest that α2-MAC is a multifunctional protein.

There are at least two distinct receptors for α2-MAC. The first is α2MR/LRP, a scavenger receptor [25]. The second is α2-macroglobulin signaling receptor (α2MSR), which activates G-protein coupled signaling cascades [26–28]. So far, little information is available about α2MSR in AD. In contrast, many studies have indicated that α2MR/LRP is linked to AD pathology.

α2MR/LRP has been purified from rat liver [29] and human placenta [30, 31]. The sequence analysis indicates that the α2-MAC receptor is identical to low density lipoprotein receptor-related protein (LRP) [32, 33]. α2MR/LRP consists of an a-chain of about 500 kDa and a 85 kDa β-chain [25]. The α-chain contains complement-type repeats.

α2MR/LRP is a multifunctional receptor for a wide variety of ligands including APP [34]. These ligands are listed in Table 1. Among the ligands, the receptor-associated protein (RAP) copurifies with α2MR/LRP [35] and special attention has been paid to its role as a molecular chaperone of α2MR/LRP [36]. RAP binds to multiple sites in the α-chain of α2MR/LRP and inhibits the binding of other ligands. An electron microscopic study has shown that RAP is a resident protein of endoplasmic reticulum (ER) [36]. Thus, RAP may inhibit the binding of ligands to α2MR/LRP in the ER, may prevent the proteolysis of the receptor, and may regulate functional expression of α2MR/LRP [37, 38].

Expression of α2-MAC and α2MR/LRP in human brain

Previous studies have shown that the mRNA for α2-MAC can be detected in the brain and spinal cord [39, 40]. Studies using cultured brain cells have indicated that α2-MAC is synthesized by astrocytes [40–42]. Astrocytic expression of α2-MAC is stimulated by inflammatory cytokines such as IL-6 [40, 43]. Neuronal and microglial expression of α2-MAC was not detected in untreated cell culture [42]. However, Ganter et al. [44] reported that IL-6 induced the expression of α2-MAC in cultured neuroblastoma cells (SH-SY5Y). This may be an important finding because α2-MAC has been detected in neurons in postmortem brain samples from AD patients [10].

In neurologically normal human brains at autopsy, the expression of α2-MAC is below detection levels [10, 45]. In AD brain, however, α2-MAC is detected in senile plaques [10, 45], neurons [10] and activated glial cells [45]. α2MR/LRP has also been localized in the human brain, with several independent groups reporting simi-

Table 1 - Ligands of α2-macroglobulin receptor/LDL-receptor related protein (α2MR/LRP)

Ligands	Refs.
α2-macroglobulin-proteinase complexes	18–20, 30, 31
complexes of α2-macroglobulin and cytokines	19–21
complexes of α2-macroglobulin and amyloid β peptide	23, 24, 52
pregnancy zone protein complexes	58
tissue-type plasminogen activator (tPA)	59
urinary-type plasminogen activator (uPA)	60
complexes of tPA or uPA with plasminogen activator inhibitor type 1	61–63
apolipoprotein E	64
apolipoprotein E-enriched lipoproteins	65
lipoprotein lipase	66
lactoferrin	63
receptor associated protein (RAP)	35, 36
secreted amyloid precursor protein	34

lar findings [11, 12, 46–48]. In neurologically normal patients, α2MR/LRP is mainly localized in neurons (Fig. 1A). In AD, the expression of α2MR/LRP is upregulated in neurons and activated glial cells, mainly reactive astrocytes and partly reactive microglia, as well as pericytes. In addition, intense deposition of α2MR/LRP is detected in senile plaques (Fig. 1B). Interestingly, many ligands of α2MR/LRP, such as α2-MAC [10, 45], apolipoprotein E [11, 49, 50], lactoferrin [51], lipoprotein lipase [47], plasminogen activators [47], plasminogen activator inhibitor complex [47], RAP [47] and APP are also detected in senile plaques. Such results suggest that α2MR/LRP may be closely associated with senile plaque formation.

An immunoelectron microscopic study revealed that α2MR/LRP-positive reaction products are localized to ribosomes, plasma membranes, endosomes, lysosomes and lipofuscin granules [48]. The subcellular distribution patterns suggest that α2MR/LRP has a function in receptor-mediated endocytosis, lysosomal uptake and degradation of ligands.

Interaction of α2-MAC and Aβ peptide

It is well known that 39–43 amino acid Aβ peptides are generated from APP. Multiple forms of APP are synthesized by alternative splicing. The major isoforms in the brain are APP695, APP751 and APP770. The extracellular regions of APP751 and APP770 contain a Kunitz proteinase inhibitor domain, and are secreted as a pro-

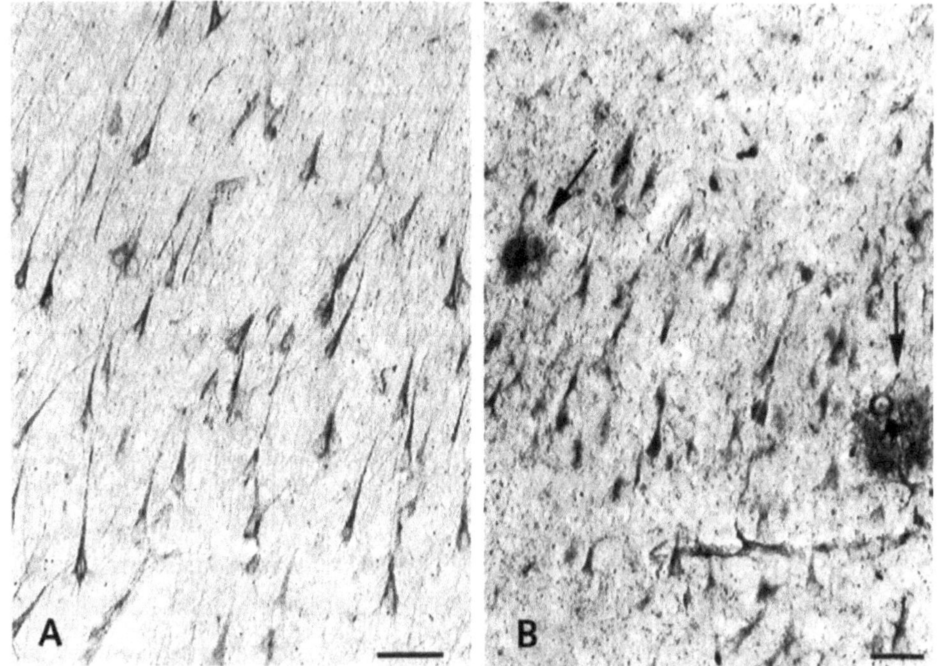

Figure 1
Immunohistochemistry for α2MR/LRP in the hippocampus of a control (A) and an Alzheimer (B) case.
(A): Pyramidal neurons are stained for α2MR/LRP.
(B): α2MR/LRP-immunoreactivity is detected in senile plaques (arrows). The monoclonal antibody gainst α2MR/LRP (A2MRα2) was kindly provided by Dr. S.K. Moestrup and Dr. J. Gliemann. Bars = 50 μm.

teinase nexin II. Kounnas et al. [34] has shown that APP 770 binds directly to α2MR/LRP and is then taken up and degraded. This pathway may occur in normal brain and could involve interaction with other ligands of α2MR/LRP such as apolipoprotein E.

In contrast to APP, there is no evidence that Aβ binds directly to α2MR/LRP. However, several lines of evidence have suggested that α2-MAC is an Aβ peptide-binding protein [24, 25, 52] and that the complex of α2-MAC and Aβ binds to α2MR/LRP [52]. Interactions between α2-MAC and Aβ may therefore play several important roles in AD pathophysiology. One such role may be clearance of extracellular Aβ in the brain. The complex of α2-MAC and Aβ is taken up and degraded *via* α2MR/LRP expressed on glioblastoma cells and fibroblasts [52]. Serine proteases for the degradation of Aβ may also be complexed with α2-MAC [53]. Interestingly, Paresce et al. [54] have shown that the aggregated Aβ uncomplexed by α2-MAC is not removed by α2MR/LRP, but is instead taken up by a scavenger receptor on microglia. Narita et al. [52] therefore proposed that there may be two pathways for Aβ degradation: (1) an α2MR/LRP-mediated pathway for the complex of α2-MAC and Aβ; and (2) an α2MR/LRP-independent pathway for free Aβ. Since many ligands for α2MR/LRP, as well as α2MR/LRP itself, have been detected in senile plaques, the α2MR/LRP-mediated clearance pathway may be impaired in the brains of AD patients [47].

Another role for α2-MAC is as a molecular chaperone for Aβ. α2-MAC inhibits β-sheet formation, amyloid aggregation and fibril formation [24]. Its potency in this regard is similar to that of apolipoprotein J [24]. Moreover, preincubation of α2-MAC and Aβ peptide (1–40) reduces neurotoxicity in rat neuronal cultures [55]. Recently, however, Fabrizi et al. [56] reported that activated α2-MAC increases Aβ peptide (25–35)-induced neurotoxicity by removing TGFβ, another ligand of α2-MAC. This result reminds us that α2-MAC is a multifunctional protein.

Other roles of α2-MAC in Alzheimer's disease

The expression of α2-MAC is at a very low level in normal brain and is upregulated in AD. α2-MAC expression is induced by inflammatory cytokines. α2-MAC and α2MR/LRP constitute a clearance system to remove a wide variety of proteinases and cytokines. Therefore, the regulatory roles of α2-MAC in neuroinflammation cannot be neglected. Recent evidence suggests that inflammation may accelerate neuronal death [57]. α2-MAC and α2MR/LRP may therefore play a role in suppressing dangerous inflammatory reactions in the AD brain.

References

1 Glenner GG, Wong CW (1984) Alzheimer's disease: Initial report of the purification and characterization of a novel cerebrovascular amyloid protein. *Biochem Biophys Res Commun* 120: 885–890

2 Masters CL, Simms G, Weinman NA, Multhaup G, McDonald BL, Beyreuther K (1985) Amyloid plaque core protein in Alzheimer disease and Down syndrome. *Proc Natl Acad Sci USA* 82: 4245–4249

3 Selkoe DJ (1994) Alzheimer's disease: a central role for amyloid. *J Neuropathol Exp* Neurol 53: 438–447

4 Selkoe DJ (1996) Amyloid β-protein and the genetics of Alzheimer's disease. *J Biol Chem* 271: 18295–18298

5 Sisodia SS, Price DL (1995) Role of the β-amyloid protein in Alzheimer's disease. *FASEB J* 9: 366–370

6 Kirschner DA, Inouye H, Duffy LK, Sinclair A, Lind M, Selkoe DJ (1987) Synthetic peptide homologous to β protein from Alzheimer disease forms amyloid-like fibrils *in vitro*. *Proc Natl Acad Sci USA* 84: 6953–6957

7 Barrow CJ, Yasuda A, Kenny PTM, Zagorski MG (1992) Solution conformations and aggregational properties of synthetic amyloid β-peptides of Alzheimer's disease. Analysis of circular dichroism spectra. *J Mol Biol* 225: 1075–1093

8 Pike CJ, Walencewicz AJ, Glabe CG, Cotman CW (1991) *In vitro* aging of β-amyloid protein causes peptide aggregation and neurotoxicity. *Brain Res* 563: 311–314

9 Mattson MP, Tomaselli KJ, Rydel RE (1993) Calcium-destabilizing and neurodegenerative effects of aggregated β-amyloid peptide are attenuated by basic FGF. *Brain Res* 621: 35–49

10 Bauer J, Strauss S, Schreiter-Gasser U, Ganter U, Schlegel P, Witt I, Yolk B, Berger M (1991) Interleukin-6 and α-2-macroglobulin indicate an acute-phase state in Alzheimer's disease cortices. *FEBS Lett* 285: 111–114

11 Rebeck GW, Harr SD, Strickland DK, Hyman BT (1993) Apolipoprotein E in sporadic Alzheimer's disease: allelic variation and receptor interactions. *Neuron* 11: 575–580.

12 Tooyama I, Kawamata T, Akiyama H, Moestrup SK, Gliemann J, McGeer PL (1993) Immunohistochemical study of α2 macroglobulin receptor in Alzheimer and control post mortem human brain. *Mol Chem Neuropathol* 18: 153–160

13 Blacker D, Wilcox MA, Laird NM, Rodes L, Horvath SM, Go RC, Perry R, Watson B Jr, Bassett SS, McInnis MG et al (1998) Alpha-2 macroglobulin is genetically associated with Alzheimer disease. *Nat Genet* 19: 357–360

14 Kang DE, Saitoh T, Chen X, Xia Y, Masliah E, Hansen LA, Thomas RG, Thal LJ, Katzman R (1997) Genetic association of the low-density lipoprotein receptor-related protein gene (LRP), an apolipoprotein E receptor, with late-onset Alzheimer's disease. *Neurology* 49: 56–61

15 Hollenbach E, Ackermann S, Hyman BT, Rebeck GW (1998) Confirmation of an association between a polymorphism in exon 3 of the low density lipoprotein receptor-related protein gene and Alzheimer's disease. *Neurology* 50: 1905–1907

16 Beffert U, Arguin C, Poirier J (1999) The polymorphism in exon 3 of the low density lipoprotein receptor-related protein gene is weakly associated with Alzheimer's disease. *Neurosci Lett* 259: 29–32

17 Harrison RA (1984) The family of proteins having internal thiol ester bonds. *Recent Adv Immunol* 17: 87–100

18 Sottrup-Jensen L (1989) α2-Macroglobulins: structure, shape and mechanism of proteinase complex formation. *J Biol Chem* 264: 11539–11542

19 Chu CT, Pizzo SV (1994) α2-Macroglobulin, complement, and biological defense: antigens, growth factors, microbial proteases, and receptor ligation. *Lab Invest* 71: 792–812

20 Borth W (1992) α2-Macroglobulin, a multifunctional binding protein with targeting characteristics. *FASEB J* 6: 3345–3353

21 LaMarre J, Wollenberg GK, Gonias SL, Hayes AM (1991) Cytokine binding and clearance properties of proteinase-activated α2-macroglobulin. *Lab Invest* 65: 3–14

22 Chu CT, Howard GC, Misra UK, Pizzo SV (1994) α2-Macroglobulin: a sensor for proteolysis. *Ann NY Acad Sci* 737: 291–307

23 Du Y, Ni B, Glim M, Dodel RC, Bales KR, Zhang Z, Hyslop PA, Paul SM (1997) α2-Macroglobulin as a β-amyloid peptide-binding plasma protein. *J Neurochem* 69: 299–305

24 Hughes SR, Khorkova O, Goyal S, Knaeblein J, Heroux J, Riedel NG, Sahasrabudhe S (1998) α2-macroglobulin associates with β-amyloid peptide and prevents fibril formation. *Proc Natl Acad Sci USA* 95: 3275–3280

25 Gliemann J, Nykjær A, Petersen MC, Jørgensen KE, Nielsen M, Andreasen Christensen EI, Lookene A, Olivecrona G, Moestrup SK (1994) The multiligand α2-macroglobulin receptor/low density lipoprotein receptor-related protein (α2MR/LRP). Binding and endocytosis of fluid phase and membrane-associated ligands. *Ann NY Acad Sci* 737: 14–38

26 Misra UK, Chu CT, Gawdi G, Pizzo SV (1994) Evidence for a second α2-macroglobulin receptor. *J Biol Chem* 269: 12541–12547

27 Misra UK, Chu CT, Gawdi G, Pizzo SV (1994) The relationship between low density lipoprotein-related protein/α2-macroglobulin receptors and the newly described α2M signaling receptor. *J Biol Chem* 269: 18303–18306

28 Misra UK, Pizzo SV (1998) Binding of receptor-recognized forms of α2-macroglobulin to the α2-macroglobulin signaling receptor activates phosphatidylinositol 3-kinase. *J Biol Chem* 273: 13399–13402

29 Moestrup SK, Gliemann J (1989) Purification of the rat hepatic α2-macroglobulin receptor as an approximately 440-kDa single chain polypeptide. *J Biol Chem* 264: 15574–15577

30 Jensen PH, Moestrup SK, Gliemann J (1989) Purification of the human placental α2-macroglobulin receptor. *FEBS Lett* 255: 275–280

31 Ashcom JD Tiller SE, Dickerson K, Cravens JL, Argraves WS, Strickland DK (1990) The human α2-macroglobulin receptor: identification of a 420-kD cell surface glycoprotein specific for the activated conformation of α2-macroglobulin. *J Cell Biol* 110: 1041–1048

32 Strickland DK, Ashcom JD, Williams S, Burgess WH, Migliorini M, Argraves WS (1990) Sequence identity between the α2-macroglobulin receptor and low density lipoprotein receptor-related protein suggests that this molecule is a multifunctional receptor. *J Biol Chem* 265: 17401–17404

33 Kristensen TS, Moestrup SK, Gliemann J, Bendtsen L, Sand O, Sorttrup-Jensen L (1990) Evidence that the newly cloned LRP is the α2-macroglobulin receptor. *FEBS Lett* 276: 151–155

34 Kounnas MZ, Moir RD, Rebeck GW, Bush AI, Argraves WS, Tanzi RE, Hyman BT, Strickland DK (1995) LDL-receptor-related protein, a multifunctional ApoE receptor,

binds secreted β-amyloid precursor protein and mediates its degradation. *Cell* 82: 331–340
35 Strickland DK, Ashcom JD, Williams S, Battey F, Behre E, McTigue K, Battey JF, Argraves WS (1991) Primary structure of α2-macroglobulin receptor-associated protein: human homologue of a Heymann nephritis antigen. *J Biol Chem* 266: 13364–13369
36 Bu G, Geuze HJ, Strous GJ, Schwartz AL (1995) 39 kDa receptor-associated protein is an ER resident protein and molecular chaperone for LDL receptor-related protein. *EMBO J* 14: 2269–2280
37 Willnow TE, Armstrong SA, Hammer RE, Herz J (1995) Functional expression of low density lipoprotein receptor-related protein is controlled by receptor-associated protein *in vivo*. *Proc Natl Acad Sci USA* 92: 4537–4541
38 Willnow TE, Rohlmann A, Horton J, Otani H, Braun JR, Hammer RE, Herz J (1996) RAP, a specialized chaperone, prevents ligand-induced ER retention and degradation of LDL receptor-related endocytic receptors. *EMBO J* 15: 2632–2639
39 Kodelja V, Heisig M, Northermann W, Heinrich PC, Zimmerman W (1986) α2-Macroglobulin gene expression during rat development studied by *in situ* hybridization. *EMBO J* 5: 3151–3156
40 Higuchi M, Ito T, Imai Y, Iwaki T, Hattori M, Kohsaka S, Niho Y, Sakaki Y (1994) Expression of the alpha-2-macroglobulin-encoding gene in rat brain and cultured astrocytes. *Gene* 142: 155–162
41 Gebicke-Haerter PJ, Bauer J, Brenner A, Gerok W (1987) α2-Macroglobulin synthesis in an astrocyte subpopulation. *J Neurochem* 49: 1139–1145
42 Saitoh S, Iijima N, Ikeda M, Nakajima K, Kimura M, Katsuki M, Mori T, Kohsaka S (1992) De novo production of α2-macroglobulin in cultured astroglia from rat brain. *Mol Brain Res* 12: 155–161
43 Hong-Brown LQ, Brown CR (1994) Cytokine and insulin regulation of alpha 2 macroglobulin, angiotensinogen, and hsp 70 in primary cultured astrocytes. *Glia* 12: 211–218
44 Ganter U, Strauss S, Jonas U, Weidemann A, Beyreuther K, Volk B, Berger M, Bauer J (1991) Alpha 2-macroglobulin synthesis in interleukin-6-stimulated human neuronal (SH-SY5Y neuroblastoma) cells. *FEBS Lett* 282: 127–131
45 Van Gool D, De Strooper V, Van Leuven F, Triau E, Dom R (1993) α2-Macroglobulin expression in neuritic-type plaques in patients with Alzheimer's disease. *Neurobiol Aging* 14: 233–237
46 Wolf BB, Lopes MBS, VandenBerg SR, Gonias SL (1992) Characterization and Immunohistochemical localization of α2-macroglobulin receptor (low-density lipoprotein receptor-related protein) in human brain. *Am J Pathol* 141: 37–42
47 Rebeck GW, Harr SD, Strickland DK, Hyman BT (1995) Multiple, diverse senile plaque-associated proteins are ligands of an apolipoprotein E receptor, the α2-macroglobulin receptor/low-density-lipoprotein receptor-related protein. *Ann Neurol* 37: 211–217
48 Tooyama I, Kawamata T, Akiyama H, Kimura H, Moestrup SK, Gliemann J, Matsuo A,

McGeer PL (1995) Subcellular localization low density lipoprotein receptor-related protein (α2-macroglobulin receptor) in human brain. *Brain Res* 691: 235–238
49 Namba Y, Tomonaga M, Kawasaki H, Ootomo E, Ikeda K (1991) Apolipoprotein E immunoreactivity in cerebral amyloid deposits and neurofibrillary tangles in Alzheimer's disease and kuru plaque amyloid in Creutzfeldt-Jakob disease. *Brain Res* 541: 163–166
50 Wisniewski T, Frangione B (1992) Apolipoprotein E: a pathological chaperone protein in patients with cerebral and systemic amyloid. *Neurosci Lett* 135: 235–238
51 Kawamata T, Tooyama I, Yamada T, Walker DG, McGeer PL (1991) Lactotransferrin immunocytochemistry in Alzheimer and normal human brain. *Am J Pathol* 142: 1574–1585
52 Narita M, Holtzman DM, Schwartz AL, Bu G (1997) α2-Macroglobulin complexes with and mediates the endocytosis of β-amyloid peptide *via* cell surface low-density lipoprotein receptor-related protein. *J Neurochem* 69:1904–1911
53 Qiu WQ, Borth W, Ye Z, Haass C, Teplow DB, Selkoe DJ (1996) Degradation of amyloid β-protein by a serine protease-α2-macroglobulin complex. *J Biol Chem* 271: 8443–8451
54 Paresce DM, Ghosh RN, Maxfield FR (1996) Microglial cells internalize aggregates of the Alzheimer's disease amyloid β-protein *via* a scavenger receptor. *Neuron* 17: 553–565
55 Du Y, Bales KR, Dodel RC, Liu X, Glinn MA, Horn JW, Little SP, Paul SM (1998) α2-Macroglobulin attenuates β-amyloid peptide 1–40 fibril formation and associated neurotoxicity of cultured fetal rat cortical neurons. *J Neurochem* 70: 1182–1188
56 Fabrizi C, Businaro R, Lauro GM, Starace G, Fumagalli L (1999) Activated α2 macroglobulin increases β-amyloid (25–35)-induced toxicity in LAN5 human neuroblastoma cells. *Exp Neurol* 155: 252–259
57 McGeer PL, McGeer EG (1995) The inflammatory response system of brain: implications for therapy of Alzheimer and other neurodegenerative diseases. *Brain Res Rev* 21: 195–218
58 Van Leuven F, Cassiman JJ, Van Den Berghe H (1986) Human pregnancy zone protein and α2-macroglobulin: high-affinity binding of complexes to the same receptor on fibroblasts and characterization of monoclonal antibodies. *J Biol Chem* 261: 16622–16625
59 Bu G, Williams S, Strickland DK, Schwartz AL (1992) Low density lipoprotein receptor-related protein/α2-macroglobulin receptor is an hepatic receptor for tissue-type plasminogen activator. *Proc Natl Acad Sci USA* 89: 7427–7431
60 Kounnas MZ, Henkin J, Argraves WS, Strickland DK (1993) Low density lipoprotein receptor-related protein/α2-macroglobulin receptor mediates cellular uptake of pro-urokinase. *J Biol Chem* 268: 21862–21867
61 Orth K, Madisoon EL, Gething M-J, SAmbrook JF, Herz J (1992) Complexes of tissue-type plasminogen activator and its serpin inhibitor plasminogen-activator inhibitor type 1 are internalized by means of the low density lipoprotein receptor-related protein/α2-macroglobulin receptor. *Proc Natl Acad Sci USA* 89: 7422–7426
62 Nykjær A, Petersen CM, Møller B, Jensen PH, Moestrup SK, Holtet TL, Etzerodt M,

Thøgersen HC, Munch M, Andreasen PA et al (1992) Purified α2-macroglobulin receptor/LDL receptor-related protein binds urokinase plasminogen activator inhibitor type 1 complex: evidence that the α2-macroglobulin receptor mediates cellular degradation of urokinase receptor-bound complexes. *J Biol Chem* 267: 14543–14546

63 Willnow TE, Goldstein JL, Orth K, Brown MS, Herz J (1992) LDL receptor related protein and gp330 bind similar ligands, including plasminogen activator-inhibitor complexes and lactoferrin, an inhibitor of chylomicron remnant clearance. *J Biol Chem* 267: 26172–26180

64 Beisiegel U, Weber W, Ihrke G, Herz J, Stanley KK (1989) The LDL-receptor-related protein, LRP is an apolipoprotein E binding protein. *Nature* 341: 162–164

65 Kowal RC, Herz J, Goldstein JL, Esser V, Brown MS (1989) Low density lipoprotein receptor-related protein mediates uptake of cholesteryl esters derived from apolipoprotein E-enriched lipoproteins. *Proc Natl Acad Sci USA* 86: 5810–5814

66 Chappell DA, Fry GL, Waknitz MA, Iverius P-H, Williams SE, Strickland DK (1992) The low density lipoprotein receptor-related protein/α2-macroglobulin receptor binds and mediates catabolism of bovine milk lipoprotein lipase. *J Biol Chem* 267: 25764–25767

Proinflammatory actions of derivatives of the β amyloid precursor protein

Steven W. Barger

Departments of Geriatrics, Anatomy, and Internal Medicine, University of Arkansas for Medical Sciences; Geriatric Research Education Clinical Center, Central Arkansas Veterans Healthcare System, Little Rock, AR 72205, USA

Introduction

The first genetic lesions associated with Alzheimer's disease were in the coding sequence of the β amyloid precursor protein (βAPP) [1]. Although these mutations account for a small proportion of familial Alzheimer (FAD) cases, they conceptually solidified the link between this protein and the pathology of the disease. As the source of the amyloid β peptide (Aβ) that accumulates in plaques, βAPP had garnered attention for several years. The mutations were immediately presumed to contribute to disease by modifying Aβ production, but increased understanding of the bioactivities of βAPP itself have led to models that do not depend on Aβ for Alzheimer pathogenesis. Both Aβ and non-amyloidogenic derivatives of βAPP can have an impact on proinflammatory glial activation. Indeed, the role of inflammatory reactions in Alzheimer's has been lent additional credence by indications of such reactions in mice transgenic for βAPP. These interactions will be reviewed and discussed here in the context of cell biology; protein-protein interactions between Aβ and α2-macroglobulin or components of the complement cascade are addressed in accompanying chapters of this volume.

βAPP expression and processing

Full-length βAPP is predominantly a glycosylated transmembrane protein expressed ubiquitously in and out of the nervous system. There are multiple splice variants, and the 695 amino acid form (βAPP_{695}) is found only in neurons. The complementary cell type-specificity (i.e. exclusive of neurons) has been documented for variants lacking exon 15, named L-APP for their original discovery in leukocytes [2]. The longest variants, βAPP_{751} and βAPP_{770} are the most predominant forms containing the Kunitz serine protease inhibitor (KPI) domain. Injury and stresses in the nervous

Neuroinflammatory Mechanisms in Alzheimer's Disease: Basic and Clinical Research,
edited by Joseph Rogers

system cause rapid elevation of βAPP expression (below), and the KPI-containing forms of the protein account for most of the increased protein.

Generation of Aβ from βAPP requires two proteolytic cleavages by the activities termed β- and γ-secretase (Fig. 1). The β-secretase activity, generating the aminoterminus of Aβ, is poorly characterized with respect to the responsible protease. It is modified by the "Swedish" FAD mutation of βAPP ($K^{670} \rightarrow N$, $M^{671} \rightarrow L$), which encodes a protein that apparently serves as a more efficient substrate. The γ-secretase activity is also mysterious, but intriguing data suggest that it may reside in the presenilins [3, 4], protein products of genes associated with a large proportion of FAD lineages [1]. The carboxyterminus of Aβ varies and some data suggest that the predominant Aβ species, ending at amino acid 40, are generated through γ-secretases and subcellular locales distinct from those creating the minor species ending at amino acid 42 or 43 [5, 6]; though other data suggest a single γ-secretase [7]. Mutations in the presenilins or the "London" mutations of βAPP (V^{717}) can elevate the proportion of $A\beta_{42/43}$ relative to $A\beta_{40}$ [1]. This has been proposed to contribute to disease through the faster fibrillogenesis demonstrated by longer species of Aβ [8, 9]. Most data indicate that β-secretase activity occurs before γ-secretase [10, 11] and the intermediate (sometimes termed C99, as it is comprised of the carboxyterminal 99 amino acids of βAPP) can be found in considerable quantity in many cells and tissues.

A cleavage event alternative to β-secretase exists that severs βAPP after amino acid 16 of the Aβ sequence. Termed α-secretase, this cleavage precludes production of full-length Aβ and liberates the aminoterminal two-thirds of βAPP into the extracellular space or vesicular lumens of the secretory pathway. This secreted APP (sAPPα) has been attributed with multiple biological effects, many of which are neuroprotective or neuromodulatory (reviewed in [12]). Its counterpart resulting from β-secretase cleavage (sAPPβ) is liberated from the cell as well, but it appears to lack some of the bioactivity of sAPPα, presumably due to its carboxyterminal truncation. It is useful for further discussion to point out that the carboxyterminal remnant of α-secretase cleavage is also a substrate for γ-secretase, producing a 24–27 amino acid peptide often referred to as p3.

The levels of βAPP expression are altered by conditions of stress. Specifically, expression is elevated by acute [13] and chronic [14] ischemia, traumatic brain injury [15], and excitotoxins [16–18]. More relevant to this volume, Alzheimer brains show by immunohistochemistry a striking elevation of βAPP levels in dystrophic neurites surrounding senile plaques [19–21]. Recent data have documented a translational regulation point mediated by an IL-1-responsive sequence element in the 5' untranslated region of βAPP mRNA [22]. However, forms of the protein containing the KPI splicing insert specifically account for most of the βAPP elevated by neuronal stress [16, 23–26], indicating that some of the increase must rely on transcriptional events. The promoter for the βAPP gene contains several defined regulatory elements, including AP-1, NF-κB, USF, and Sp-1 binding sites; and its activity is responsive to interleukin-1 (IL-1) and other cytokines [27–29].

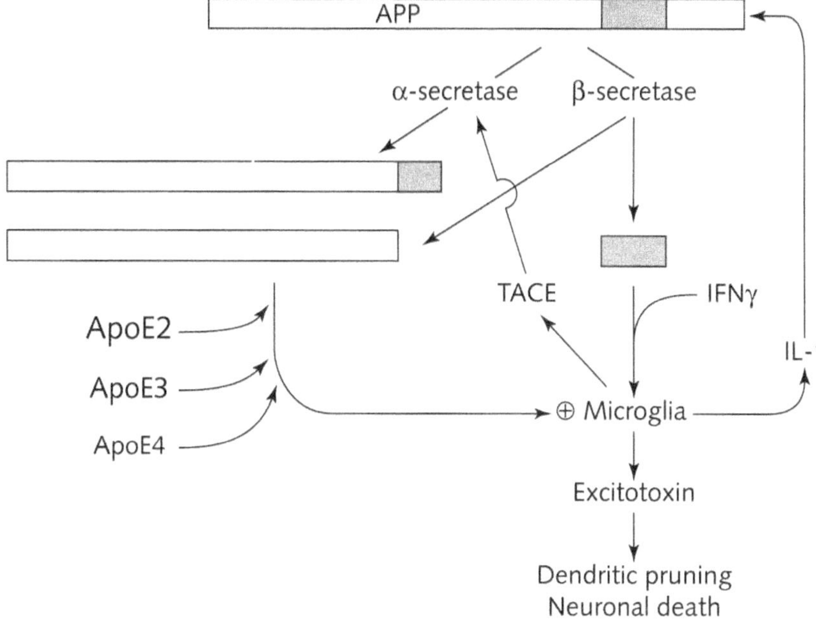

Figure 1
Schematic representation of the proinflammatory pathways stimulated by the major fragments of βAPP. The holoprotein, containing the Aβ peptide sequence (hatching), is processed primarily by α-secretase to generate sAPPα. When β-secretase cleavage occurs, the sAPP moeity (sAPPβ) is truncated carboxyterminally, and an amyloidogenic fragment is left for processing by γ-secretase and generation of Aβ. All these fragments can activate microglia, but most studies have indicated that Aβ has a corequirement for IFNγ or other cytokines. Activation of microglia results in the production of excitotoxins which can have subtle (synaptic or dendritic toxicity) or dramatic (neuron cell death) consequences. Activated microglia also secrete elevated levels of IL-1 which can promote positive feedback through the induction of βAPP expression. ApoE can inhibit the proinflammatory activity of sAPP, but with a potency that differs between the genetic variants.

Some of the specific stimuli that elevate βAPP expression also can affect its processing. For example, IL-1 increases secretion of an APP moeity, likely to be sAPPα [30–33]. Glutamate has a similar effect, apparently mediated by metabotropic receptors [34]. This is consistent with similar results with other signalling events coupled to phosphatidyinositol hydrolysis, such as mucscarinic acetylcholine receptor stimulation [30, 35]. Stimulated secretion of sAPPα has been attributed to the metalloprotease disintegrin, tumor necrosis factor (TNF)α converting enzyme (TACE) [36, 37]. Together with the regulation of βAPP expression by IL-1 and other proinflammatory cytokines, this finding invites speculation about the role of sAPPα in coordinated inflammatory responses.

Glial activation by Aβ

As detailed elsewhere in this volume, amyloid plaques are associated with distinctly activated glial components. Astrocytes with elevated expression of glial fibrillary acidic protein (GFAP) surround the plaque, and microglia overexpressing IL-1 appear within the amyloid deposit [38]. These associations have led investigators to explore the effects of Aβ on cultured glial cells. When applied to astrocytes, Aβ creates a complex array of responses. Among the effects noted are changes in morphology [39-41], elevation of GFAP and fibroblast growth factor expression [42], elevation of inducible nitric oxide synthase (iNOS) expression [40, 43], and inhibition of glucose and glutamate uptake [44]. Aβ also stimulates the exocytosis of formazen by astrocytes, which has complicated the use of MTT as a survival measure in these cells [45].

Microglia have also been treated with Aβ in culture. The first report of activation of cultured microglia by Aβ described a dependency on costimulation with interferon (IFN)γ [46]. Subsequently, several other costimuli were identified that were capable of making microglia competent to respond to Aβ with an inflammatory profile; these include macrophage-colony stimulating factor (M-CSF) [43], IL-1β [47, 48], and TNFα [48]. In combination with IFNγ or other costimuli, micromolar concentrations of Aβ stimulate rodent microglia to elevate their expression of iNOS, TNFα [46], IL-6, IL-1β [43], and complement factor C3 [49]. Aβ also stimulates release of reactive oxygen species [50, 51] and glutamate [52].

Structural considerations have been important to the plethora of studies that focused on Aβ neurotoxicity. Pike et al. [53] first delineated the connection between the aggregation of Aβ into a β-sheet conformation and its neurotoxicity. This was satisfying conceptually, as clinical symptoms are associated with the presence of plaques containing Aβ in a suitable conformation for staining with Congo red, i.e. β-sheet. Likewise, some studies of glial activation have sought to determine the relevant structural issues. Many studies have been performed with a peptide containing only amino acids 25–35 of Aβ. Historically, this was an expeditious peptide in neurotoxicity studies because it was one of the smallest sequences evoking cell death [54], though it is not detected in human brain under normal or pathological conditions. $A\beta_{25-35}$ is capable of stimulating reactions from both astrocytes and microglia. Nevertheless, other reports have linked the ability to activate microglia with the aminoterminal 16 amino acids of Aβ [51], which contains a putative heparin-binding site. The p3 peptide, which lacks these amino acids, is deficient at inducing morphological changes, neurotoxin production, or iNOS expression in astrocytes [40, 55]. The aminoterminal residues also appear necessary for the ability of Aβ to fix complement, as p3 is inactive in these assays as well [56, 57]. As a product of α-secretase, p3 would be logically harmless *in vivo*; at least two of the βAPP mutations leading to FAD actually decrease the ratio of p3:Aβ. Indeed, persons with Down's syndrome live with p3 deposits for many years before the onset of more classical signs of AD [58, 59]. Even in Alzheimer's disease, the nominatively asymptomatic deposits in the cerebellum are comprised largely of p3 [59]. However, this peptide contains all the sequence of $A\beta_{25-35}$, aggregates quite readily, and demonstrates fulminate neurotoxicity when tested in culture [60]. Together, these data call into question the relevance of *in vitro* neurotoxicity of Aβ and, more importantly, suggest that the distinction between the clinical presentation of a person with significant p3 deposition and that of an individual with congophilic amyloid is due to activities residing in the aminoterminal heparin-binding residues.

The mechanisms involved in microglial activation by Aβ are being explored, but are still somewhat controversial. In several models, the receptor for advanced glycation end-products (RAGE) appears to mediate the effects of Aβ on microglia [61]. Some confusion was generated by the use of soluble Aβ in such assays of binding to a specific receptor, which appeared inconsistent with the correlations between the formation of insoluble amyloid fibrils and disease. However, the other major class of defined receptors implicated in Aβ glial activation, the scavenger receptors, can bind to immobilized amyloid [62]. Such results indicate that Aβ need not be soluble to bind and activate receptors. Nevertheless, Aβ has been reported to activate mitogen-activated protein kinases (MAPKs) (below), an effect that other ligands of either RAGE or scavenger receptors cannot duplicate [63]. Indeed, the role of scavenger receptors is drawn into question by irrelevance of class A receptors in a transgenic mouse model [64]. Some data suggest that Aβ's actions on microglia reflect indirect mechanisms, whereby Aβ first induces proinflammatory cytokines in cells other than microglia. For instance, Aβ can elevate expression of M-CSF in peripheral neuroblastoma cells [65]; if the same is true of CNS neurons, it could provide an important stimulus or co-stimulus. Similarly, Aβ has been shown to elevate CD-40 expression on microglia [66], offering a scenario that would depend on CD-40 ligand (CD-40L) produced by other cells (e.g. endothelial cells or lymphocytes). An important role for CD-40 is apparent in this latter model as a βAPP transgenic mouse line produced a diminished microglial response and neurofibrillary aberrancy when crossed with a CD-40L-deficient line [67].

Intracellularly, the mechanisms of glial activation by Aβ are beginning to be elucidated. In microglia, Aβ triggers an activation of kinase cascades associated with the MAPK family. For instance, Erk 1, Erk 2, and p38 MAPKs were activated by Aβ in multiple reports [63, 68, 69]; however, there is disagreement as to whether the Jun N-terminal kinase (JNK) responds to Aβ ([68], cf. [63]). Combs et al. [69] suggest an elaborate scheme involving at least three kinases and a release of intracellular calcium stores before the classical Ras-Erk pathway is encountered. The involvement of Ras and the Erks is consistent with similar results after activation of RAGE receptors [70], and responses to lipopolysaccharide (LPS) mirrored those to Aβ in at least one study [68]. Tyrosine kinase activity is required for Aβ-induced microglial superoxide production [50] and chemotaxis [71]. In contrast, morphological reactions of astrocytes to Aβ are not affected by inhibitors of tyrosine kinases or phosphatases and depended instead on serine/threonine phosphatases [72].

Microglia vs astrocytes: accidental antagonists in Aβ clearance?

The activation of microglia by Aβ can include a stimulation of phagocytic activity [73, 74], perhaps indicating a beneficial role for microglia clearance of Aβ aggregates. It has been suggested that compromises in such a tonic clearance process may even be the root cause of amyloid accumulation in disease or normal aging. Deductive quantitations suggest that plaques are in an equilibrium of formation and clearance in Alzheimer's disease [75]. Interestingly, Aβ antigenicity was apparent in presumptive microglia in mice innoculated against Aβ [76], suggesting that the immunization may have accentuated Aβ phagocytosis and/or digestion by microglia.

Intriguing studies have been performed with a paradigm designed to mimic the deposition of Aβ that seeds a plaque [73, 77, 78]. In this approach, a solution of Aβ peptide is spotted onto a tissue culture surface and allowed to dry before the plating of various cell cultures. If microglia are cultured in this setting, they will phagocytose the Aβ deposit; this result may involve the ability of activated phagocytes to produce insulin-degrading enzyme [79], a metalloprotease that can degrade Aβ. However, if astrocytes are allowed to grow on the plate prior to the addition of microglia, the phagocytosis is severely inhibited, even if the astrocytes have been killed [77, 78]. This effect apparently depends on the ability of the astrocytes to deposit chondroitin sulfate proteoglycans [78], the production of which is elevated by contact with Aβ [77]. The presence of proteoglycans in amyloid plaques [80] suggests that similar sequelae may occur *in vivo*. Microglia and astrocytes generally have different strategies for dealing with parenchymal abnormalities: phagocytic microglia attempt to remove the foreign or damaged material, whereas astrocytes wall it off with a barrier that includes proteoglycans. It is possible that the amyloid thus protected by astrocyte-produced proteoglycan allows an unproductive activation of the nearby microglia that is thus persistent and capable of greater by-stander damage of the adjacent neuronal elements than would be the case if the amyloid could be cleared quickly.

Glial activation by sAPP

The neuroprotective activity of sAPPα has been correlated with the protein's ability to stimulate the activity of a transcription factor that binds κB enhancer elements [81]. This led to the speculation that sAPPα might activate *bona fide* NF-κB in glial cells, along with the commensurate proinflammatory outcomes. We tested this possibility in primary cultures of rat microglia and in a mouse microglial cell line. At doses in the low nanomolar range, sAPPα activated DNA-binding activity that was identified as NF-κB by DNA-specificity and reactivity with antibodies [82]. sAPPα also induced the expression of IL-1β and iNOS in microglia. Finally, microglia treated with sAPPα expressed neurotoxicity when combined with hippocampal neurons in cocultures. Interestingly, sAPPβ also activated microglia with similar potency and efficacy. This is meaningful because the compromised neuroprotective activity of sAPPβ has been incorporated into an hypothesis speculating that shifts in the α-secretase:β-secretase processing ratios could leave neurons vulnerable to incipient stresses [83]. The proinflammatory activity of sAPPβ only adds to this risk by maintaining the potential stress of microglial activation under conditions of increased β-secretase activity. Although sAPP levels are reportedly decreased in Alzheimer cerebrospinal fluid [84], βAPP is elevated in the vicinity of microglia-laden plaques [85]. Notably, an unusual FAD-associated mutation in βAPP results in increased sAPP production and decreased total Aβ production [86].

Previous studies had shown that sAPPα can interact physically and functionally with apolipoprotein E (ApoE) [87]. The latter protein has been implicated in Alzheimer pathogenesis by genetic analyses demonstrating an earlier age of onset in populations with the ε4 allele of the ApoE gene [88, 89]. ApoE binds sAPP in solution, and the protein encoded by the ε4 allele sequence (ApoE4) appears to have a lower affinity for sAPP [87]. A deletion mutant of sAPP that is diminished in proinflammatory activity is also deficient in binding ApoE. This structural relationship suggests that ApoE may bind at or near amino acid residues involved in proinflammatory stimulation. Consistent with this idea, incubation of sAPP with ApoE lessens its ability to activate microglia, and ApoE4 is less effective in this regard than are other forms of the protein [82].

The physiological relevance of the proinflammatory actions of sAPP is supported by work focusing on endogenously produced sAPP. In one model, medium from neuronal cells cultured under conditions of stress activates microglial cells, and this effect is blocked with anti-APP antibody [90]. Similarly, we found that embyonic neurons cultured from βAPP-transgenic mice released into their medium a proinflammatory activity that could be inhibited by anti-APP antibody or antisense oligonucleotides (Fig. 2). βAPP overexpressed *in vivo* by virally-mediated transfer also induces microglial activation *via* a mechanism exclusive of Aβ deposits [91].

In pursuit of the mechanisms mediating neurotoxicity of activated microglia, we have considered the possibility of excitotoxicity. Microglia exposed to amyloid plaques produce an uncharacterized excitotoxin [92], and Aβ can stimulate glutamate release from monocytes [93]. Microglia activated by sAPP also appears to produce an excitotoxin [94]. Conditioned medium from sAPP-treated microglia specifically causes a large increase in intracellular calcium levels ($[Ca^{2+}]_i$) when applied to hippocampal neurons (Fig. 3A). This $[Ca^{2+}]_i$ elevation is sensitive to a glutamate receptor antagonist. This medium also contains substantial concentrations of glutamate (Fig. 3B). Preliminary studies have shown that NOS inhibitors with specificity for neuronal NOS are more potent than those specific for iNOS at inhibiting the neurotoxicity generated by activated microglia. Neuronal NOS is activated post-translationally by calcium/calmodulin, suggesting that the elevation of neuronal $[Ca^{2+}]_i$ by microglia-produced excitotoxins makes a more important contribution to neurotoxicity than does microglia-produced NO.

Feedforward reactions: inflammatory induction of βAPP expression and processing

Inflammatory reactions include several steps through which negative feedback may be activated to limit the duration and scope of potential harm to host tissues. Destructive inductions of inflammation often involve a perpetual activation or positive feedback that allows the system to reach harmful levels of by-stander damage. Among many other possibilities, inflammatory stimuli can elevate the expression of βAPP. One of the first factors determined to activate the promoter of the βAPP gene was IL-1, which often evokes transcriptional effects through the NF-κB transcription factor. Although there are putative NF-κB binding sites in the βAPP promoter, the only ones analyzed appear to bind a p50 homodimer [17], which is a transcriptional repressor in most systems. This is consistent with data suggesting that the actions of IL-1 on βAPP transcription involve AP-1 and heat-shock elements [27,

Figure 2
Proinflammatory activity in APP-transgenic cultures is dependent upon secretion of sAPP from neuronal cultures. Neuronal cultures were established from the neocortex of mice transgenic for a V^{717} mutant of human βAPP.
(A) APP was detected in unconcentrated conditioned medium from Tg or wildtype cultures when analyzed by western blotting. In one set of cultures, the sAPP was immunodepleted by immunoprecipitation with anti-APP antibody. In another set, expression of βAPP was suppressed with antisense oligonucleotides directed against the βAPP transgene (APP-AS). In the last set, astrocytes were allowed to grow to ~30% of total cells.
(B) Conditioned medium was collected from Tg or wildtype neuronal cultures treated with the various manipulations of sAPP described in (A). The medium then was applied to primary microglial cultures and nitrite levels were measured after 24 h. ($^*p < 0.5$)

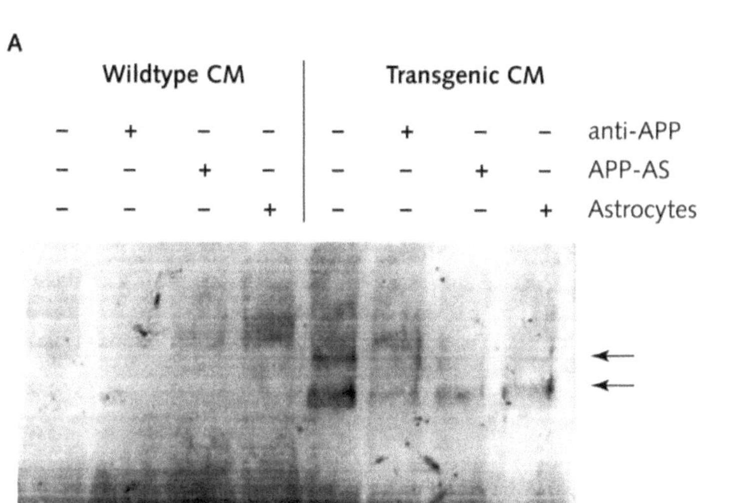
A
Wildtype CM
Transgenic CM
anti-APP
APP-AS
Astrocytes

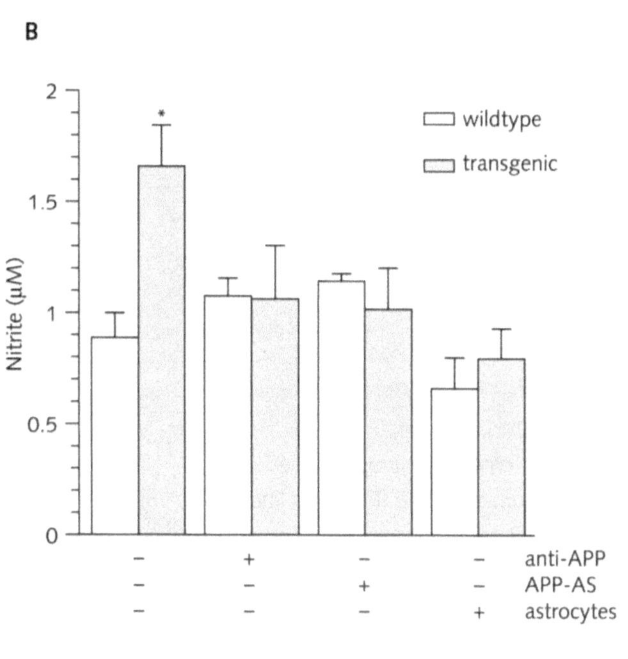
B
Nitrite (μM)
2
1.5
1
0.5
0
wildtype
transgenic
anti-APP
APP-AS
astrocytes

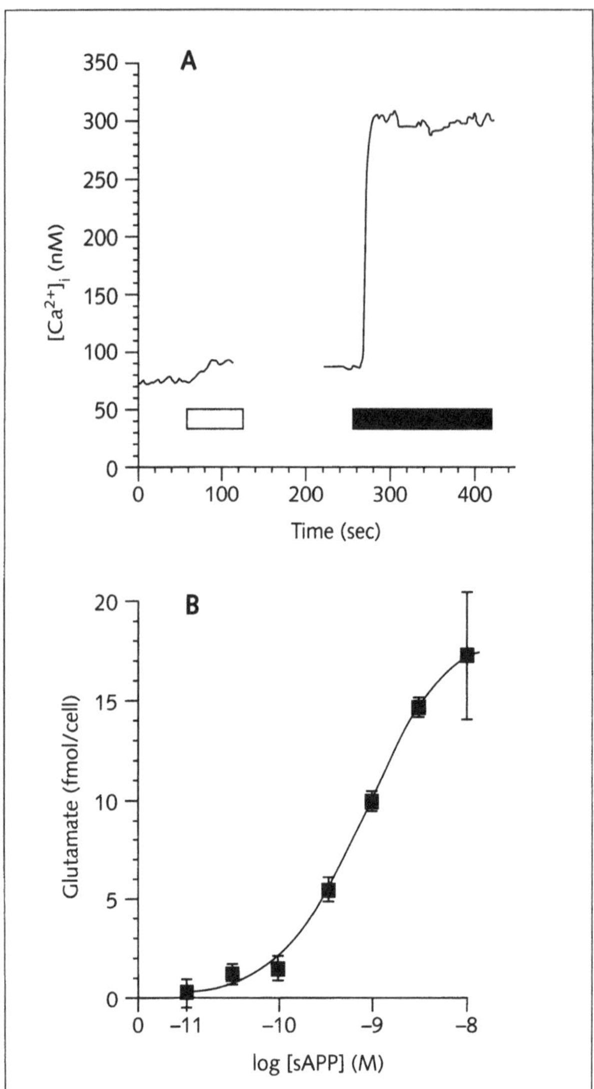

Figure 3
Glutamate release by sAPP-activated microglia.
(A) Intracellular, ionic calcium concentration was monitored in rat primary hippocampal neurons by ratiometric fura-2 microfluorescence. The neurons were exposed to conditioned medium from rat primary microglia (1:25 dilution) that had been incubated for 20 h either alone (open bar) or with 10 nM sAPPβ (filled bar). The break in the trace represents a wash.
(B) Glutamate levels were measured by HPLC in conditioned medium of primary microglia treated for 16 h with the indicated concentrations of sAPPα. Values represent the mean ± SEM for quadruplicate cultures.

95, 96] and that the promoter is unresponsive to reactive oxygen species [96]. Besides these transcriptional regulatory events, IL-1 appears to activate βAPP translation through effects on a sequence in the 5' untranslated region of the βAPP mRNA [22].

In addition to elevating the expression of βAPP, IL-1 can have effects on βAPP processing. While most studies have determined that IL-1 promotes α-secretase processing of βAPP [30, 31], it promotes the generation of potentially amyloidogenic βAPP fragments in endothelial cells [97]. When the total pools of these molecules are considered, Aβ and sAPPα secretion are not strictly reciprocal [31, 97, 98]. Therefore, cytokines may elevate sAPPα release without compromising Aβ production, a scenario that would lead to an even greater degree of inflammatory stimulation.

Conclusions

Aβ and other derivatives of βAPP have been a focus of Alzheimer's disease research for some time due to their connections to the genetics and neuropathology of the disease. Recently, data has accumulated that allows the incorporation of these polypeptides into inflammation-related hypotheses. Activation of microglia and astrocytes by Aβ may reflect initial attempts to clear or confine amyloid deposits. Mounting evidence, however, suggests that the sustained accumulation of these reactive cells can cause damage to neuronal elements. Besides the other common toxins contributing to by-stander damage in the periphery, glutamate and other excitotoxins are likely mediators of glial-mediated neurotoxicity in the CNS. Thus, direct neuromodulatory or neuroprotective strategies may be added to the therapeutic initiatives already focused on suppression of amyloid production/aggregation and dampening of inflammatory responses.

Acknowledgements
Much thanks to Dr. Anthony S. Basile (NIDDK) for HPLC measurements of glutamate. This work was supported by funds from NIH (NS35872) and the Alzheimer's Association (RG1-96-076).

References

1 Hardy J (1997) Amyloid, the presenilins and Alzheimer's disease. *Trends Neurosci* 20: 154–159
2 Konig G, Monning U, Czech C, Prior R, Banati R, Schreiter-Gasser U, Bauer J, Masters CL, Beyreuther K (1992) Identification and differential expression of a novel alternative

splice isoform of the beta A4 amyloid precursor protein (APP) mRNA in leukocytes and brain microglial cells. *J Biol Chem* 267: 10804–10809

3 De Strooper B, Annaert W, Cupers P, Saftig P, Craessaerts K, Mumm JS, Schroeter EH, Schrijvers V, Wolfe MS, Ray WJ et al (1999) A presenilin-1-dependent gamma-secretase-like protease mediates release of Notch intracellular domain. *Nature* 398: 518–522

4 Wolfe MS, Xia W, Ostaszewski BL, Diehl TS, Kimberly WT, Selkoe DJ (1999) Two transmembrane aspartates in presenilin-1 required for presenilin endoproteolysis and gamma-secretase activity. *Nature* 398: 513–517

5 Citron M, Diehl TS, Gordon G, Biere AL, Seubert P, Selkoe DJ (1996) Evidence that the 42- and 40-amino acid forms of amyloid beta protein are generated from the beta-amyloid precursor protein by different protease activities. *Proc Natl Acad Sci USA* 93: 13170–13175

6 Figueiredo-Pereira ME, Efthimiopoulos S, Tezapsidis N, Buku A, Ghiso J, Mehta P, Robakis NK (1999) Distinct secretases, a cysteine protease and a serine protease, generate the C termini of amyloid beta-proteins Abeta1–40 and Abeta1–42, respectively. *J Neurochem* 72: 1417–1422

7 Durkin JT, Murthy S, Husten EJ, Trusko SP, Savage MJ, Rotella DP, Greenberg BD, Siman R (1999) Rank-order of potencies for inhibition of the secretion of abeta40 and abeta42 suggests that both are generated by a single gamma-secretase. *J Biol Chem* 274: 20499–20504

8 Jarrett JT, Berger EP, Lansbury PT, Jr. (1993) The carboxy terminus of the beta amyloid protein is critical for the seeding of amyloid formation: implications for the pathogenesis of Alzheimer's disease. *Biochemistry* 32: 4693–4697

9 Snyder SW, Ladror US, Wade WS, Wang GT, Barrett LW, Matayoshi ED, Huffaker HJ, Krafft GA, Holzman TF (1994) Amyloid-beta aggregation: selective inhibition of aggregation in mixtures of amyloid with different chain lengths. *Biophys J* 67: 1216–1228

10 Selkoe DJ, Yamazaki T, Citron M, Podlisny MB, Koo EH, Teplow DB, Haass C (1996) The role of APP processing and trafficking pathways in the formation of amyloid β-protein. *Ann NY Acad Sci* 777: 57–64

11 Paganetti PA, Lis M, Klafki HW, Staufenbiel M (1996) Amyloid precursor protein truncated at any of the gamma-secretase sites is not cleaved to beta-amyloid. *J Neurosci Res* 46: 283–293

12 Mattson MP (1997) Cellular actions of β-amyloid precursor protein, and its soluble and fibrillogenic peptide derivatives. *Physiol Rev* 77: 1081–1132

13 Nukina N, Kanazawa I, Mannen T, Uchida Y (1992) Accumulation of amyloid precursor protein and beta-protein immunoreactivities in axons injured by cerebral infarct. *Gerontology* 38: 10–14

14 Suenaga T, Ohnishi K, Nishimura M, Nakamura S, Akiguchi I, Kimura J (1994) Bundles of amyloid precursor protein-immunoreactive axons in human cerebrovascular white matter lesions. *Acta Neuropathol* 87: 450–455

15 Blumbergs PC, Scott G, Manavis J, Wainwright H, Simpson DA, McLean AJ (1994)

Staining of amyloid precursor protein to study axonal damage in mild head injury. *Lancet* 344: 1055–1056

16 Sola C, Garcia-Ladona FJ, Mengod G, Probst A, Frey P, Palacios JM (1993) Increased levels of the Kunitz protease inhibitor-containing beta APP mRNAs in rat brain following neurotoxic damage. *Brain Res Mol Brain Res* 17: 41–52

17 Grilli M, Goffi F, Memo M, Spano P (1996) Interleukin-1β and glutamate activate the NF-κB/Rel binding site from the regulatory region of the amyloid precursor protein gene in primary neuronal cultures. *J Biol Chem* 271: 15002–15007

18 Chen ST, Garey LJ, Patel AJ, Malik Q, Jen LS (1998) Factors that affect the expression of β-amyloid precursor protein immunoreactivity in the rat retina. *J Neuropathol Exp Neurol* 57: 16–20

19 Shoji M, Hirai S, Yamaguchi H, Harigaya Y, Kawarabayashi T (1990) Amyloid beta-protein precursor accumulates in dystrophic neurites of senile plaques in Alzheimer-type dementia. *Brain Res* 512: 164–168

20 Joachim C, Games D, Morris J, Ward P, Frenkel D, Selkoe D (1991) Antibodies to non-beta regions of the beta-amyloid precursor protein detect a subset of senile plaques. *Am J Pathol* 138: 373–384

21 Cras P, Kawai M, Lowery D, Gonzalez-DeWhitt P, Greenberg B, Perry G (1991) Senile plaque neurites in Alzheimer disease accumulate amyloid precursor protein. *Proc Natl Acad Sci USA* 88: 7552–7556

22 Rogers JT, Leiter LM, McPhee J, Cahill CM, Zhan SS, Potter H, Nilsson LN (1999) Translation of the Alzheimer amyloid precursor protein mRNA is up-regulated by interleukin-1 through 5'-untranslated region sequences. *J Biol Chem* 274: 6421–6431

23 Koistinaho J, Pyykonen I, Keinanen R, Hokfelt T (1996) Expression of beta-amyloid precursor protein mRNAs following transient focal ischaemia. *Neuroreport* 7: 2727–2731

24 Siman R, Card JP, Nelson RB, Davis LG (1989) Expression of beta-amyloid precursor protein in reactive astrocytes following neuronal damage. *Neuron* 3: 275–285

25 Willoughby DA, Johnson SA, Pasinetti GM, Tocco G, Najm I, Baudry M, Finch CE (1992) Amyloid precursor protein mRNA encoding the Kunitz protease inhibitor domain is increased by kainic acid-induced seizures in rat hippocampus. *Exp Neurol* 118: 332–339

26 Palacios G, Mengod G, Tortosa A, Ferrer I, Palacios JM (1995) Increased beta-amyloid precursor protein expression in astrocytes in the gerbil hippocampus following ischaemia: association with proliferation of astrocytes. *Eur J Neurosci* 7: 501–510

27 Goldgaber D, Harris HW, Hla T, Maciag T, Donnelly RJ, Jacobsen JS, Vitek MP, Gajdusek DC (1989) Interleukin-1 regulates synthesis of amyloid β-protein precursor mRNA in human endothelial cells. *Proc Natl Acad Sci USA* 86: 7606–7610

28 Lahiri DK, Nall C (1995) Promoter activity of the gene encoding the β-amyloid precursor protein is up-regulated by growth factors, phorbol ester, retinoic acid and interleukin-1. Mol *Brain Res* 32: 233–240

29 Ringheim GE, Szczepanik AM, Petko W, Burgher KL, Zhu SZ, Chao CC (1998) En-

hancement of beta-amyloid precursor protein transcription and expression by the soluble interleukin-6 receptor/interleukin-6 complex. *Brain Res* Mol *Brain Res* 55: 35–44

30 Buxbaum JD, Oishi M, Chen HI, Pinkas-Kramarski R, Jaffe EA, Gandy SE, Greengard P (1992) Cholinergic agonists and interleukin 1 regulate processing and secretion of the Alzheimer β/A4 amyloid protein precursor. *Proc Natl Acad Sci USA* 89: 10075–10078

31 Vasilakos JP, Carroll RT, Emmerling MR, Doyle PD, Davis RE, Kim KS, Shivers BD (1994) Interleukin-1β dissociates β-amyloid precursor protein and β-amyloid peptide secretion. *FEBS Lett* 354: 289–292

32 Dash PK, Moore AN (1995) Enhanced processing of APP induced by IL-1 beta can be reduced by indomethacin and nordihydroguaiaretic acid. *Biochem Biophys Res Commun* 208: 542–548

33 Seguchi K, Kataoka H, Uchino H, Nabeshima K, Koono M (1999) Secretion of protease nexin-II/amyloid beta protein precursor by human colorectal carcinoma cells and its modulation by cytokines/growth factors and proteinase inhibitors. *Biol Chem* 380: 473–483

34 Jolly-Tornetta C, Gao ZY, Lee VM, Wolf BA (1998) Regulation of amyloid precursor protein secretion by glutamate receptors in human Ntera 2 neurons. *J Biol Chem* 273: 14015–14021

35 Nitsch RM, Slack BE, Wurtman RJ, Growdon JH (1992) Release of Alzheimer amyloid precursor derivatives stimulated by activation of muscarinic acetylcholine receptors. *Science* 258: 304–307

36 Buxbaum JD, Liu KN, Luo Y, Slack JL, Stocking KL, Peschon JJ, Johnson RS, Castner BJ, Cerretti DP, Black RA (1998) Evidence that tumor necrosis factor alpha converting enzyme is involved in regulated alpha-secretase cleavage of the Alzheimer amyloid protein precursor. *J Biol Chem* 273: 27765–27767

37 Merlos-Suarez A, Fernandez-Larrea J, Reddy P, Baselga J, Arribas J (1998) Pro-tumor necrosis factor-alpha processing activity is tightly controlled by a component that does not affect notch processing. *J Biol Chem* 273: 24955–24962

38 Griffin WS, Sheng JG, Royston MC, Gentleman SM, McKenzie JE, Graham DI, Roberts GW, Mrak RE (1998) Glial-neuronal interactions in Alzheimer's disease: the potential role of a 'cytokine cycle' in disease progression. *Brain Pathol* 8: 65–72

39 Salinero O, Moreno-Flores MT, Ceballos ML, Wandosell F (1997) beta-Amyloid peptide induced cytoskeletal reorganization in cultured astrocytes. *J Neurosci Res* 47: 216–223

40 Hu J, Akama KT, Krafft GA, Chromy BA, Van Eldik LJ (1998) Amyloid-beta peptide activates cultured astrocytes: morphological alterations, cytokine induction and nitric oxide release. *Brain Res* 785: 195–206

41 Meske V, Hamker U, Albert F, Ohm TG (1998) The effects of beta/A4-amyloid and its fragments on calcium homeostasis, glial fibrillary acidic protein and S100beta staining, morphology and survival of cultured hippocampal astrocytes. *Neuroscience* 85: 1151–1160

42 Pike CJ, Cummings BJ, Monzavi R, Cotman CW (1994) Beta-amyloid-induced changes

in cultured astrocytes parallel reactive astrocytosis associated with senile plaques in Alzheimer's disease. *Neuroscience* 63: 517–531
43 Murphy GM, Jr., Yang L, Cordell B (1998) Macrophage colony-stimulating factor augments beta-amyloid-induced interleukin-1, interleukin-6, and nitric oxide production by microglial cells. *J Biol Chem* 273: 20967–20971
44 Parpura-Gill A, Beitz D, Uemura E (1997) The inhibitory effects of beta-amyloid on glutamate and glucose uptakes by cultured astrocytes. *Brain Res* 754: 65–71
45 Abe K, Saito H (1998) Amyloid beta protein inhibits cellular MTT reduction not by suppression of mitochondrial succinate dehydrogenase but by acceleration of MTT formazan exocytosis in cultured rat cortical astrocytes. *Neurosci Res* 31: 295–305
46 Meda L, Cassatella MA, Szendrei GI, Otvos L Jr., Baron P, Villalba M, Ferrari D, Rossi F (1995) Activation of microglial cells by β-amyloid protein and interferon-γ. *Nature* 374: 647–650
47 Gitter BD, Cox LM, Rydel RE, May PC (1995) Amyloid β peptide potentiates cytokine secretion by interleukin-1β-activated human astrocytoma cells. *Proc Natl Acad Sci USA* 92 (23): 10738–10741
48 Rossi F, Bianchini E (1996) Synergistic induction of nitric oxide by β-amyloid and cytokines in astrocytes. *Biochem Biophys Res Commun* 225: 474–478
49 Haga S, Ikeda K, Sato M, Ishii T (1993) Synthetic Alzheimer amyloid beta/A4 peptides enhance production of complement C3 component by cultured microglial cells. *Brain Res* 601: 88–94
50 McDonald DR, Brunden KR, Landreth GE (1997) Amyloid fibrils activate tyrosine kinase-dependent signaling and superoxide production in microglia. *J Neurosci* 17: 2284–2294
51 Van Muiswinkel FL, Raupp SF, de Vos NM, Smits HA, Verhoef J, Eikelenboom P, Nottet HS (1999) The amino-terminus of the amyloid-beta protein is critical for the cellular binding and consequent activation of the respiratory burst of human macrophages. *J Neuroimmunol* 96: 121–130
52 Noda M, Nakanishi H, Akaike N (1999) Glutamate release from microglia *via* glutamate transporter is enhanced by amyloid-beta peptide. *Neuroscience* 92: 1465–1474
53 Pike CJ, Burdick D, Walencewicz AJ, Glabe CG, Cotman CW (1993) Neurodegeneration induced by β-amyloid peptides *in vitro*: the role of peptide assembly state. *J Neurosci* 13: 1676–1687
54 Yankner BA, Duffy LK, Kirschner DA (1990) Neurotrophic and neurotoxic effects of amyloid beta protein: reversal by tachykinin neuropeptides. *Science* 250: 279–282
55 Giulian D, Haverkamp LJ, Yu JH, Karshin W, Tom D, Li J, Kirkpatrick J, Kuo LM, Roher AE (1996) Specific domains of beta-amyloid from Alzheimer plaque elicit neuron killing in human microglia. *J Neurosci* 16: 6021–6037
56 Velazquez P, Cribbs DH, Poulos TL, Tenner AJ (1997) Aspartate residue 7 in amyloid beta-protein is critical for classical complement pathway activation: implications for Alzheimer's disease pathogenesis. *Nat Med* 3: 77–79

57 Webster S, Bonnell B, Rogers J (1997) Charge-based binding of complement component C1q to the Alzheimer amyloid beta-peptide. *Am J Pathol* 150: 1531–1536
58 Lalowski M, Golabek A, Lemere CA, Selkoe DJ, Wisniewski HM, Beavis RC, Frangione B, Wisniewski T (1996) The "nonamyloidogenic" p3 fragment (amyloid beta17-42) is a major constituent of Down's syndrome cerebellar preamyloid. *J Biol Chem* 271: 33623–33631
59 Kida E, Wisniewski KE, Wisniewski HM (1995) Early amyloid-β deposits show different immunoreactivity to the amino- and carboxy-terminal regions of β-peptide in Alzheimer's disease and Down's syndrome brain. *Neurosci Lett* 193: 105–108
60 Pike CJ, Overman MJ, Cotman CW (1995) Amino-terminal deletions enhance aggregation of β-amyloid peptides *in vitro*. *J Biol Chem* 270: 23895–23898
61 Yan SD, Chen X, Fu J, Chen M, Zhu H, Roher A, Slattery T, Zhao L, Nagashima M, Morser J et al (1996) RAGE and amyloid-β peptide neurotoxicity in Alzheimer's disease. *Nature* 382: 685–691
62 El Khoury J, Hickman SE, Thomas CA, Cao L, Silverstein SC, Loike JD (1996) Scavenger receptor-mediated adhesion of microglia to β-amyloid fibrils. *Nature* 382: 716–719
63 McDonald DR, Bamberger ME, Combs CK, Landreth GE (1998) beta-Amyloid fibrils activate parallel mitogen-activated protein kinase pathways in microglia and THP1 monocytes. *J Neurosci* 18: 4451–4460
64 Huang F, Buttini M, Wyss-Coray T, McConlogue L, Kodama T, Pitas RE, Mucke L (1999) Elimination of the class A scavenger receptor does not affect amyloid plaque formation or neurodegeneration in transgenic mice expressing human amyloid protein precursors. *Am J Pathol* 155: 1741–1747
65 Du Yan S, Zhu H, Fu J, Yan S, Roher A, Tourtellotte WW, Rahavashisth T, Chen X, Godman GC, Stern D et al (1997) Amyloid-β peptide-receptor for advanced glycation endproduct interaction elicits neuronal expression of macrophage-colony stimulating factor: a proinflammatory pathway in Alzheimer disease. *Proc Natl Acad Sci USA* 94: 5296–5301
66 Tan J, Town T, Paris D, Suo Z, Song S, Yu H, Kundtz A, Crawford F, Mullan M (1998) Ligation of a specific CD molecule initiates activation of microglial cells by Alzheimer's β-amyloid peptides. *Soc Neurosci Abstr* 24: 1752
67 Tan J, Town T, Paris D, Mori T, Suo Z, Crawford F, Mattson MP, Flavell RA, Mullan M (1999) Microglial activation resulting from CD40-CD40L interaction after β-amyloid stimulation. *Science* 286: 2352–2355
68 Pyo H, Jou I, Jung S, Hong S, Joe EH (1998) Mitogen-activated protein kinases activated by lipopolysaccharide and beta-amyloid in cultured rat microglia. *Neuroreport* 9: 871–874
69 Combs CK, Johnson DE, Cannady SB, Lehman TM, Landreth GE (1999) Identification of microglial signal transduction pathways mediating a neurotoxic response to amyloidogenic fragments of beta-amyloid and prion proteins. *J Neurosci* 19: 928–939
70 Lander HM, Tauras JM, Ogiste JS, Hori O, Moss RA, Schmidt AM (1997) Activation

of the receptor for advanced glycation end products triggers a p21(ras)-dependent mitogen-activated protein kinase pathway regulated by oxidant stress. *J Biol Chem* 272: 17810–17814
71 Nakai M, Hojo K, Taniguchi T, Terashima A, Kawamata T, Hashimoto T, Maeda K, Tanaka C (1998) PKC and tyrosine kinase involvement in amyloid beta (25-35)-induced chemotaxis of microglia. *Neuroreport* 9: 3467–3470
72 Salinero O, Moreno-Flores MT, Wandosell F (1997) Okadaic acid modulates the cytoskeleton changes induced by amyloid peptide (25-35) in cultured astrocytes. *Neuroreport* 8: 3333–3338
73 Ard MD, Cole GM, Wei J, Mehrle AP, Fratkin JD (1996) Scavenging of Alzheimer's amyloid beta-protein by microglia in culture. *J Neurosci Res* 43: 190–202
74 Kopec KK, Carroll RT (1998) Alzheimer's beta-amyloid peptide 1–42 induces a phagocytic response in murine microglia. *J Neurochem* 71: 2123–2131
75 Cruz L, Urbanc B, Buldyrev SV, Christie R, Gomez-Isla T, Havlin S, McNamara M, Stanley HE, Hyman BT (1997) Aggregation and disaggregation of senile plaques in Alzheimer disease. *Proc Natl Acad Sci USA* 94: 7612–7616
76 Schenk D, Barbour R, Dunn W, Gordon G, Grajeda H, Guido T, Hu K, Huang J, Johnson-Wood K, Khan K et al (1999) Immunization with amyloid-beta attenuates Alzheimer-disease-like pathology in the PDAPP mouse. *Nature* 400: 173–177
77 Hoke A, Canning DR, Malemud CJ, Silver J (1994) Regional differences in reactive gliosis induced by substrate-bound beta-amyloid. *Exp Neurol* 130: 56–66
78 Shaffer LM, Dority MD, Gupta-Bansal R, Frederickson RC, Younkin SG, Brunden KR (1995) Amyloid β protein (Aβ) removal by neuroglial cells in culture. *Neurobiol Aging* 16: 737–745
79 Qiu WQ, Walsh DM, Ye Z, Vekrellis K, Zhang J, Podlisny MB, Rosner MR, Safavi A, Hersh LB, Selkoe DJ (1998) Insulin-degrading enzyme regulates extracellular levels of amyloid beta-protein by degradation. *J Biol Chem* 273: 32730–32738
80 Snow AD, Mar H, Nochlin D, Kimata K, Kato M, Suzuki S, Hassell J, Wight TN (1988) The presence of heparan sulfate proteoglycans in the neuritic plaques and congophilic angiopathy in Alzheimer's disease. *Am J Pathol* 133: 456–463
81 Barger SW, Mattson MP (1996) Induction of neuroprotective κB-dependent transcription by secreted form of the Alzheimer's β-amyloid precursor. *Mol Brain Res* 40: 116–126
82 Barger SW, Harmon AD (1997) Microglial activation by secreted Alzheimer amyloid precursor protein and modulation by apolipoprotein E. *Nature* 388: 878–881
83 Furukawa K, Sopher BL, Rydel RE, Begley JG, Pham DG, Martin GM, Fox M, Mattson MP (1996) Increased activity-regulating and neuroprotective efficacy of α-secretase-derived secreted amyloid precursor protein conferred by a c-terminal heparin-binding domain. *J Neurochem* 67: 1882–1896
84 Van Nostrand WE, Wagner SL, Shankle WR, Farrow JS, Dick M, Rozemuller JM, Kuiper MA, Wolters EC, Zimmerman J, Cotman CW (1992) Decreased levels of solu-

ble amyloid β-protein precursor in cerebrospinal fluid of live Alzheimer disease patients. *Proc Natl Acad Sci USA* 89: 2551–2555

85 Griffin WS, Sheng JG, Roberts GW, Mrak RE (1995) Interleukin-1 expression in different plaque types in Alzheimer's disease: significance in plaque evolution. *J Neuropathol Exp Neurol* 54: 276–281

86 Ancolio K, Dumanchin C, Barelli H, Warter JM, Brice A, Campion D, Frebourg T, Checler F (1999) Unusual phenotypic alteration of β amyloid precursor protein (βAPP) maturation by a new Val-715 → Met βAPP-770 mutation responsible for probable early-onset Alzheimer's disease. *Proc Natl Acad Sci USA* 96: 4119–4124

87 Barger SW, Mattson MP (1997) Isoform-specific modulation by apolipoprotein E of the activities of secreted β-amyloid precursor protein. *J Neurochem* 69: 60–67

88 Roses AD (1996) Apolipoprotein E alleles as risk factors in Alzheimers disease. *Annu Rev Med* 47: 387–400

89 Meyer MR, Tschanz JT, Norton MC, Welsh-Bohmer KA, Steffens DC, Wyse BW, Breitner JC (1998) APOE genotype predicts when – not whether – one is predisposed to develop Alzheimer disease. *Nat Genet* 19: 321–322

90 Li Y, Liu L, Kang J, Sheng JG, Barger SW, Mrak RE, Griffin WST (2000) Neuronal-glial interactions mediated by interleukin-1 enhance neuronal acetylcholinesterase activity and mRNA expression. *J Neurosci* 20: 149–155

91 Nishimura I, Uetsuki T, Dani SU, Ohsawa Y, Saito I, Okamura H, Uchiyama Y, Yoshikawa K (1998) Degeneration *in vivo* of rat hippocampal neurons by wild-type Alzheimer amyloid precursor protein overexpressed by adenovirus-mediated gene transfer. *J Neurosci* 18: 2387–2398

92 Giulian D, Haverkamp LJ, Li J, Karshin WL, Yu J, Tom D, Li X, Kirkpatrick JB (1995) Senile plaques stimulate microglia to release a neurotoxin found in Alzheimer brain. *Neurochem Int* 27: 119–137

93 Klegeris A, McGeer PL (1997) β-amyloid protein enhances macrophage production of oxygen free radicals and glutamate. *J Neurosci Res* 49: 229–235

94 Barger SW, Basile AS (2001) Activation of microglia by secreted amyloid precursor protein evokes release of glutamate by cystine exchange. *J Neurochem* 78: 846–854

95 Donnelly RJ, Friedhoff AJ, Beer B, Blume AJ, Vitek MP (1990) Interleukin-1 stimulates the beta-amyloid precursor protein promoter. *Cell Mol Neurobiol* 10: 485–495

96 Yang Y, Quitschke WW, Brewer GJ (1998) Upregulation of amyloid precursor protein gene promoter in rat primary hippocampal neurons by phorbol ester, IL-1 and retinoic acid, but not by reactive oxygen species. *Brain Res Mol Brain Res* 60: 40–49

97 Schmitt TL, Steiner E, Klinger P, Sztankay A, Grubeck-Loebenstein B (1996) The production of an amyloidogenic metabolite of the Alzheimer amyloid beta precursor protein (APP) in thyroid cells is stimulated by interleukin 1 beta, but inhibited by interferon gamma. *J Clin Endocrinol Metab* 81: 1666–1669

98 Dyrks T, Monning U, Beyreuther K, Turner J (1994) Amyloid precursor protein secretion and beta A4 amyloid generation are not mutually exclusive. *FEBS Lett* 349: 210–214

The involvement of glial cell-derived reactive oxygen and nitrogen species in Alzheimer's disease

Douglas G. Walker[1], *Lih-Fen Lue*[1], *Andis Klegeris*[2] *and Patrick L. McGeer*[2]

[1]Sun Health Research Institute, 10515 West Santa Fe Drive, Sun City, AZ 85351, USA; [2]Kinsmen Laboratory of Neurological Research, University of British Columbia, 2255 Wesbrook Mall, Vancouver, B.C., V6T 1Z3 Canada

Introduction

Alzheimer's disease (AD) is a neurodegenerative disorder characterized by adult-onset progressive dementia and mainly affects the elderly. Pathologically, the brains of AD patients are characterized by the presence of neurofibrillary tangles (NFTs), amyloid β peptide (Aβ)-containing senile plaques (SPs) and synaptic and neuronal cell loss. Most research on AD has focused on the mechanisms that result in the formation of these insoluble NFTs and SPs [1, 2]. NFTs represent the insoluble filamentous remnants of the cytoskeleton of affected neurons, with a major component being phosphorylated forms of the microtubule-associated protein tau. SPs primarily contain aggregated Aβ peptide fragments derived from the amyloid precursor protein (APP). In AD brains, both SPs and NFTs, as well as vulnerable neurons, have been shown to undergo a number of modifications indicative of ongoing oxidative stress [3–12].

A central feature of this article is an examination of the mechanisms and consequences of excess free radical production. A free radical is a molecule that contains one or more unpaired electrons. An unpaired electron is one that is alone in an orbital. The energy to pair electrons confers a high degree of reactivity to free radicals. They oxidize nearby molecules by stripping electrons. This can be very damaging to proteins, lipids and DNA [14]. There are two main potential sources of toxic free radical production. Firstly, increased amounts of reactive oxygen species can be produced by any cell type, including neurons, as a result of impaired electron transport chain functioning during mitochondrial oxidative metabolism. Secondly, phagocytic cells (neutrophils and monocytes/macrophages) can produce large amounts of reactive oxygen species as a result of activation of their NADPH oxidase complex. Different biochemical pathways result in the formation of reactive oxygen species, but all could lead to the presence of similar modifications in tissue samples. It should be noted that reactive oxygen species can also be produced by different cells as a result of the action of cyclooxygenases, lipoxygenases, xanthine oxidase, certain microsomal enzymes, and from the conversion of catecholamines and

Neuroinflammatory Mechanisms in Alzheimer's Disease: Basic and Clinical Research,
edited by Joseph Rogers

indolamines by monoamine oxidase or from the non-enzymatic auto-oxidation of catecholamines [15]. These latter pathways will not be considered in this article. The production of excess reactive nitrogen species by glial cells and their reaction with cellular structures will be considered as a form of oxidative stress.

Oxidative stress and neurodegeneration

There have been a number of reviews that have considered the role of oxidative stress in AD [4, 6, 14, 16–21] and other neurodegenerative diseases, including Parkinson's disease (PD) [23, 24], Down's syndrome (DS), Huntington's disease [25], AIDS dementia [26], stroke [27] and amyotrophic lateral sclerosis [28, 29]. In relation to AD, the emphasis of much recent research has been on the types of oxidative stress that the Aβ peptide might be inducing on vulnerable neurons [30–36]. Also, there have been a number of reports describing the presence of chemical modifications in AD brain tissues, which are indicative of oxidative stress [3–13]. The major focus of this article will be a consideration of the evidence that activated glial cells may be producing increased amounts of reactive oxygen and nitrogen species and that these could be causing some of the pathology in the AD brain.

Inflammation and Alzheimer's disease

There is evidence that a chronic inflammatory state exists in the AD-affected brain. As there have been a number of review articles documenting the reactive microglia and astrocyte responses, and other inflammatory-associated reactions occurring in the AD brain, the nature of these changes will not be reiterated in this article [37–40]. Activated glial cells, especially microglia, have been shown *in vitro* to express a large array of potentially damaging products, including reactive oxygen and nitrogen species [41–44]. Although it has not been possible to directly demonstrate that glial-derived reactive oxygen and nitrogen species are causing damage in AD brains, cumulative data have shown that activated glia appear to contribute to the pathogenic processes in AD.

Sources of reactive oxygen species in cells and tissues

The brain is particularly susceptible to oxidative stress due to its high content of unsaturated lipids, high rate of oxygen consumption, relative shortage of antioxidant enzymes compared to other tissues, and the high overall concentration of catalytic iron [14, 18]. Reactive oxygen species are produced by mitochondria as a consequence of normal oxidative metabolism. The cell can detoxify free radicals *via* its antioxidant defense system. This system includes the enzymes superoxide dismutase, glutathione peroxidase, glutathione reductase and catalase. However, it has been shown that the brain is relatively deficient in these antioxidant enzymes compared to other tissues [4, 14]. If the mitochondrial electron transport chain becomes impaired with aging, either for genetic or environmental reasons (accumulation of toxins or Aβ peptide), gradually increasing cycles of oxidative damage may accumulate, resulting in the damage and death of neurons [14]. The pathways involved in reactive oxygen species production by mitochondria are shown in Figure 1. Impaired electron transport chain function also leads to decreased ATP production resulting in an energy deficit. Elevated reactive oxygen species can also lead to cell membrane compromise, chromosomal damage, abnormal gene transcription, and the induction of apoptosis or necrosis. Much work over recent years in this area has been carried out by Mattson and colleagues, and Behl and colleagues, who have identified mechanisms of oxidative stress induced *in vitro* by Aβ peptide on neurons [22, 31, 35, 45–51] and by Smith, Perry and colleagues who have extensively characterized types of oxidative modifications that are found in AD-affected brain tissue [7–9, 11–13, 52–58]. In particular, these latter authors were prominent in characterizing the contribution that advanced glycation endproducts, one of the hallmarks of oxidative stress, may have to AD pathology [57, 58].

Characterization of oxidative damage in brain

Oxygen free radicals can be very damaging to cells, causing the oxidation of essential cellular constituents including proteins, lipids and DNA. Such oxidation can also result in protein cross-linking, which has been identified in both Aβ plaques and NFTs [59, 60]. DNA oxidation can result in strand breakage, which has been detected in increased amounts in brain cells in AD cases [61]. Markers for some of these reactions can be detected *in vivo* by analysis for malondialdehyde [4, 13], 8-hydroxy-deoxyguanosine [8], 4-hydroxynonenal [5, 7, 62, 63], nitrotyrosine [3, 56, 64] and advanced glycation endproducts [57, 58, 60, 65, 66]. Increased amounts of these products have been detected chemically or by demonstrating increased immunoreactivity in the characteristic AD lesions.

Could the oxidative stress occurring in AD be caused by activated microglia?

The markers of oxidative damage found in AD brains could be caused by excess free radicals produced from any of the sources mentioned including activated microglia and astrocytes. Most of the data suggesting that phagocytic cells contribute to oxidative tissue damage in AD tissue have come indirectly from *in vitro* studies. Pos-

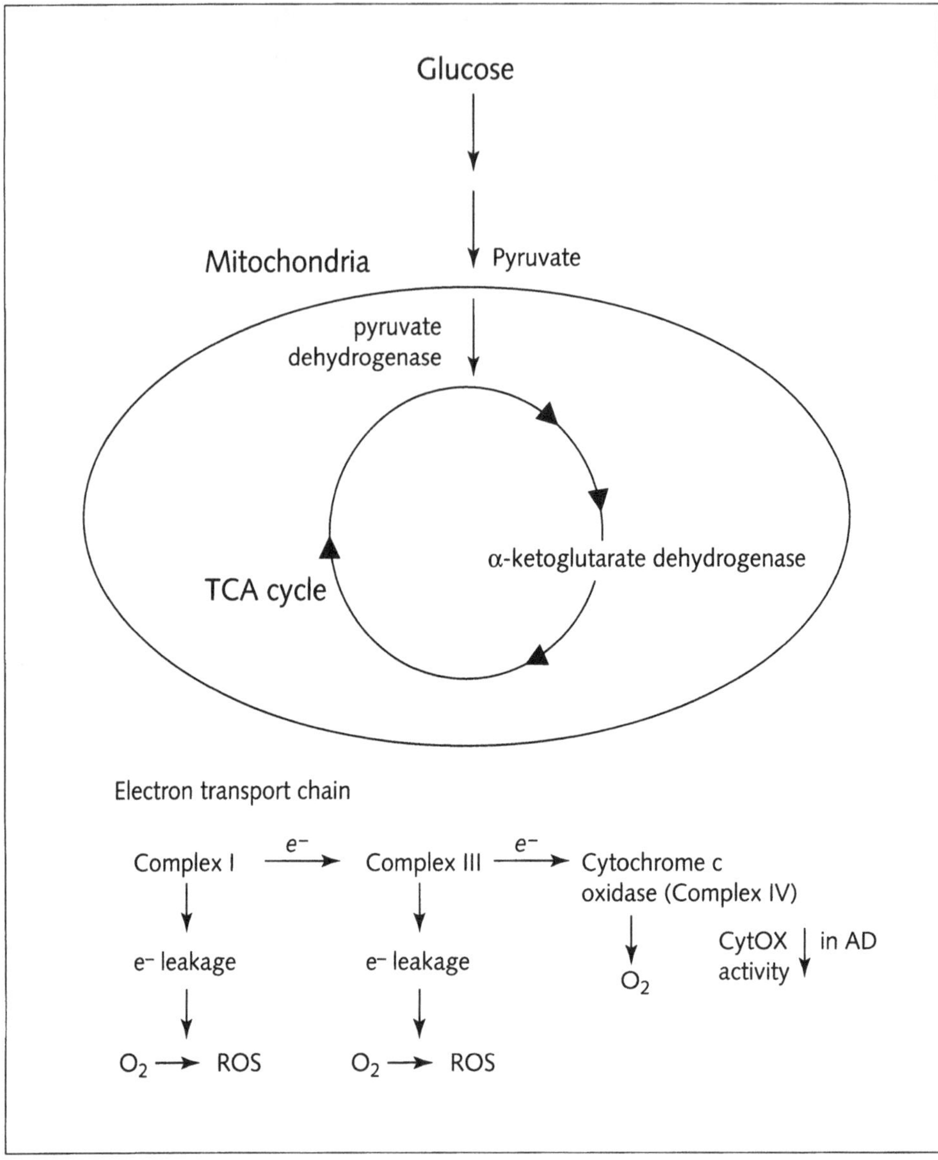

Figure 1
Pathway of oxidative metabolism indicating stages of mitochondrial free radical generation
Diagram summarizing the main pathway for energy metabolism and the stages in the process where free radicals can be generated. Two key rate limiting enzymes in the process are shown (pyruvate dehydrogenase and α-ketoglutarate dehydrogenase). A decrease in α-ketoglutarate dehydrogenase activity has been demonstrated in AD brains. Leakage of electrons (e^-) occurs in this process in all cells, but increases with aging and in AD because of decreased cytochrome c oxidase activity.

session of the components of the NADPH oxidase complex is a feature of professional phagocytic cells (macrophages/microglia and neutrophils) [67, 68]. Formation of an active NADPH oxidase results in the production of superoxide ($O_2^{-\cdot}$) by the reduction of oxygen using NADPH as the electron donor. This reaction is shown in Figure 2A. A diagrammatic scheme of the components and mechanism of activation of the NADPH oxidase complex is shown in Figure 2B. The major pathways for the metabolism and detoxification of superoxide is shown in Figure 3 (reactive oxygen pathways) with the essential components being superoxide dismutase (SOD) and catalase. Also involved in this process are glutathione (GSH) and glutathione peroxidase (GSHPx). Activation of the components of the NADPH oxidase complex to form a functional enzyme is a relatively rapid process and is not dependent on the synthesis of new proteins. The consequence of activation of this complex, namely the rapid production of superoxide radicals, has been designated the "respiratory burst" of phagocytic cells. Superoxide and other oxygen radicals are highly effective at killing invading microorganisms. Individuals with genetic defects in this pathway, characterized as chronic granulomatous disease, are prone to recurrent bacterial infections [69].

The core components of the NADPH oxidase complex are five proteins designated $p40^{PHOX}$, $p47^{PHOX}$, $p67^{PHOX}$, $p22^{PHOX}$ and $gp91^{PHOX}$. The $p22^{PHOX}$ and $gp91^{PHOX}$ cells exist as a dimeric flavohemoprotein known as cytochrome b_{558} in membranes, while in resting cells the $p40^{PHOX}$, $p47^{PHOX}$ and $p67^{PHOX}$ components exists in the cytosol as a complex. Upon activation by a wide range of stimuli that include Aβ peptides, opsonized zymosan and complement C3bi fragment, the $p47^{PHOX}$ becomes highly phosphorylated. As a result of this, the complex migrates to the membrane where it forms the active NADPH oxidase after association with cytochrome b_{558}. The critical step in this process is the transportation of the cytosolic complex, which is dependent on the phosphorylation of $p47^{PHOX}$ [70]. Although indispensable in the NADPH oxidase complex, the function of $p67^{PHOX}$ is still unresolved but is believed to be involved in electron transport [67]. The $p40^{PHOX}$ subunit appears to have an inhibitory role in the oxidase activating system [67]. The surface locale from which superoxide radicals are released into the extracellular space is still uncertain. Colocalization of $p47^{PHOX}/p67^{PHOX}$ with flavocytochrome b_{558} was found to be restricted to the phagosomal membrane and not intracellular granules [68].

Inappropriate activation of phagocyte NADPH oxidase has the potential to do damage to healthy tissue. The following experimental evidence suggests that this process could be involved in neurodegenerative diseases such as AD. Using rat peritoneal macrophages, we demonstrated that the Aβ peptide could directly activate the NADPH oxidase complex [71]. Addition of Aβ peptide 1–40 or the neurotoxic Aβ peptide subfragment 25–35 caused a significant increase in oxygen consumption and luminol-dependent chemiluminescence in treated cells. In a follow-up study, where the production of superoxide was directly measured using the cytochrome c

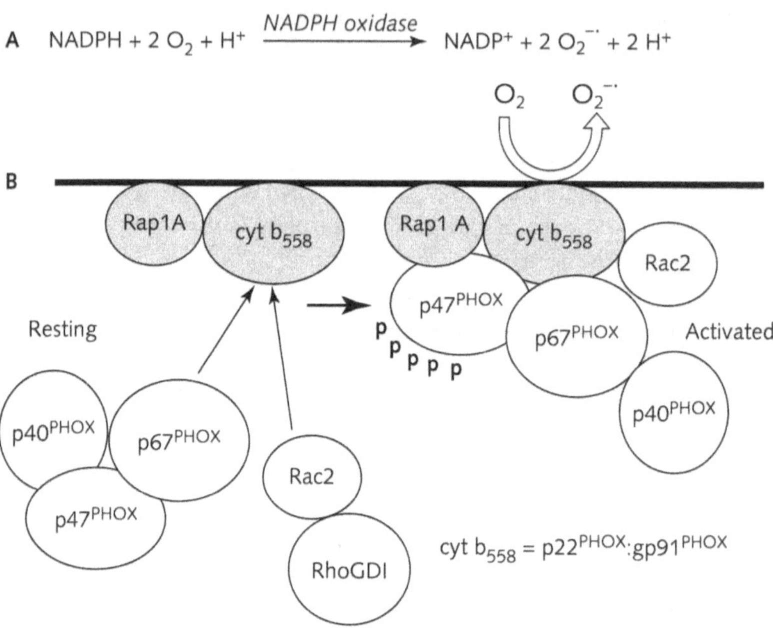

Figure 2
Schematic diagram showing the features of NADPH oxidase activation.
(A) Reaction catalyzed by NADPH oxidase.
(B) Schematic diagram showing the key features of the activation of microglial NADPH oxidase. In the resting state, the $p67^{PHOX}$, $p47^{PHOX}$, $p40^{PHOX}$ and rac2 components are present in the cytosol, whereas $gp91^{PHOX}$ and $p22^{PHOX}$ (cytochrome b_{558}) are on the membranes. Activation results in the phosphorylation of $p47^{PHOX}$ which brings about the cytosolic components binding on the membrane with cytochrome b_{558} and forming active NADPH oxidase.

reduction assay, these earlier results were confirmed [72]. Also, it was shown that pretreatment of rat peritoneal macrophages with these Aβ peptides significantly increased the amount of NADPH oxidase activation in cells subsequently treated with the protein kinase C activator phorbol myristate acetate (PMA) [72]. This indicated that the Aβ peptides were able to prime the respiratory burst response of the macrophages. Similarly, it was demonstrated using the cytochrome c reduction assay that $A\beta_{1-40}$ treatment of rodent microglia could enhance (prime) the production of superoxide induced by PMA [73]. These authors have since shown that activation of the NADPH oxidase complex in human macrophages involves the binding of Aβ peptide subfragment (amino acids 1–16) to these cells. It was shown that $A\beta_{1-16}$ did

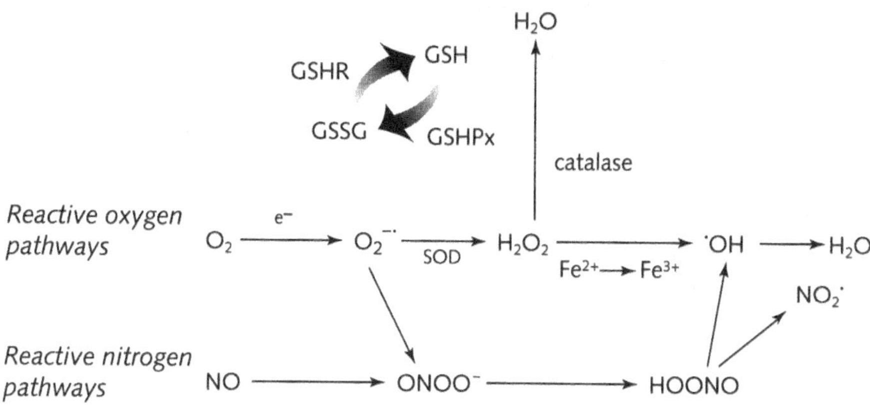

Figure 3
Key pathways of reactive oxygen and nitrogen generation, interaction and metabolism. O_2^-, superoxide; SOD, superoxide dismutase: OH˙, hydroxyl radical; NO, nitric oxide; $ONOO^-$, peroxynitrite anion; H_2O_2, hydrogen peroxide; HOONO, peroxynitrite; NO_2˙, nitrogen dioxide; GSSG, oxidized glutathione; GSH, reduced glutathione; GSHPx, glutathione peroxidase.

not cause the activation of NADPH oxidase, but did block the activation caused by $A\beta_{1-42}$ [74]. Interestingly, this observation is similar to the findings of Giulian who showed that the Aβ region 11–16 was required for microglia to produce a small molecule neurotoxin in response to full length $A\beta_{1-40}$ or $_{1-42}$ [75]. In the earlier report [74], it was clearly shown that $A\beta_{25-35}$ was not effective in inducing NADPH oxidase activation. This finding is in conflict with several other studies [71, 76, 77]. Increased superoxide production and tyrosine kinase activity were observed in human THP-1 monocytes and rat microglia after treatment with either $A\beta_{1-42}$ or Aβ subfragment 25–35 [76]. In addition, in a recent study it was shown that $A\beta_{25-35}$ was as effective as $A\beta_{1-42}$ in activating the respiratory burst in rodent microglia and human monocytes and neutrophils [77]. Two important sets of experiments were carried out by these authors to show that the increased production of superoxide was due to activation of NADPH oxidase and not due to one of the other pathways. Firstly, they demonstrated that there was translocation of the $p67^{PHOX}$, $p47^{PHOX}$ and $p40^{PHOX}$ proteins to the cell membrane after the cells were treated with Aβ. Secondly, these authors failed to observe the Aβ activation effect with neutrophils and monocytes derived from chronic granulomatous disease patients. These patients had genetic defects in the cytochrome b_{558} component or the $p47^{PHOX}$ of the NADPH oxidase complex [77]. NADPH oxidase activation induced by Aβ peptides was considerably potentiated if the cells were primed by pretreatment with either interferon-γ (IFNγ) or tumor necrosis factor-α (TNFα). These authors have suggested that the enhanced respiratory burst that was observed by pretreatment of phagocytic cells with these cytokines for 4–5 days was due to the synthesis of increased amounts of the NADPH oxidase components [77, 78]. Inhibition of NADPH oxidase activity was observed in cells treated with a src-tyrosine kinase inhibitor, a phosphatidylinositol-3 kinase inhibitor or dibutyryl cyclic AMP. This is in agreement with another report [76]. Inhibition of NADPH oxidase activation has also been observed in human monocytes treated with vitamin E (α-tocopherol) [80]. This effect was partly due to attenuation of $p47^{PHOX}$ phosphorylation and membrane translocation, and appeared independent from its action as a free radical scavenger [80]. We showed that rat brain microglia and peritoneal macrophages demonstrated similar NADPH-dependent respiratory burst responses to different activation stimuli [81].

As mentioned previously, the activation of the NADPH oxidase complex is not dependent on new cellular protein synthesis. All resting phagocytic cells have the potential to produce an NADPH-oxidase mediated respiratory response if a suitable agent activates them. Direct demonstration of microglial superoxide production in such tissue is unlikely to be possible due to the short-lived nature of these reactive oxygen species. Experiments were carried out to characterize $p47^{PHOX}$ protein expression in human brain microglia by immunoblot analysis. A representative western blot is shown in Figure 4. This demonstrated that there was no increase in $p47^{PHOX}$ protein expression in human microglia stimulated for 24 h with $A\beta_{1-42}$ peptide. It was also demonstrated that there was an approximately four-fold greater amount of $p47^{PHOX}$ present in human microglia (Fig. 4, lanes 1 and 2) compared to THP-1 monocyte/macrophage cells. Equivalent amounts of protein were applied to each lane on the immunoblot. This result does not tend to agree with the finding of Meda et al. [78] who reported a two-fold increase in $p47^{PHOX}$ protein in monocytes (not microglia) that were stimulated with $A\beta_{25-35}$ (not $A\beta_{1-42}$). Western blots of microglia lysates demonstrated that both the $gp91^{PHOX}$ and $p22^{PHOX}$ NADPH oxidase subunits are present in unstimulated and stimulated microglia [82]. It was recently demonstrated that there were significantly increased levels of membrane-associated $p47^{PHOX}$ and $p67^{PHOX}$ in AD brain extracts compared to ND brain extracts. This was interpreted as evidence for increased and persistent activation of the microglial NADPH oxidase complex in AD brains [140]. Enhanced expression of $p22^{PHOX}$ has also been identified in AD brain tissue [83]. There have been no reports to date on the localization of the NADPH oxidase complex components at the cellular level in AD brain tissues.

Although it is not possible to directly observe activation of NADPH oxidase in microglia in AD brain tissue, there has been extensive demonstration of the presence of activated microglia in AD brains [84–86]. These cells have generally been characterized by the demonstration of increased expression of the major histocompati-

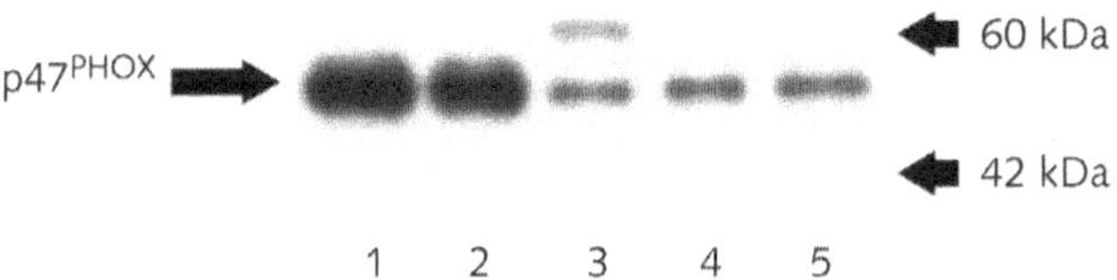

Figure 4
Comparison of $p47^{PHOX}$ expression in human microglia and THP-1 monocyte/macrophages. Immunoblot showing relative amounts of $p47^{PHOX}$. Lane 1) Unstimulated human post-mortem brain-derived microglia; lane 2) Aβ-stimulated (10 μM/24 h) human brain microglia; lane 3) THP-1 monocytes; lane 4) unstimulated THP-1 macrophages; lane 5) IFNγ stimulated THP-1 macrophages. Each lane contained 20 μg of cellular protein. Aβ-stimulation did not increase $p47^{PHOX}$ protein levels in microglia.

bility complex protein HLA-DR [87]. These activated cells are found in increased numbers in close association with the Aβ plaques and neurofibrillary tangles that show oxidative modifications [65, 66].

Sources of reactive nitrogen species in cells and tissues

Different reactive nitrogen species can be produced in living cells. The major forms of reactive nitrogen species and their metabolism are shown in Figure 3 (reactive nitrogen pathways). A possible involvement of toxic forms of nitric oxide in AD has been suggested by the demonstration of increased amounts of nitrated residues of tyrosine in neurofibrillary tangles, and in neurons showing evidence of DNA damage [3, 56, 64, 88]. The presence of nitrotyrosine-modified proteins is direct evidence for the action of peroxynitrite. Increased production of nitric oxide (NO), along with its interaction with superoxide, can result in the formation of peroxynitrite, a highly reactive product (Fig. 3). This can oxidize proteins resulting in the formation of carbonyl groups, as well as modify tyrosine residues to form nitrotyrosine [3, 7, 56, 64]. Increased amounts of nitrotyrosine residues were detected by high performance liquid chromatography along with electrochemical detection in affected regions of AD brains [89]. Furthermore, increased amounts of nitrotyrosine-modified proteins were localized by immunohistochemistry using nitrotyrosine-specific antibodies in the regions of brains from AD cases that had pathological changes [3, 56, 64]. In addition to demonstrating that increased amounts of nitrotyrosine-modified proteins were present on neurofibrillary tangles in AD brains [3], two other studies showed nitrotyrosine-modified proteins in many cortical and hippocampal neurons in AD brains that did not have tangles [56, 64]. Similar changes were not observed in control brains. It was demonstrated that there was increased nuclear fragmentation in most neurons that showed nitrotyrosine immunoreactivity [64].

There are three different nitric oxide synthase (NOS) enzymes present in different cells of the brain. NOS type I is found in neurons, NOS type III is found mainly in endothelial cells, while NOS type II (also called inducible NOS-iNOS) is induced in astrocytes and microglia in response to inflammatory stimuli [42, 90–94]. It is thus possible that the increased synthesis of NO could be derived from cells other than glia, but activated glial cells can produce large amounts of NO relative to neurons or endothelial cells. It has been demonstrated that microglia from rodents can be stimulated to produce large amounts of NO as a result of stimulation of expression of the inducible NOS gene [95, 96]. However, it appears that human microglia do not readily express inducible NOS [97, 98]. In culture, human microglia do not respond to the same stimuli that evoke NO production by rodent microglia [42, 93, 100, 101]. In particular, we showed that Aβ peptide cannot activate NO production by human microglia derived from postmortem human brains [101]. A similar failure to induce NO production in adult human microglia has been demonstrated by others [102]. Production of NO by human microglia is still a subject of some controversy [103,104]. There have been studies indicating that cytokine-stimulated human microglia do produce NO, though they have not been widely replicated. In another study, apolipoprotein E, but not Aβ, induced NO production by human macrophages (microglia were not tested) that had been primed with polyinosinic-polycytidilic acid [105]. This agent is commonly used to mimic the cellular consequences of viral exposure. It has been shown that there are differences in the structure of the human iNOS promoter compared to the mouse iNOS gene promoter. This difference makes the human gene hyporesponsive to lipopolysaccharide and IFNγ [106]. There have been reports that iNOS immunoreactivity has been localized to microglia in brain tissue of Parkinson's disease, multiple sclerosis and AIDS cases [107–109]. Overall, this would indicate that inducing stimuli encountered *in vivo* have not been fully tested in *in vitro* experiments. However, in AD brain tissue sections, iNOS was only localized in astrocytes that were closely associated with plaques; microglia were not immunoreactive for iNOS [110].

In comparison to human microglia, human astrocytes can be stimulated by inflammatory cytokines to produce NO [111]. This has been demonstrated using both human fetal astrocytes and human adult astrocytes [93, 102]. Astrocyte expression of iNOS is most strongly induced by the synergistic interaction of IFNγ combined with IL-1β, followed in potency by IL-1β with TNFα, and then by IL-1β alone [93, 112]. IL-1 receptor antagonist protein and IFNβ effectively block IFNγ/IL-1β induction of iNOS expression by astrocytes [94, 112, 113]. NO derived from activated astrocytes can also be neurotoxic to human neurons [90, 114]. *In vitro* studies have shown that astrocyte-produced NO can induce apoptosis in neurons co-cultured with the astrocytes. The neurotoxic effect can be blocked by coincubation of stimulated astrocytes with a NOS inhibitor [114]. As astrocytes expressing iNOS have been observed associated with plaques in AD brains, this provides evidence for the possible contribution of astrocyte-derived nitric oxide to AD pathogenesis [110].

Similarities in pathogenic mechanisms between AD and acquired immunodeficiency syndrome (AIDS)-associated dementia may exist. There is evidence that glial-produced nitric oxide and superoxide contribute to the neurotoxicity observed in the brains of AIDS patients that develop a dementia syndrome [108, 115]. These patients are of interest for studying mechanisms of neurodegenerative pathology as they can be compared to AIDS patients that do not develop the dementia. One recent study showed that in the group of AIDS patients that showed dementia, there was increased expression of superoxide dismutase in brain microglia, especially in those cells that were infected with HIV. Inducible NOS immunoreactivity was detected in both astrocytes and microglia in the brains of these patients [115]. Stronger immunoreactivity for nitrotyrosine-modified proteins was detectable in the AIDS patients with dementia compared to those without dementia [115]. As these patients show evidence of synaptic and neuronal loss, but not the plaques and tangles of AD, it is good evidence that glial-produced free radicals are responsible for these changes.

Role of microglial-derived myeloperoxidase in Alzheimer's disease (and multiple sclerosis)

Direct demonstration of microglial-derived free radicals in AD-affected brain tissue has not been possible. As mentioned above, evidence for increased oxidative stress in AD tissue due to reactive glia is indirect. The activation of the microglial NADPH oxidase system can be hypothesized to occur in AD based on a number of *in vitro* cell culture experiments. Recently, a role for microglial-derived myeloperoxidase (MPO) in AD and multiple sclerosis has been identified [116, 117]. MPO catalyses a reaction between hydrogen peroxide, produced by the action of NADPH oxidase then superoxide dismutase, and chloride to generate hypochlorous acid, a potent oxidizing agent. Hypochlorous acid can further react with other molecules to generate different reactive oxygen species, including singlet oxygen. The reactions catalyzed by MPO are illustrated in Figure 5.

MPO is readily detectable in circulating neutrophils and monocytes; however, its expression is downregulated in cells that have differentiated into macrophages. Similarly, mature microglia do not appear to express myeloperoxidase [116–118]. This has been demonstrated in human brain tissue. Recent studies have demonstrated that MPO immunoreactivity can be detected in some tissue microglia and that MPO gene expression can be induced in cultured microglia. MPO immunoreactivity was demonstrated in microglial-like cells in active MS lesions [117]. Similarly, MPO

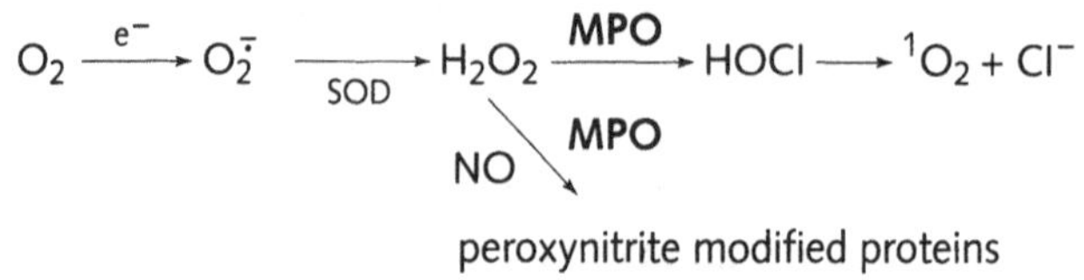

$$O_2 \xrightarrow{e^-} O_2^{\bar{\cdot}} \xrightarrow[SOD]{} H_2O_2 \xrightarrow{MPO} HOCl \longrightarrow {}^1O_2 + Cl^-$$

NO + H_2O_2 $\xrightarrow{MPO}$ peroxynitrite modified proteins

Figure 5
Pathways catalyzed by myeloperoxidase. $O_2^{-}\bullet$, superoxide; SOD, superoxide dismutase; H_2O_2, hydrogen peroxide; MPO, myeloperoxidase; HOCl, hypochlorous acid; NO, nitric oxide; ${}^1O_2$, singlet oxygen; Cl^-, chloride ion.

immunoreactivity has been detected in microglia localized around Aβ immunoreactive plaques in AD brains [116]. Expression of MPO was not detected in non-plaque-containing brain regions or in control brains, except within the lumen of the cerebral vessels. This is consistent with the antibody identifying MPO within circulating monocytes or neutrophils. The diffuse nature of the plaque-associated MPO immunoreactivity is consistent with this enzyme being released by microglia in an active form. *In vitro* studies demonstrated the expression of MPO mRNA in rodent and human adult microglia, with increased expression occurring in rodent microglia that had been exposed to aggregated Aβ peptide [116]. Interestingly, it was shown that a significantly greater number of AD and MS female patients had the SpSp MPO alleles compared with the SpN alleles [116, 117]. The difference in the alleles occurs in the promoter region of the MPO gene, and the Sp allele is associated with a higher expression of MPO mRNA resulting from the stronger SP1 transcription factor binding site [116]. It is not clear why the effect of the different alleles in increasing the incidence of both AD and MS is only observed in female patients. However, this finding is in line with the well established fact that these diseases are more prevalent in females.

Role of MPO in the generation of reactive nitrogen species

Recent studies have shown that MPO can be involved in the generation of reactive nitrogen species [119, 120]. As mentioned above, the interaction of microglial-derived superoxide and nitric oxide, with the formation of peroxynitrite, might be responsible for the formation of the nitrotyrosine-modified proteins that have been identified in NFTs and/or non-tangle containing neurons in AD brains. However, recent studies have indicated that peroxynitrite is not efficient in modifying tyrosine residues *in vivo* at physiological pH. An alternative pathway for the formation of nitrotyrosine-modified proteins has been proposed [119, 120]. MPO in combination with hydrogen peroxide and nitrite (the autoxidation product of nitric oxide) was capable of inducing protein nitrosation of apoB-100 and induction of low-density lipoprotein lipid peroxidation [121]. This modification was sufficient to induce the uptake of LDL by macrophages and transform them into atherogenic foam cells. This was not observed if the nitrite was not included in the reaction. A similar mechanism may be occurring in the brain under conditions where neurodegenerative stimuli cause activation of MPO in microglia/macrophages, and where the stimuli also cause the induction of NO production by activated glial cells. The consequence of this could be the formation of nitrotyrosine-modified proteins. These new findings also indicated that NO-modified proteins might be more potent at activating microglia and thus further exacerbating the inflammatory processes in the brain [121].

Therapeutic avenues for antioxidants/anti-inflammatory agents

A range of agents have been tested or proposed as therapy for AD based on their antioxidant or anti-inflammatory properties. A clinical trial of indomethacin and long term prospective epidemiological studies have shown the possible effectiveness of cyclooxygenase inhibitors in treating AD [122, 123]. The cellular target in the AD brain for such agents has not been determined. Most cells have the capacity to express cyclooxygenase type 1 or 2 (including astrocytes and neurons); however, cyclooxygenase inhibitors are known to have anti-inflammatory actions on phagocytic cells. Recently it has been suggested that the non-steroidal anti-inflammatory class of drugs may mediate their anti-inflammatory action (in part) as agonists of the peroxisome proliferator-activated receptor-γ [124, 125].

Vitamin E (α-tocopherol) has been proposed as therapy for AD [126, 127]. This is based on its potency as a free radical scavenger. However, in a clinical trial there was only a very small effect on inhibiting the progression of AD following administration of vitamin E [128]. *In vitro*, it has been demonstrated that vitamin E had a significant effect on inhibiting the respiratory burst of human monocytes by blocking the translocation of $p47^{PHOX}$ to the membrane. This was due to vitamin E inhibiting its phosphorylation by protein kinase C [80].

An epidemiological study of leprosy patients in Japan has shown that those continuously treated with dapsone or its didextrose sulfonate derivative had a considerably decreased prevalence of AD [129]. This protection was weaker in those cases where the drugs were administered intermittently, thus suggesting that the drug use rather than underlying pathology was responsible for this observation. Dapsone is known to suppress inflammation in a number of animal models [130]. One of its main mechanisms of action in peripheral tissues is thought to be inhibition of leukocyte myeloperoxidase [131, 132]. In light of the recent observation of myeloperoxidase involvement in AD [116], this inhibitory property could also explain the apparent anti-dementia action of dapsone.

The agent propentofylline, a xanthine derivative, has also been tested as a treatment for AD. Its principal mode of action is as an adenosine reuptake inhibitor and phosphodiesterase inhibitor. This agent has shown effectiveness in inhibiting superoxide production by activated macrophages and microglia [133–135]. One small clinical trial showed that propentofylline was effective in slowing the rate of cognitive decline in AD patients [136, 137]. Thus, this agent may be an effective AD therapy as it might not only inhibit microglial activation and reduce the amount of microglia free radical production but also stimulate nerve growth factor production by astrocytes [138, 139].

Conclusions

There is good evidence of increased oxidative stress occurring in human brains affected by AD. Activated glial cells have been shown to produce a number of the agents that can mediate oxidative stress. It is well established that there is a considerable increase in the numbers of activated microglia and astrocytes in human brains affected by AD. Since other mechanisms for the increased oxidative stress have been identified, at present it is not possible to determine the relative contribution of different sources of the free radicals that are causing the oxidative damage in AD brains. This important problem needs to be researched. Once answered, it will allow the design of a more targeted therapy for AD based on inhibiting free radical production. To date, data indicate that anti-inflammatory therapies are more effective than anti-oxidants as a treatment for AD, though the two features may be interrelated to some extent.

References

1 Dodart JC, Mathis C, Ungerer A (2000) The beta-amyloid precursor protein and its derivatives: from biology to learning and memory processes. *Rev Neurosci* 11: 75–93

2 Braak E, Griffing K, Arai K, Bohl J, Bratzke H, Braak H (1999) Neuropathology of Alzheimer's disease: what is new since A. Alzheimer? *Eur Arch Psychiatry Clin Neurosci* 249 (Suppl 3): 14–22

3 Good PF, Werner P, Hsu A, Olanow CW, Perl DP (1996) Evidence of neuronal oxidative damage in Alzheimer's disease. *Am J Pathol* 149: 21–28

4 Markesbery WR (1997) Oxidative stress hypothesis in Alzheimer's disease. *Free Radic Biol Med* 23: 134–147

5 Markesbery WR, Lovell MA (1998) Four-hydroxynonenal, a product of lipid peroxidation, is increased in the brain in Alzheimer's disease. *Neurobiol Aging* 19: 33–36

6 Markesbery WR, Carney JM (1999) Oxidative alterations in Alzheimer's disease. *Brain Pathol* 9: 133–146
7 Smith MA, Sayre LM, Anderson VE, Harris PL, Beal MF, Kowall N, Perry G (1998) Cytochemical demonstration of oxidative damage in Alzheimer disease by immunochemical enhancement of the carbonyl reaction with 2,4-dinitrophenylhydrazine. *J Histochem Cytochem* 46: 731–735
8 Nunomura A, Perry G, Pappolla MA, Wade R, Hirai K, Chiba S, Smith MA (1999) RNA oxidation is a prominent feature of vulnerable neurons in Alzheimer's disease. *J Neurosci* 19: 1959–1964
9 Raina AK, Templeton DJ, Deak JC, Perry G, Smith MA (1999) Quinone reductase (NQO1), a sensitive redox indicator, is increased in Alzheimer's disease. *Redox Rep* 4: 23–27
10 Sayre LM, Perry G, Smith MA (1999) *In situ* methods for detection and localization of markers of oxidative stress: application in neurodegenerative disorders. *Methods Enzymol* 309: 133–152
11 Sayre LM, Perry G, Harris PL, Liu Y, Schubert KA, Smith MA (2000) *In situ* oxidative catalysis by neurofibrillary tangles and senile plaques in Alzheimer's disease: a central role for bound transition metals. *J Neurochem* 74: 270–279
12 Smith MA, Vasak M, Knipp M, Castellani RJ, Perry G (1998) Dimethylargininase, a nitric oxide regulatory protein, in Alzheimer disease. *Free Radic Biol Med* 25: 898–902
13 Smith MA, Rudnicka-Nawrot M, Richey PL, Praprotnik D, Mulvihill P, Miller CA, Sayre LM, Perry G (1995) Carbonyl-related posttranslational modification of neurofilament protein in the neurofibrillary pathology of Alzheimer's disease. *J Neurochem* 64: 2660–2666
14 Cassarino DS, Bennett JP (1999) An evaluation of the role of mitochondria in neurodegenerative diseases: mitochondrial mutations and oxidative pathology, protective nuclear responses, and cell death in neurodegeneration. *Brain Res Rev* 29: 1–25
15 Singer TP, Ramsay PR (1995) Monoamine oxidases: old friends hold many surprises. *FASEB J* 9: 605–610
16 Benzi G, Moretti A (1995) Are reactive oxygen species involved in Alzheimer's disease? *Neurobiol Aging* 16: 661–674
17 Multhaup G, Ruppert T, Schlicksupp A, Hesse L, Beher D, Masters CL, Beyreuther K (1997) Reactive oxygen species and Alzheimer's disease. *Biochem Pharmacol* 54: 533–39
18 Behl C (1999) Alzheimer's Disease and Oxidative stress: Implications for novel therapeutic approaches. *Prog Neurobiol* 57: 301–323
19 Prasad KN, Cole WC, Hovland AR, Prasad KC, Nahreini P, Kumar B, Edwards-Prasad J, Andreatta CP (1999) Multiple antioxidants in the prevention and treatment of neurodegenerative disease: analysis of biologic rationale. *Curr Opin Neurol* 12: 761–770
20 Perry G, Smith MA (1998) Is oxidative damage central to the pathogenesis of Alzheimer disease? *Acta Neurol Belg* 98: 175–179

21 Perry G, Raina AK, Nunomura A, Wataya T, Sayre LM, Smith MA (2000) How important is oxidative damage? Lessons from Alzheimer's disease. *Free Radic Biol Med* 28: 831–834

22 Mattson MP, Pedersen WA, Duan W, Culmsee C, Camandola S (1999) Cellular and molecular mechanisms underlying perturbed energy metabolism and neuronal degeneration in Alzheimer's and Parkinson's diseases. *Ann NY Acad Sci* 893: 154–175

23 Youdim MB, Lavie L (1994) Selective MAO-A and B inhibitors, radical scavengers and nitric oxide synthase inhibitors in Parkinson's disease. *Life Sci* 55: 2077–2082

24 Jenner P (1998) Oxidative mechanisms in nigral cell death in Parkinson's disease. *Mov Disord* 13 (Suppl 1): 24–34

25 Browne SE, Ferrante RJ, Beal MF (1999) Oxidative stress in Huntington's disease. *Brain Pathol* 9: 147–163

26 Israel N, MA (1997) Oxidative stress in human immunodeficiency virus infection. *Cell Mol Life Sci* 53: 864–870

27 Love S (1999) Oxidative stress in brain ischemia. *Brain Pathol* 9: 119–131

28 Liu D, Wen J, Liu J, Li L (1999) The roles of free radicals in amyotrophic lateral sclerosis: reactive oxygen species and elevated oxidation of protein, DNA, and membrane phospholipids. *FASEB J* 13: 2318–2328

29 Cookson MR, Shaw PJ (1999) Oxidative stress and motor neurone disease. *Brain Pathol* 9: 165–186

30 Choi-Miura NH, Oda T (1996) Relationship between multifunctional protein "clusterin" and Alzheimer disease. *Neurobiol Aging* 17: 717–722

31 Fu W, Luo H, Parthasarathy S, Mattson MP (1998) Catecholamines potentiate amyloid beta-peptide neurotoxicity: involvement of oxidative stress, mitochondrial dysfunction, and perturbed calcium homeostasis. *Neurobiol Dis* 5: 229–243

32 Guo Q, Sebastian L, Sopher BL, Miller MW, Ware CB, Martin GM, Mattson MP (1999) Increased vulnerability of hippocampal neurons from presenilin-1 mutant knock-in mice to amyloid beta-peptide toxicity: central roles of superoxide production and caspase activation. *J Neurochem* 72: 1019–1029

33 Mattson MP, Goodman Y, Luo H, Fu W, Furukawa K (1997) Activation of NF-kappaB protects hippocampal neurons against oxidative stress-induced apoptosis: evidence for induction of manganese superoxide dismutase and suppression of peroxynitrite production and protein tyrosine nitration. *J Neurosci* Res 49: 681–697

34 Yatin SM, Aksenov M, Butterfield DA (1999) The antioxidant vitamin E modulates amyloid beta-peptide-induced creatine kinase activity inhibition and increased protein oxidation: implications for the free radical hypothesis of Alzheimer's disease. *Neurochem Res* 24: 427–435

35 Mattson MP (1997) Central role of oxyradicals in the mechanism of amyloid beta peptide cytotoxicity. *Alz Dis Rev* 2: 1–14

36 Mattson MP, Pedersen WA (1998) Effects of amyloid precursor protein derivatives and oxidative stress on basal forebrain cholinergic systems in Alzheimer's disease. *Int J Dev Neurosci* 16: 737–753

37 McGeer PL, McGeer EG (1995) The inflammatory response system of brain: implications for therapy of Alzheimer and other neurodegenerative diseases. *Brain Res Rev* 21: 195–218
38 McGeer PL, McGeer EG (1998) Mechanisms of cell death in Alzheimer disease – immunopathology. *J Neural Transm Suppl* 54: 159–166
39 Gehrmann J, Matsumoto Y, Kreutzberg GW (1995) Microglia: intrinsic immuneffector cell of the brain. *Brain Res Brain Res Rev* 20: 269–287
40 McGeer EG, McGeer PL (1998) The importance of inflammatory mechanisms in Alzheimer disease. *Exp Gerontol* 33: 371–378
41 Banati RB, Gehrmann J, Schubert P, Kreutzberg GW (1993) Cytotoxicity of microglia. *Glia* 7: 111–118
42 Colton C, Wilt S, Gilbert D, Chernyshev O, Snell J, Dubois-Dalcq M (1996) Species differences in the generation of reactive oxygen species by microglia. *Mol Chem Neuropathol* 28: 15–20
43 McDonald DR, Brunden KR, Landreth GE (1997) Amyloid fibrils activate tyrosine kinase-dependent signaling and superoxide production in microglia. *J Neurosci* 17: 2284–2294
44 Brosnan CF, Battistini L, Raine CS, Dickson DW, Casadevall A, Lee SC (1994) Reactive nitrogen intermediates in human neuropathology: an overview. *Dev Neurosci* 16: 152–161
45 Guo ZH, Mattson MP (2000) Neurotrophic factors protect cortical synaptic terminals against amyloid and oxidative stress-induced impairment of glucose transport, glutamate transport and mitochondrial function. *Cereb Cortex* 10: 50–57
46 Mattson MP, Partin J, Begley JG (1998) Amyloid beta-peptide induces apoptosis-related events in synapses and dendrites. *Brain Res* 807: 167–176
47 Bruce-Keller AJ, Begley JG, Fu W, Butterfield DA, Bredesen DE, Hutchins JB, Hensley K, Mattson MP (1998) Bcl-2 protects isolated plasma and mitochondrial membranes against lipid peroxidation induced by hydrogen peroxide and amyloid beta-peptide. *J Neurochem* 70: 31–39
48 Behl C, Davis JB, Klier FG, Schubert D (1994) Amyloid beta peptide induces necrosis rather than apoptosis. *Brain Res* 645: 253–264
49 Behl C, Davis JB, Lesley R, Schubert D (1994) Hydrogen peroxide mediates amyloid beta protein toxicity. *Cell* 77: 817–827
50 Sagara Y, Dargusch R, Klier FG, Schubert D, Behl C (1996) Increased antioxidant enzyme activity in amyloid beta protein-resistant cells. *J Neurosci* 16: 497–505
51 Schubert D, Behl C, Lesley R, Brack A, Dargusch R, Sagara Y, Kimura H (1995) Amyloid peptides are toxic *via* a common oxidative mechanism. *Proc Natl Acad Sci USA* 92: 1989–1993
52 Castellani RJ, Smith MA, Nunomura A, Harris PL, Perry G (1999) Is increased redox-

active iron in Alzheimer disease a failure of the copper-binding protein ceruloplasmin? *Free Radic Biol Med* 26: 1508–1512

53 Munch G, Schinzel R, Loske C, Wong A, Durany N, Li JJ, Vlassara H, Smith MA, Perry G, Riederer P (1998) Alzheimer's disease – synergistic effects of glucose deficit, oxidative stress and advanced glycation endproducts. *J Neural Transm* 105: 439–461

54 Raina AK, Takeda A, Nunomura A, Perry G, Smith MA (1999) Genetic evidence for oxidative stress in Alzheimer's disease. *Neuroreport* 10: 1355–1357

55 Russell RL, Siedlak SL, Raina AK, Bautista JM, Smith MA, Perry G (1999) Increased neuronal glucose-6-phosphate dehydrogenase and sulfhydryl levels indicate reductive compensation to oxidative stress in Alzheimer disease. *Arch Biochem Biophys* 370: 236–239

56 Smith MA, Richey HP, Sayre LM, Beckman JS, Perry G (1997) Widespread peroxynitrite-mediated damage in Alzheimer's disease. *J Neurosci* 17: 2653–2657

57 Yan SD, Yan SF, Chen X, Fu J, Chen M, Kuppusamy P, Smith MA, Perry G, Godman GC, Nawroth P (1995) Non-enzymatically glycated tau in Alzheimer's disease induces neuronal oxidant stress resulting in cytokine gene expression and release of amyloid beta-peptide. *Nat Med* 1: 693–99

58 Yan SD, Chen X, Schmidt AM, Brett J, Godman G, Zou YS, Scott CW, Caputo C, Frappier T, Smith MA (1994) Glycated tau protein in Alzheimer disease: a mechanism for induction of oxidant stress. *Proc Natl Acad Sci USA* 91: 7787–7791

59 Munch G, Mayer S, Michaelis J, Hipkiss AR, Riederer P, Muller R, Neumann A, Schinzel R, Cunningham AM (1997) Influence of advanced glycation end-products and AGE-inhibitors on nucleation-dependent polymerization of beta-amyloid peptide. *Biochim Biophys Acta* 1360: 17–29

60 Munch G, Thome J, Foley P, Schinzel R, Riederer P (1997) Advanced glycation endproducts in ageing and Alzheimer's disease. *Brain Res Brain Res Rev* 23: 134–143

61 Gabbita SP, Lovell MA, Markesbery WR (1998) Increased nuclear DNA oxidation in the brain in Alzheimer's disease. *J Neurochem* 71: 2034–2040

62 Ando Y, Brannstrom T, Uchida K, Nyhlin N, Nasman B, Suhr O, Yamashita T, Olsson T, El Salhy M, Uchino M et al (1998) Histochemical detection of 4-hydroxynonenal protein in Alzheimer amyloid. *J Neurol Sci* 156: 172–176

63 Montine KS, Reich E, Neely MD, Sidell KR, Olson SJ, Markesbery WR, Montine TJ (1998) Distribution of reducible 4-hydroxynonenal adduct immunoreactivity in Alzheimer disease is associated with APOE genotype. *J Neuropathol Exp Neurol* 57: 415–425

64 Su JH, Deng G, Cotman CW (1997) Neuronal DNA damage precedes tangle formation and is associated with up- regulation of nitrotyrosine in Alzheimer's disease brain. *Brain Res* 774: 193–199

65 Dickson DW, Sinicropi S, Yen SH, Ko LW, Mattiace LA, Bucala R, Vlassara H (1996) Glycation and microglial reaction in lesions of Alzheimer's disease. *Neurobiol Aging* 17: 733–743

66 Takeda A, Yasuda T, Miyata T, Goto Y, Wakai M, Watanabe M, Yasuda Y, Horie K,

Inagaki T, Doyu M, et al (1998) Advanced glycation end products co-localized with astrocytes and microglial cells in Alzheimer's disease brain. *Acta Neuropathol (Berlin)* 95: 555–558

67 Babior BM (1999) NADPH oxidase: an update. *Blood* 93: 1464–1476

68 DeLeo FR, Allen LA, Apicella M, Nauseef WM (1999) NADPH oxidase activation and assembly during phagocytosis. *J Immunol* 163: 6732–6740

69 Kume A, Dinauer MC (2000) Gene therapy for chronic granulomatous disease. *J Lab Clin Med* 135: 122–128

70 Johnson JL, Park JW, Benna JE, Faust LP, Inanami O, Babior BM (1998) Activation of p47(PHOX), a cytosolic subunit of the leukocyte NADPH oxidase. Phosphorylation of ser-359 or ser-370 precedes phosphorylation at other sites and is required for activity. *J Biol Chem* 273: 35147–35152

71 Klegeris A, Walker DG, McGeer PL (1994) Activation of macrophages by Alzheimer β amyloid peptide. *Biochem Biophys Res Comm* 199: 984–991

72 Klegeris A, McGeer PL (1997) β-amyloid protein enhances macrophage production of oxygen free radicals and glutamate. *J Neurosci* Res 49: 229–235

73 Van Muiswinkel FL, Veerhuis R, Eikelenboom P (1996) Amyloid beta protein primes cultured rat microglial cells for an enhanced phorbol 12-myristate 13-acetate-induced respiratory burst activity. *J Neurochem* 66: 2468–2476

74 Van Muiswinkel FL, Raupp SF, de Vos NM, Smits HA, Verhoef J, Eikelenboom P, Nottet HS (1999) The amino-terminus of the amyloid-beta protein is critical for the cellular binding and consequent activation of the respiratory burst of human macrophages. *J Neuroimmunol* 96: 121–130

75 Giulian D, Haverkamp LJ, Yu JH, Karshin W, Tom D, Li J, Kirkpatrick J, Kuo YM, Roher AE (1996) Specific domains of beta-amyloid from Alzheimer plaque elicit neuron killing in human microglia. *J Neurosci* 16: 6021–6037

76 McDonald DR, Brunden KR, Landreth GE (1997) Amyloid fibrils activate tyrosine kinase-dependent signaling and superoxide production in microglia. *J Neurosci* 17: 2284–2294

77 Della-Bianca V, Dusi S, Bianchini E, Dal-Pra I, Rossi F (1999) β amyloid activates the O_2 forming NADPH oxidase in microglia, monocytes and neutrophils. A possible inflammatory mechanism of neuronal damage in Alzheimer's disease. *J Biol Chem* 274: 15493–15499

78 Meda L, Bonaiuto C, Baron P, Otvos LJ, Rossi F, Cassatella MA (1996) Priming of monocyte respiratory burst by beta-amyloid fragment (25-35). *Neurosci Lett* 219: 91–94

79 Cassatella MA, Bazzoni F, Flynn RM, Dusi S, Trinchieri G, Rossi F (1990) Molecular basis of interferon-gamma and lipopolysaccharide enhancement of phagocyte respiratory burst capability. Studies on the gene expression of several NADPH oxidase components. *J Biol Chem* 265: 20241–20246

80 Cachia O, Benna JE, Pedruzzi E, Descomps B, MA, Leger CL (1998) Alpha-tocopherol

inhibits the respiratory burst in human monocytes. Attenuation of p47(phox) membrane translocation and phosphorylation. *J Biol Chem* 273: 32801–32805

81 Klegeris A, McGeer PL (1994) Rat brain microglia and peritoneal macrophages show similar responses to respiratory burst stimulants. *J Neuroimmunol* 53: 83–90

82 Sankarapandi S, Zweier JL, Mukherjee G, Quinn MT, Huso DL (1998) Measurement and characterization of superoxide generation in microglial cells: evidence for an NADPH oxidase-dependent pathway. *Arch Biochem Biophys* 353: 312–321

83 Van Muiswinkel FL (1999) Enhanced expression of microglial NADPH oxidase (p22-PHOX) in Alzheimer's disease. *Alzheimer Dis Assoc Disord* 451–455

84 McGeer PL, Kawamata T, Walker DG, Akiyama H, Tooyama I, McGeer EG (1993) Microglia in degenerative neurological disease. *Glia* 7: 84–92

85 Carpenter AF, Carpenter PW, Markesbery WR (1993) Morphometric analysis of microglia in Alzheimer's disease. *J Neuropathol Exp Neurol* 52: 601–608

86 Griffin WS, Sheng JG, Roberts GW, Mrak RE (1995) Interleukin-1 expression in different plaque types in Alzheimer's disease: significance in plaque evolution. *J Neuropathol Exp Neurol* 54: 276–281

87 McGeer PL, Itagaki S, Tago H, McGeer EG (1988) Occurrence of HLA-DR reactive microglia in Alzheimer's disease. *Ann NY Acad Sci* 540: 319–323

88 Su JH, Deng G, Cotman CW (1997) Neuronal DNA damage precedes tangle formation and is associated with up- regulation of nitrotyrosine in Alzheimer's disease brain. *Brain Res* 774: 193–199

89 Hensley K, Maidt ML, Yu Z, Sang H, Markesbery WR, Floyd RA (1998) Electrochemical analysis of protein nitrotyrosine and dityrosine in the Alzheimer brain indicates region-specific accumulation. *J Neurosci* 18: 8126–8132

90 Chao CC, Hu S, Sheng WS, Bu D, Bukrinsky MI, Peterson PK (1996) Cytokine-stimulated astrocytes damage human neurons *via* a nitric oxide mechanism. *Glia* 16: 276–84

91 Chao CC, Lokensgard JR, Sheng WS, Hu S, Peterson PK (1997) IL-1-induced iNOS expression in human astrocytes *via* NF-kappa B. *Neuroreport* 8: 3163–3166

92 Ii M, Sunamoto M, Ohnishi K, Ichimori Y (1996) beta-Amyloid protein-dependent nitric oxide production from microglial cells and neurotoxicity. *Brain Res* 720: 93–100

93 Lee SC, Dickson DW, Liu W, Brosnan CF (1993) Induction of nitric oxide synthase activity in human astrocytes by interleukin-1 beta and interferon-gamma. *J Neuroimmunol* 46: 19–24

94 Liu J, Zhao ML, Brosnan CF, Lee SC (1996) Expression of type II nitric oxide synthase in primary human astrocytes and microglia: role of IL-1beta and IL-1 receptor antagonist. *J Immunol* 157: 3569–3576

95 McCann SM, Licinio J, Wong ML, Yu WH, Karanth S, Rettorri V (1998) The nitric oxide hypothesis of aging. *Exp Gerontol* 33: 813–826

96 Dawson VL, Dawson TM (1998) Nitric oxide in neurodegeneration. Prog *Brain Res* 118: 215–29

97 Hu S, Chao CC, Khanna KV, Gekker G, Peterson PK, Molitor TW (1996) Cytokine and free radical production by porcine microglia. *Clin Immunol Immunopathol* 78: 93–96

98 Colton C, Wilt S, Gilbert D, Chernyshev O, Snell J, Dubois-Dalcq M (1996) Species differences in the generation of reactive oxygen species by microglia. *Mol Chem Neuropathol* 28: 15–20
99 Ding M, St.Pierre BA, Parkinson JF, Medberry P, Wong JL, Rogers NE, Ignarro LJ, Merrill JE (1997) Inducible nitric-oxide synthase and nitric oxide production in human fetal astrocytes and microglia. A kinetic analysis. *J Biol Chem* 272: 11327–11335
100 Lee SC, Brosnan CF (1996) Cytokine Regulation of iNOS Expression in human glial cells. *Methods* 10: 31–37
101 Walker DG, Kim SU, McGeer PL (1995) Complement and cytokine gene expression in cultured microglia derived from postmortem human brains. *J Neurosci* Res 40: 478–493
102 Zhao ML, Liu JS, He D, Dickson DW, Lee SC (1998) Inducible nitric oxide synthase expression is selectively induced in astrocytes isolated from adult human brain. *Brain Res* 813: 402–405
103 Colasanti M, Persichini T, Di Pucchio T, Gremo F, Lauro GM (1995) Human ramified microglial cells produce nitric oxide upon Escherichia coli lipopolysaccharide and tumor necrosis factor alpha stimulation. *Neurosci Lett* 200: 144–146
104 Colasanti M, Persichini T, Menegazzi M, Mariotto S, Giordano E, Caldarera CM, Sogos V, Lauro GM, Suzuki H (1995) Induction of nitric oxide synthase mRNA expression. Suppression by exogenous nitric oxide. *J Biol Chem* 270: 26731–26733
105 Vitek MP, Snell J, Dawson H, Colton CA (1997) Modulation of nitric oxide production in human macrophages by apolipoprotein-E and amyloid-beta peptide. *Biochem Biophys Res Commun* 240: 391–394
106 Zhang X, Laubach VE, Alley EW, Edwards KA, Sherman PA, Russell SW, Murphy WJ (1996) Transcriptional basis for hyporesponsiveness of the human inducible nitric oxide synthase gene to lipopolysaccharide/interferon-gamma. *J Leukoc Biol* 59: 575–585
107 Hunot S, Dugas N, Faucheux B, Hartmann A, Tardieu M, Debre P, Agid Y, Dugas B, Hirsch EC (1999) FcepsilonRII/CD23 is expressed in Parkinson's disease and induces, *in vitro*, production of nitric oxide and tumor necrosis factor-alpha in glial cells. *J Neurosci* 19: 3440–3447
108 Vincent VA, De Groot CJ, Lucassen PJ, Portegies P, Troost D, Tilders FJ, Van Dam AM (1999) Nitric oxide synthase expression and apoptotic cell death in brains of AIDS and AIDS dementia patients. *AIDS* 13: 317–326
109 Oleszak EL, Zaczynska E, Bhattacharjee M, Butunoi C, Legido A, Katsetos CD (1998) Inducible nitric oxide synthase and nitrotyrosine are found in monocytes/macrophages and/or astrocytes in acute, but not in chronic, multiple sclerosis. *Clin Diagn Lab Immunol* 5: 438–445
110 Wallace MN, Geddes JG, Farquhar DA, Masson MR (1997) Nitric oxide synthase in reactive astrocytes adjacent to beta-amyloid plaques. *Exp Neurol* 144: 266–272
111 Lee SC, Brosnan CF (1996) Cytokine Regulation of iNOS Expression in Human Glial Cells. *Methods* 10: 31–37
112 Hu S, Sheng WS, Peterson PK, Chao CC (1995) Differential regulation by cytokines of human astrocyte nitric oxide production. *Glia* 15: 491–494

113 Hua LL, Liu JS, Brosnan CF, Lee SC (1998) Selective inhibition of human glial inducible nitric oxide synthase by interferon-beta: implications for multiple sclerosis. *Ann Neurol* 43: 384–387

114 Chao CC, Hu S, Ehrlich L, Peterson PK (1995) Interleukin-1 and tumor necrosis factor-alpha synergistically mediate neurotoxicity: involvement of nitric oxide and of N-methyl-D-aspartate receptors. Brain Behav Immun 9: 355–365

115 Boven LA, Gomes L, Hery C, Gray F, Verhoef J, Portegies P, Tardieu M, Nottet HS (1999) Increased peroxynitrite activity in AIDS dementia complex: implications for the neuropathogenesis of HIV-1 infection. *J Immunol* 162: 4319–4327

116 Reynolds WF, Rhees J, Maciejewski D, Paladino T, Sieburg H, Maki RA, Masliah E (1999) Myeloperoxidase polymorphism is associated with gender specific risk for Alzheimer's disease. *Exp Neurol* 155: 31–41

117 Nagra RM, Becher B, Tourtellotte WW, Antel JP, Gold D, Paladino T, Smith RA, Nelson JR, Reynolds WF (1997) Immunohistochemical and genetic evidence of myeloperoxidase involvement in multiple sclerosis. *J Neuroimmunol* 78: 97–107

118 Ulvestad E, Williams K, Mork S, Antel J, Nyland H (1994) Phenotypic differences between human monocytes/macrophages and microglial cells studied *in situ* and *in vitro*. *J Neuropathol Exp Neurol* 53: 492–501

119 Hazen SL, Zhang R, Shen Z, Wu W, Podrez EA, MacPherson JC, Schmitt D, Mitra SN, Mukhopadhyay C, Chen Y, et al (1999) Formation of nitric oxide-derived oxidants by myeloperoxidase in monocytes: pathways for monocyte-mediated protein nitration and lipid peroxidation *in vivo*. *Circ Res* 85: 950–958

120 van Dalen CJ, Winterbourn CC, Senthilmohan R, Kettle AJ (2000) Nitrite as a Substrate and Inhibitor of Myeloperoxidase. Implications for nitration and hypochlorous acid production at sites of inflammation. *J Biol Chem* 275: 11638–11644

121 Podrez EA, Schmitt D, Hoff HF, Hazen SL (1999) Myeloperoxidase-generated reactive nitrogen species convert LDL into an atherogenic form *in vitro*. *J Clin Invest* 103: 1547–1560

122 Rogers J, Kirby LC, Hempelman SR, Berry DL, McGeer PL, Kaszniak AW, Zalinski J, Cofield M, Mansukhani L, Willson P (1993) Clinical trial of indomethacin in Alzheimer's disease. *Neurology* 43: 1609–1611

123 McGeer PL, Schulzer M, McGeer EG (1996) Arthritis and anti-inflammatory agents as possible protective factors for Alzheimer's disease: a review of 17 epidemiologic studies. *Neurology* 47: 425–432

124 Ricote M, Li AC, Willson TM, Kelly CJ, Glass CK (1998) The peroxisome proliferator-activated receptor-gamma is a negative regulator of macrophage activation. *Nature* 391: 79–82

125 Combs CK, Johnson DE, Karlo C, Cannady SB, Landreth GE (2000) Inflammatory mechanisms in Alzheimer's disease: Inhibition of β-amyloid stimulated proinflammatory responses and neurotoxicity by PPAR-γ agonists. *J Neurosci* 20: 558–567

126 Behl C (1999) Vitamin E and other antioxidants in neuroprotection. *Int J Vitam Nutr Res* 69: 213–219

127 Grundman M (2000) Vitamin E and Alzheimer disease: the basis for additional clinical trials. *Am J Clin Nutr* 71: 630S–636S
128 Sano M, Ernesto C, Thomas RG, Klauber MR, Schafer K, Grundman M, Woodbury P, Growdon J, Cotman CW, Pfeiffer E et al (1997) A controlled trial of selegiline, alpha-tocopherol, or both as treatment for Alzheimer's disease. The Alzheimer's Disease Cooperative Study. *N Engl J Med* 336: 1216–1222
129 McGeer PL, Harada N, Kimura H, McGeer EG, Schulzer M (1992) Prevalence of dementia amongst elderly Japanese with leprosy: apparent effect of chronic drug therapy. *Dementia* 3: 146–149
130 Lewis AJ, Gemmell DK, Stimson WH (1978) The anti-inflammatory profile of dapsone in animal models of inflammation. *Agents Actions* 8: 578–586
131 Bozeman PM, Learn DB, Thomas EL (1992) Inhibition of the human leukocyte enzymes myeloperoxidase and eosinophil peroxidase by dapsone. *Biochem Pharmacol* 44: 553–563
132 Kettle AJ, Winterbourn CC (1991) Mechanism of inhibition of myeloperoxidase by anti-inflammatory drugs. *Biochem Pharmacol* 41: 1485–1492
133 Banati RB, Schubert P, Rothe G, Gehrmann J, Rudolphi K, Valet G, Kreutzberg GW (1994) Modulation of intracellular formation of reactive oxygen intermediates in peritoneal macrophages and microglia/brain macrophages by propentofylline. *J Cereb Blood Flow Metab* 14: 145–149
134 Si QS, Nakamura Y, Kataoka K (1997) Adenosine inhibits superoxide production in rat peritoneal macrophages *via* elevation of cAMP level. *Immunopharmacology* 36: 1–7
135 Si Q, Nakamura Y, Ogata T, Kataoka K, Schubert P (1998) Differential regulation of microglial activation by propentofylline *via* cAMP signaling. *Brain Res* 812: 97–104
136 Kittner B, Rossner M, Rother M (1997) Clinical trials in dementia with propentofylline. *Ann NY Acad Sci* 826: 307–316
137 Rother M, Erkinjuntti T, Roessner M, Kittner B, Marcusson J, Karlsson I (1998) Propentofylline in the treatment of Alzheimer's disease and vascular dementia: a review of phase III trials. *Dement Geriatr Cogn Disord* 9 (Suppl 1): 36–43
138 Schubert P, Ogata T, Rudolphi K, Marchini C, McRae A, Ferroni S (1997) Support of homeostatic glial cell signaling: a novel therapeutic approach by propentofylline. *Ann NY Acad Sci* 826: 337–347
139 Yamada K, Nitta A, Hasegawa T, Fuji K, Hiramatsu M, Kameyama T, Furukawa Y, Hayashi K, Nabeshima T (1997) Orally active NGF synthesis stimulators: potential therapeutic agents in Alzheimer's disease. *Behav Brain Res* 83: 117–122
140 Shimohama S, Tanino H, Kawakami N, Okamura N, Kodama H, Yamaguchi T, Hayakawa T, Nunomura A, Chiba S, Perry G, Smith MA (2000) Activation of NADPH oxidase in Alzheimer's disease brains. *Biochem Biophys Res Commun* 273: 5–9

The role of cyclooxygenase in Alzheimer's disease neurodegeneration

Giulio Maria Pasinetti

Neuroinflammation Research Laboratories, Department of Psychiatry, Mount Sinai School of Medicine, One Gustave L. Levy Place, New York, NY 10029, USA

Introduction

In the past few years, many epidemiological studies have addressed directly the possible protective effect of anti-inflammatory drug use with regard to AD. As recently reviewed [1], the great majority of these studies suggest that non-steroidal anti-inflammatory drugs (NSAIDs) do have a protective effect. Perhaps the most convincing of these clinical efforts is the Baltimore Longitudinal Study of Aging, which utilized data collected prospectively, thereby minimizing recall bias issues; again the results indicated a protective effect with NSAID use [2]. One small controlled trial of indomethacin, a potent NSAID, suggested that the drug slowed cognitive deterioration in AD [3].

While the mechanism of action of NSAIDs is not entirely clear, it is generally assumed that their effects are mediated by competitive inhibition of cyclooxygenase (COX) catalytic activity, thus reducing the production of inflammatory prostaglandins (PGs) from membrane-derived arachidonate. The apparent protective effect of NSAIDs suggests that COX might be involved in neurodegenerative mechanisms. In view of the particular interest in clinical trials of NSAIDs in AD, we and others have investigated the role of COX in neurodegeneration. More recently, three pharmaceutical companies have begun pursuing clinical trials of selective COX-2 inhibitors in order to prevent and/or treat AD. In addition, the NIA-funded Alzheimer's Disease Cooperative Study consortium is about to begin a multicenter trial comparing the efficacy of non-selective NSAIDs to a selective COX-2 inhibitor in attenuating the rate of disease progression.

Cyclooxygenase: the target of NSAIDs

In recent years it has been established that COX exists in two isoforms coded by distinct genes on different chromosomes [4–6]. The two isoforms share about 80% homology and have similar catalytic activity, but are physiologically distinct. COX-

Neuroinflammatory Mechanisms in Alzheimer's Disease: Basic and Clinical Research,
edited by Joseph Rogers

2 is inducible in inflammatory cells in response to inflammatory signals such as cytokines and lipopolysaccharide, and is down-regulated by glucocorticoids, while COX-1 is generally constitutive. It thus appears that COX-2 mediates inflammatory activity, while COX-1 has housekeeping functions, including gastric cytoprotection. Traditional NSAIDs are non-selective COX inhibitors; their beneficial effects derive from COX-2 inhibition, while gastrointestinal, renal and platelet toxicity is likely mediated by COX-1 inhibition. The use of newly developed highly selective COX-2 inhibitors holds promise for increased efficacy with vastly reduced toxicity [7].

Neuronal COX-2 and its expression in AD brain

Immunocytochemical evidence indicates that COX-2 expression is elevated in AD brain. We [8] and others [9–11] found that COX-2 protein content is increased in postmortem AD brain and that the elevation of COX-2 signal is localized primarily to neuronal cells. The evidence showing the regulation of COX-2 mRNA in AD brain is equivocal [8, 9, 12] which may be in part due to the fact that COX-2 mRNA is an unstable short-lived RNA species with a half-life of approximately 3–5 h [12]. Thus, COX-2 mRNA may not be the appropriate index for assessing COX-2 regulation in human post-mortem tissues.

Recent immunocytochemical evidence shows that the increased levels of COX-2 content in subsets of neurons of the pyramidal layer of the hippocampal formation correlates with neuronal atrophy [13], consistent with previous evidence showing that in AD (and Down's syndrome), COX-2 protein content is preferentially elevated in neurons with neurofibrillary tangles (NFT) and damaged axons [10]. Again, no evidence of COX-2 expression in cells other than neurons was found. This is of high interest, especially in view of the evidence that glial and endothelial cells may also express and regulate COX-2 mRNA/protein in other neurodegenerative or inflammatory conditions *in vivo* [14–18] or *in vitro* [19–21]. Thus, this selective neuronal compartmentalization of COX-2 in AD brain suggests a potential role of COX-2 in neurodegenerative mechanisms independent of classical inflammatory cascades, as depicted in Figure 1. Consistent with this hypothesis, we have shown that primary neuron cultures derived from transgenic mice with neuronal overexpression of human (h)COX-2 are more susceptible to excitotoxic and β amyloid ($A\beta_{25-35}$)-mediated neuronal death [13, 22].

If neuronal COX-2 is the target of NSAIDs in AD, a selective COX-2 inhibitor with central nervous system penetration would be a good candidate for therapeutic trials in AD. Recently approved selective COX-2 inhibitors have been largely successful because these drugs share COX-2 inhibitory efficacy with older non-selective COX inhibitors (such as indomethacin) with remarkably fewer side effects. These drugs are now being developed for AD treatment.

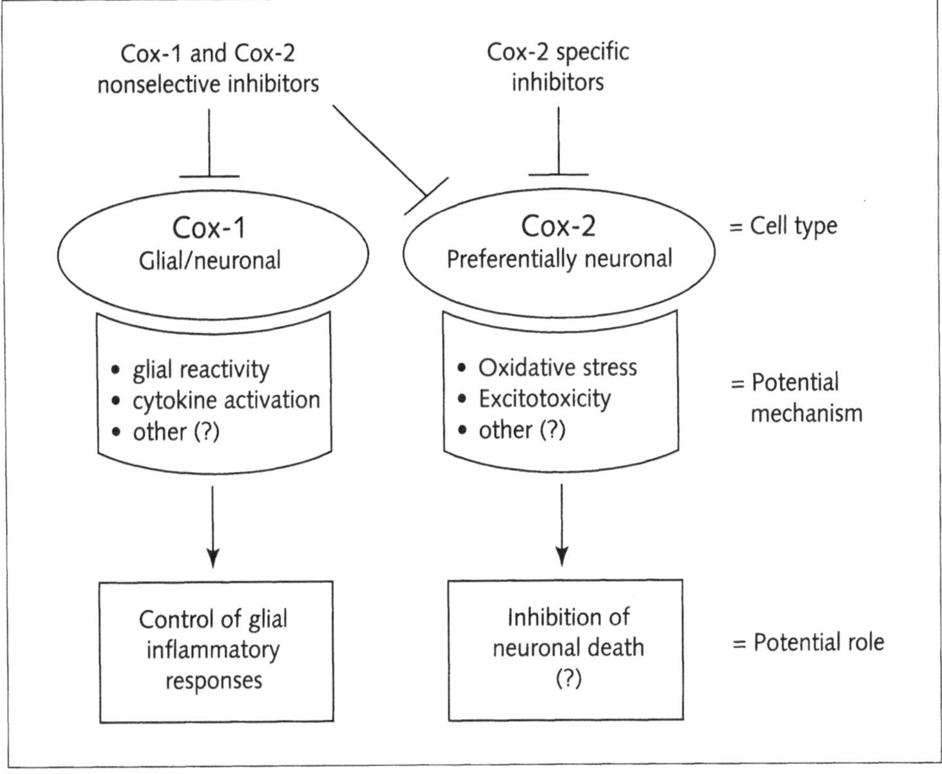

Figure 1
Hypothetical role of NSAIDs in Alzheimer's disease.

The potential role of COX-1 in glial mediated inflammatory cascades in AD

Inhibition of COX-1 expression might also be beneficial to AD neurodegeneration (Fig. 1). While the regulation of COX-1 in AD brain is still controversial [8, 9], COX-1 appears to be expressed in both glia and neurons of the AD brain [8, 23]. Little is known about the role of constitutive COX-1 expression in brain, and its expression in glia may be linked to more traditional inflammatory mechanisms. For example, there is evidence that the number of activated microglia is reduced in non-demented elderly subjects with a history of NSAID use when compared to age-matched control cases with no history of NSAID exposure [24]. Therefore, while COX-2 specific inhibitors may influence the clinical progression of AD by inhibiting COX-2 activity in neurons (modulating the enzyme's role in oxidative and excitotoxic mechanisms, as discussed below), non-selective NSAIDs might influence AD progression through simultaneous inhibition of COX-1 and COX-2-mediated responses in glia and neurons (at the cost of side effects associated with non-selective COX inhibitors).

COX and its potential role in oxidative metabolism in AD brain

The enzymatic reaction involved in PG production by activation of COX is a two step reaction: cyclooxygenase catalyzes the formation of PG from arachidonic acid, and peroxidase reduces hydroperoxides (PGG_2) and activates the cyclooxygenase (Fig. 2). The peroxidase activity of COX can also generate reactive oxygen species (ROS) [25]. While NSAIDs in general may block PG formation by competing with arachidonic acid for binding (see Fig. 2 legend), they may also indirectly affect the peroxidase activity by blocking the formation of the hydroperoxide PGG_2 [25]. Which of these activities could be responsible for neuroprotection in AD? Evidence is accumulating that points to a possible role for free radicals in the pathogenesis of AD and provides a basis for postulating a role for neuronal COX-2 peroxidase activity in AD [26]. Consistent with this evidence we recently found that the peroxidase (and cyclooxygenase) activity of COX-2 is stimulated by synthetic, aggregated $A\beta_{1-40}$ peptides in a cell free system (Pasinetti, unpublished observations). The data suggests the possibility that Aβ peptides may stimulate the peroxidase component of COX-2 in neurons leading to an increase in generation of ROS. Moreover, because Aβ peptides also contain redox-active methionine and tyrosine residues, they may also function as co-substrates for the COX-2 peroxidase component. The redox activity of COX-2 (and possibly the constitutive COX-1) in neurons may therefore represent a potential site of action for the apparent beneficial effects of NSAIDs in AD. This hypothesis is presently under investigation in our laboratory using a double transgenic mouse model in which a mutated amyloid precursor protein (APP), whose expression leads to AD type neuropathology, is co-overexpressed in neurons with human COX-2.

Neuronal COX-2 and lipid peroxidation: a lesson from transgenic mice overexpressing human COX-2 in neurons

Based on the evidence that in AD brain neuronal COX-2 is the appropriate target for NSAID regimens [8, 13], transgenic mice with neuronal overexpression of COX -2 may provide a unique method of measuring relevant brain activity of COX inhibitors. Using this transgenic mouse model, we found that overexpression of the human (h)COX-2 in neurons [22] leads to elevated brain lipid peroxidation as assessed by increased levels of malondialdehyde (MDA, Fig. 2) (Pasinetti, unpublished observation), consistent with the evidence that MDA can be generated directly through the metabolism of PGH_2 [27].

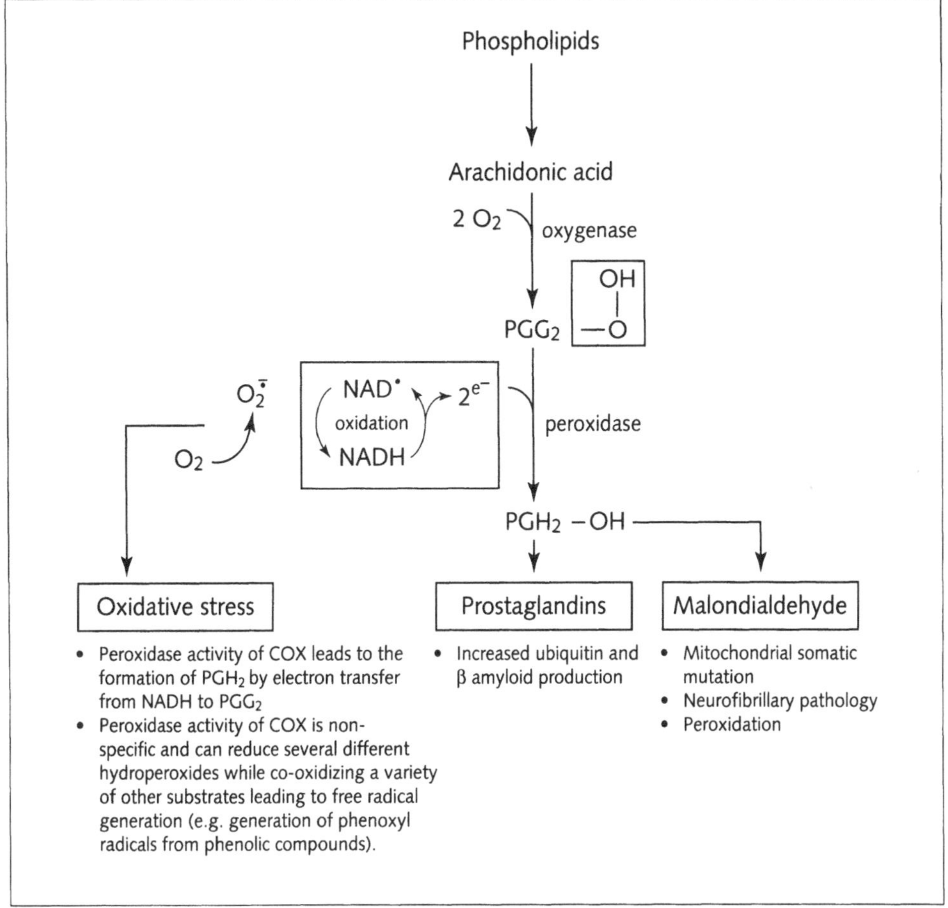

Figure 2
Hypothetical role of cycloxygenase in neurodegeneration and Alzheimer's disease.

Increased levels of MDA and other carbonyl compounds has important implications in AD neurodegeneration (Fig. 2). For example, there is evidence that carbonyl-related post-translational modification of neurofilament protein, through cross-links, might account for the biochemical properties of neurofibrillary tangles and their resistance to degradation *in vivo* [26] (Fig. 2). Morever, MDA can also be mutagenic by forming adducts to deoxyguanosine and deoxyadenosine residues and, as suggested in Figure 2, to participate in mechanisms leading to accumulation of mitochondrial somatic mutations. Based on this evidence, it is possible that the beneficial role of NSAIDs in AD is related to neuronal COX-2 inhibition with subsequent modulation of MDA-mediated responses involved in neurofibrillary pathology. Notably, there is also evidence suggesting that PGs may influence Aβ-mediated production and degradation ultimately contributing to neuronal degeneration independent of COX-mediated oxidative stress [28] (Fig. 2).

Neuronal COX-2 expression and its role in excitotoxicty

There is evidence that several of the prostanoid products of arachidonic acid metabolism by COX potentiate glutamate excitotoxicity [28, 29], representing another mechanism by which COX-2 overexpression in neurons of the AD brain might accelerate neurodegeneration. There is evidence that excitotoxicity potentiates Aβ hippocampal neurodegeneration in rats [30], and that NMDA-mediated neuronal death is diminished in a dose-dependent manner by COX-2 inhibitors in primary neuronal cultures [31]. We have used our transgenic mice overexpressing neuronal hCOX-2 in neurons to explore the role of COX-2 in excitotoxic neurodegeneration. We found that overexpression of neuronal hCOX-2 in neurons of transgenic mice potentiates the intensity and lethality of kainic-acid (KA) neurotoxicity coincidentally with potentiation of expression of the immediate early genes *c-fos* and *zif-268* [22]. These findings suggest that COX-2 expression in neurons may play a casual role in excitotoxic neuron death, possibly through control of expression of immediate early genes (Fig. 2). This formulation is also consistent with the recent hypothesis that in AD chronic excitotoxic activity may be responsible for the widespread pattern of neurodegeneration [32]. It is possible that neuronal COX-2 may potentiate Aβ-mediated toxicity by influencing glutamatergic tone through potentiation of excitotoxic mechanisms.

The role of COX-2 in complement gene expression

A novel feature of COX-2 mediated responses in inflammatory neurodegenerative mechanisms in AD may involve activities of the complement cascade. We found that the elevation of neuronal hCOX-2 in our transgenic mouse model [22] causes increased expression of the complement component C1q (C1qB) mRNA in neuronal layers of the hippocampal formation (Pasinetti, unpublished observation). This preliminary evidence is of particular interest in view of the finding that neuronal C1q expression is elevated in the AD brain [33, 34] where it may control pro-inflammatory complement cascades [35]. Moreover, there is evidence that human C1q binds to Aβ peptides [36] and potentiates Aβ aggregation [35, 37]. Ongoing studies in our laboratory are exploring the correlation between C1q expression (and other components of the complement cascade) and COX-2 in neurons of AD brain at different stages of clinical disease. These studies will explore the hypothesis that COX inhibitors modulate AD neurodegeneration in part by blocking the induction of complement activity.

There is a critically important limitation to the utility of studying the relationship between COX-2, C1q and Aβ toxicity in mice. Unlike human C1q, mouse C1q does not interact directly with Aβ fragments [38]. The absence of this link may explain, in part, the lack of neurodegeneration in mouse amyloid precursor protein (APP) transgenics, and may influence the pathogenicity of COX-2 overexpression in mice.

COX-2 inhibition may be distinct from anti-inflammatory effects

We hypothesize that NSAIDs may not necessarily neuroprotect solely by suppressing inflammation in the AD brain (i.e. cytokine-driven acute phase response in glia), but also by influencing the role of COX-2 in neurons. For example, the hypothesis that COX-2 inhibitors may influence the activity of COX-2 in neurons (e.g. blocking production of MDA in neurons at risk) may explain a paradox in the interpretation of the epidemiological data supporting a neuroprotective effect of NSAIDs in AD. Retrospective studies demonstrate a protective effect among individuals who report past use of NSAIDs, primarily ibuprofen [1], a drug with both COX-1 and COX-2 inhibitory activity. However, the majority of ibuprofen users take doses that are analgesic rather than anti-inflammatory. Daily doses of ibuprofen up to 1200 mg are analgesic, not anti-inflammatory; daily doses of 2400 mg and greater are necessary for a systemic anti-inflammatory effect in patients with rheumatoid arthritis [39]. It seems unlikely that casual use of NSAIDs could significantly suppress destructive brain inflammation. Different cell types have markedly different sensitivity to COX inhibitors; for example, platelet COX is inhibited by doses of aspirin (82 mg per day) far below the doses necessary to inhibit inflammatory cell activity (4–7 g per day). Perhaps low doses of ibuprofen, without an anti-inflammatory effect, can influence neuronal COX-2 function and limit oxidative stress (e.g. by Aβ or by the COX activity itself) to sub-threshold levels. Interestingly, we note that the level of neuronal COX-2 expression is influenced not only by inflammatory stimuli [6], but also by synaptic activity [40, 41]. As discussed above, immunodetectable hippocampal COX-2 in AD is primarily localized in neurons [8, 9, 13]. Therefore it would be expected that COX-2 inhibitors might affect neuronal metabolic activities independent of glial inflammatory (possibly COX-1-mediated) activities.

Status of anti-inflammatory drug trials in AD: implications for prevention or treatment

The characterization of inflammatory processes in the AD brain has led to efforts in developing anti-inflammatory treatment strategies to slow the rate of disease progression. The recent elucidation of the respective physiological roles of COX-2 and

COX-1 has resulted in great interest within the pharmaceutical industry in the development of selective inhibitors of COX-2 [7]. Such agents may be highly effective in suppressing inflammation in diseases such as rheumatoid arthritis and should have reduced gastrointestinal toxicity. Their safety and specificity for the COX-2 isoform, which may be involved in AD, makes these NSAIDs excellent candidates for therapeutic trials in AD.

However, because therapeutic trials of potential disease-modifying regimens select patients at one or more stages of clinical disease, the expression of COX-2 (and other inflammatory markers) in AD brain should be investigated in correlation with antemortem assessment of AD dementia. This information would be immediately relevant to the design of NSAIDs drug trials [42]. Ongoing studies in our laboratory are exploring the expression of COX-2 in brain samples from post-mortem AD cases at different clinical stages of disease identified by antemortem assessments using the Clinical Dementia Rating (CDR) and the cognitive subscale of the Alzheimer's Disease Assessment Scale (ADAScog). We have found that the COX-2 protein content in pyramidal neurons of the hippocampal formation is already elevated in cases of mild-moderate (CDR = 1–2) and severe (CDR = 4–5) dementia, but not in cases of questionable (CDR = 0.5) dementia, suggesting the possibility of preventive therapeutic interventions with COX-2 inhibitors in a population highly susceptible to progressive dementia [43]. This evidence is of high interest, especially in view of the fact that two pharmaceutical companies are now conducting large-scale trials of selective COX-2 inhibitors that slow the progression of AD. One of these trials targets the earliest stage of disease (i.e. slowing the progression from questionable to mild-moderate dementia).

In summary, studies in animal and cell culture models of AD-type neurodegeneration, studies of post-mortem AD brain tissue, as well as a large number of epidemiological studies all point to COX-2 (and possibly COX-1) as an important therapeutic target in AD.

Acknowledgments

Supported by National Institute on Aging AG13799, AG14239 and AG14766 to GMP

References

1 McGeer PL, Schulzer M, McGeer EG (1996) Arthritis and anti-inflammatory agents as possible protective factors for Alzheimer's disease: A review of 17 epidemiologic studies. *Neurology* 47: 425–432

2 Stewart WF, Kawas C, Corrada M, Metter EJ (1997) Risk of Alzheimer's disease and duration of NSAID use. *Neurology* 48: 626–632

3 Rogers J, Kirby LC, Hempelman SR, Berry DL, McGeer PL, Kaszniak AW, Zalinski J, Cofield M, Mansukhani L, Willson P et al (1993) Clinical trial of indomethacin in Alzheimer's disease. *Neurology* 43: 1609–1611
4 Kujubu DA, Fletcher BS, Varnum BC, Lim RW, Herschman HR (1991) TIS10, a phorbol ester tumor promoter-inducible mRNA from Swiss 3T3 cells encodes a novel prostaglandin synthase/cyclooxygenase homologue. *J Biol Chem* 266: 12866–12872
5 O'Banion MK, Winn VD, Young DA (1992) cDNA cloning and functional activity of a glucocorticoid-regulated inflammatory cyclooxygenase. *Proc Natl Acad Sci USA* 89: 4888–4892
6 Cao C, Matsumura K, Yamagata K, Watanabe Y (1995) Induction by lipo-polysaccharide of cyclooxygenase-2 mRNA in rat brain; its possible role in the febrile response. *Brain Res* 697: 187–196
7 Vane JR, Botting RM (1995) New insights into the mode of action of anti-inflammatory drugs. *Inflamm Res* 44: 1–10
8 Pasinetti GM, Aisen PS (1998) Cyclooxygenase-2 expression is increased in frontal cortex of Alzheimer's disease brain. *Neuroscience* 87 (2): 319–324
9 Yasojima K, Schwab C, McGeer EG, McGeer LP (1999) Distribution of cyclooxygenase-1 and cyclooxygenase-2 mRNAs and proteins in human brain and peripheral organs. *Brain Res* 830: 226–236
10 Oka A, Takashima S (1997) Induction of cyclooxygenase 2 in brains of patients with Down's syndrome and dementia of Alzheimer type: specific localization in affected neurons and axons. *Neuroreport* 8: 1161–1164
11 Kitamura Y, Shimohama S, Koike H, Kakimura J, Matsuoka Y, Nomura Y, Gebicke-Haerter PJ, Taniguchi T (1999) Increased expression of cyclooxygenases and peroxisome proliferator-activated receptor-gamma in Alzheimer's disease brains. *Biochem Biophys Res Commun* 254 (3): 582–586
12 Lukiw WJ, Bazan NG (1997) Cyclooxygenase 2 RNA message abundance stability and hypervariability in sporadic Alzheimer neocortex. *J Neurosci Res* 50: 937–945
13 Ho L, Pieroni C, Winger D, Purohit DP, Aisen P, Pasinetti GM (1999) Regional distribution of cyclooxygenase-2 in the hippocampal formation in Alzheimer's disease. *J Neurosci Res* 57:295–303
14 Collaço-Moraes Y, Aspey B, Harrison M, De Belleroche J (1996) Cyclooxygenase-2 messenger RNA induction in focal cerebral ischemia. *J Cereb Blood Flow Met* 16: 1366–1372
15 Sairanen T, Ristimäki A, Karjalainen-Lindsberg ML, Paetau A, Kaste M, Lindsberg PJ (1998) Cyclooxygenase-2 is induced globally in infracted human brain. *Ann Neurol* 43: 738–747
16 Hirst WD, Young KA Newton R, Allport VC, Marriott DR, Wilkin GP (1999) Expression of COX-2 by normal and reactive astrocytes in the adult rat central nervous system. *Mol Cell Neurosci* 13: 57–68
17 Elmquiat JK, Breder CD, Sherin JE, Scammell TE, Hickey WF, Dewitt D, Saper CB (1997) Intravenous lipopolysaccharide induced cyclooxygenase 2-like immunoreactivity

in rat brain perivascular microglia and meningeal macrophages. *J Comp Neurol* 19: 716–725

18 Cao C, Matsumura K Yamagata G, Watanabe Y (1997) Lipopolysaccharide injected into the cerebral ventricle evokes fever through induction of cyclooxygenase-2 in brain endothelial cells. *J Neurosci* 19: 716–725

19 Thore CR, Nam MJ, Busija DW (1996) Immunofluorescent localization of constitutive and inducible prostaglandin H synthase in ovine astroglia. *J Comp Neurol* 367:1–9

20 Bauer MKA, Lieb K, Schulze-Osthoff K, Berger M, Gebicke-Haerter PJ, Bauer J, Fiebich BL (1997) Expression and regulation of cyclooxygenase-2 in rat microglia. *Eur J Biochem* 243: 726–731

21 Minghetti L, Polazzi E, Nicolini A, Créminon C, Levi G (1996) Interferon gamma and nitric oxide down-regulate lipopolysaccharide-induced prostanoid production in cultured rat microglial cells by inhibiting cyclooxygenase-2 expression. *J Neurochem* 66: 1963–1970

22 Kelly K, Ho L, Winger D, Freire-Moar J, Aisen P, Borelli C, Pasinetti GM (1999) Potentiation of excitotoxicity in transgenic mice overexpressing neuronal cyclooxygenase-2. *Am J Path* 155: 1–10

23 Yermakova AV, Rollins J, Callahan LM, Rogers J, O'Banion MK (1999) Cyclooxygenase-1 in human Alzheimer's and control brain: quantitative analysis of expression by microglia and CA3 hippocampal neurons. *J Neuropathol Exp Neurol* 58 (11): 1135–1146

24 Mackenzui IRA, Munoz DG (1998) Nonsteroidal anti-inflammatory drug use and Alzheimer-type pathology in aging. *Neurology* 50: 986–990

25 Pasinetti GM (1998) Cyclooxygenase and inflammation in Alzheimer's disease: experimental approaches and clinical intervention. *J Neurosci Res* 54: 1–6

26 Smith MA, Rudnicka-Nawrot M, Richey PL, Praprotnik D, Mulvihill P, Miller CA, Sayre LM, Perry G (1995) Carbonyl-related posttranslation modification of neurofilament protein in the neurofibrillary pathology of Alzheimer's disease. *J Neurochem* 64 (6): 2660–2666

27 Halliwell B, Gutteridge JMC (1995) Lipid peroxidation: a radical chain reaction. In: B Halliwell, JMC Gutteridge (eds): *Free radicals in biology and medicine*. 3rd ed. Clarendon Press, Oxford, 188–276

28 Prasad KN, Hovland AR, La Rosa FG, Hovland PG (1998) Prostaglandins as a putative neurotoxin in Alzheimer's disease. *Proc Soc Exp Biol Med* 219 (2): 120–125

29 Kimura H, Okamoto K, Sakai Y (1985) Modulatory effects of prostaglandins D2, E2 and F2α on the postsynaptic action of inhibitory and excitatory amino acids in cerebellar Purkinje cell dendrites *in vitro*. *Brain Res* 330: 235–244

30 Morimoto K, Yoshimi K, Tonohiro T, Yamada N, Oda T and Kaneko I (1998) Co-injection of beta-amyloid with ibotenic acid induces synergistic loss of rat hippocampal neurons. *Neuroscience* 84 (2): 479–487

31 Hewett SJ, Hewett JA (1997) COX-2 contributes to NMDA-induced neuronal death in cortical cell cultures. *Society for Neuroscience Abstracts* 23: 1666

32 Olney JW, Wozniak DF, Farber NB (1997) Excitotoxic neurodegeneration in Alzheimer disease – New hypothesis and new therapeutic strategies. *Arch Neurol* 54: 1234–1240
33 Terai K, Walker DG, McGeer EG, McGeer PL (1997) Neurons express proteins of the classical complement pathway in Alzheimer disease. *Brain Res* 769: 385–390
34 Afagh A, Cummings BJ, Cribbs DH, Cotman CW, Tenner AJ (1996) Localization and cell association of C1qB in Alzheimer's disease brain. *Exp Neurology* 138: 22–32
35 Webster S, Bonnell B, Rogers J (1997) Charge-based binding of complement component C1qB to the Alzheimer amyloid β-peptide. *Am J Pathology* 150: 1531–1536
36 Velazquez P, Cribbs DH, Poulos TL, Tenner AJ (1997) Aspartate residue 7 in amyloid B-protein is critical for classical complement pathway activation: Implications for Alzheimer's disease pathogenesis. *Nat Med* 3: 77–80
37 Webster S, Lue LF, Brachova L, Tenner AJ, McGeer PL, Terai K, Walker DG, Bradt B, Cooper NR, Rogers J (1997) Molecular and cellular characterization of the membrane attack complex. C5b-9 in Alzheimer's disease. *Neurobiol Aging* 18: 415–421
38 Velazquez P, Cribbs D, Poulos T, Tenner J (1997) Aspartate residue 7 in amyloid β-protein is critical for classical complement pathway activation: Implications for Alzheimer's disease pathogenesis. *Nat Med* 3: 77–79
39 Clements PJ, Paulus HE (1993) Nonsteroidal anti-inflammatory drugs (NSAIDs). In: WN Kelley, ED Harris Jr, S Ruddy, CB Sledge (eds): *Textbook of rheumatology*. WB Saunders Company, Philadelphia, 700–730
40 Yamagata K, Andreasson KI, Kaufmann WE, Barnes CA, Worley PF (1993) Expression of a mitogen-inducible cyclooxygenase in brain neurons: regulation by synaptic activity and glucocorticoids. *Neuron* 11: 371–386
41 Tocco G, Musleh W, Sakhi S, Schreiber S, Baudry M, Pasinetti GM (1997) Complement and glutamate neurotoxicity. Genotypic influences of C5 in a mouse model of hippocampal neurodegeneration. *Mol Chem Neuropathol* 31: 1–12
42 Aisen PS, Pasinetti GM (1998) Glucocorticoids in Alzheimer's disease: the story so far. *Drugs Aging* 12: 1–6
43 Ho L, Purohit D, Haroutunran V, Luterman JD, Willis F, Naslund J, Buxbaum JD, Mohs RC, Aisen PS, Pasinetti GM (2001) Neuronal cyclooxygenase-2 expression in the hippocampal formation as a function of the clinical progression of Alzheimer's disease. *Arch Neurol* 58 (3): 487–492

Microglia

Ian R.A. Mackenzie

Department of Pathology and Laboratory Medicine, University of British Columbia, Vancouver, B.C., V6T 2B5 Canada

Introduction

The demonstration of increased levels of inflammatory and immune system proteins in Alzheimer's disease (AD) brain tissue [1–3], combined with epidemiological evidence that anti-inflammatory therapy may decrease the risk of AD [4], has led to the hypothesis that inflammation plays an important role in the disease pathogenesis. As the resident immune-competent cells in the central nervous system (CNS), microglia are the most likely candidate to orchestrate this inflammatory response, by producing and responding to a variety of immune system molecules [2, 5, 6]. As phagocytes, microglia may also be involved in either the formation or degradation of amyloid, a process important in the physical transformation of senile plaques (SP) [7]. Finally, microglia are a potential source of several neurotoxic substances which could contribute to neurodegeneration [2, 8]. Given that microglial cells may play such a central role in AD, it seems prudent to consider therapeutic strategies directed towards manipulating microglial activity in the treatment of AD.

Immune function of microglia

Although the origin of microglia has been the source of much controversy in the past, it is now believed that they are generated in bone marrow, circulate as monocytes and migrate into the CNS during fetal development, where they take up permanent residency as tissue phagocytes [5, 6]. In their normal resting state, ramified microglia form a reticular array throughout the neuropil. In response to injury, these cells become activated; they proliferate, change their morphology, migrate to the area of injury and participate in the inflammatory process by expressing a variety of surface antigens and secretory products (Tab. 1). This activated state is best demonstrated in tissue sections by increased expression of major histocompatibility complex type II cell surface glycoprotein (MHC II) [9–11] and altered morphology with increased perikaryal cytoplasm and thicker, shorter cell processes [5, 6]. The dis-

Neuroinflammatory Mechanisms in Alzheimer's Disease: Basic and Clinical Research,
edited by Joseph Rogers

Table 1 - Some secretory products and surface receptors expressed by microglia

cytokines	IL-1α, IL-1β, IL-3, IL-5, IL-6, TNFα, MCP-1, MIP-1α
complement	C1, C3, C4
eicosanoids	prostoglandin D2, leukotriene C4
surface antigens and receptors	MHC class I, II (HLA-DR, HLA-DP, HLA-DQ)
	LCA
	complement receptors (C1q,C3, C5a)
	cytokine receptors (IL-1R, IL-2R)
	chemokine receptors (CCR3, CCR5)
	Fcγ receptor
	CSF-1 receptor
	vitronectin recptor
	RAGE
growth factors	NGF, bFGF, TGFα, TGFβ
reactive oxygen intermediates	
nitric oxide	

covery that many microglia in AD brain tissue express MHC II, whereas such immunoreactivity is scant in tissue from non-demented controls, provided much of the early impetus for research into inflammatory processes in AD [1, 9–12]. MHC II is a cell surface protein that allows cells to present antigen to T-helper lymphocytes. Although the expression of MHC II itself may have little direct significance in AD, it provides an indication of the immunological capabilities of these activated microglial cells.

In culture, microglia appear capable of constitutively secreting many of the immune proteins that are elevated in AD brain tissue [2, 13–16]. Of these, the pro-inflammatory cytokines and complement proteins may have particular relevance to AD pathogenesis. Interleukin-1 (IL-1) and tumor necrosis factor α (TNFα) may be directly or indirectly neurotoxic [17], whereas IL-6 may promote neuronal survival under certain restricted conditions [18]. IL-1β stimulates the proliferation and activation of astrocytes. The astrocytes, in turn, produce colony stimulating factor (CSF), which has a reciprocal effect on microglia [19, 20]. The production of IL-1 and IL-6 by glial cells is hypothesized to be a driving force in the formation of SP [21–23]. Finally, IL-1β stimulates amyloid precursor protein (APP) production [23–26] and influences amyloid β protein (Aβ) metabolism [27].

Microglia are also capable of producing a number of complement proteins, receptors and regulators. As discussed in detail in previous chapters, there is strong evidence that the classical complement pathway is activated in AD and that this is triggered when C1q binds to the amyloid component of SP [28-30]. Both microglia and neurons are a potential source of C1q [15, 28, 29, 31, 32]. Moreover, microglia express receptors for several complement fragments, including C1q [32], C3 [33] and C5a [34,35]. The complement within SP may attract microglia [29, 32, 35] and these activated cells may then provide a local source of additional pro-inflammatory molecules, including more complement [13, 15, 32]. Therefore, although some other cell type (such as neurons) may be the initial source of complement in AD, the recruitment and activation of microglia may be a crucial step in maintaining activity of the complement system and amplifying the associated inflammatory process.

Relationship of microglia to SP

Although activated microglia are also found in affected brain regions in other neurodegenerative conditions (such as amyotrophic lateral sclerosis (ALS), dementia with Lewy bodies, Parkinson's disease, Creutzfeldt-Jakob disease (CJD) and Pick's disease) [36–40], the striking tendency of these cells to aggregate in and around SP [7, 10, 41–46], where they co-localize with other markers of inflammation, suggests this process is more specific in AD (Fig. 1).

SP are the most characteristic pathological feature of AD and several lines of evidence suggest that the formation and accumulation of SP plays a central role in the pathogenesis of this disease [47, 48]. SP consist of a focal deposit of an amyloidogenic protein (Aβ) in the neuropil, either in a nonfibrillar, "pre-amyloid" form which predominates in *diffuse* SP (DP) or as compact, fibrillar amyloid which may be associated with dystrophic neurites in *neuritic* plaques (NP). Cross-sectional studies suggest that DP are an early pathological change that may evolve (mature) into NP [49–53]. This transformation from DP to NP is likely a crucial step, since it is the presence of numerous NP that is most diagnostic of AD [54]. The specific mechanism by which Aβ is deposited in the brain and how SP evolve from one morphological subtype to another is uncertain, but the close physical association of microglia with SP suggests that these cells may be involved [7, 10, 42–46].

Microglia may be involved in the formation of SP

The initial event in SP formation is thought to be the deposition of Aβ protein in the neuropil as DP [46–48]. Although neurons are most often suggested as the origin of this protein, cultured microglia have been shown to synthesize APP and metabolize it in such a way that would favour Aβ production [55, 56]. Against such a primary role *in vivo* is the finding that microglia in AD brain do not express APP mRNA [57]. In addition, several studies have shown that microglia aggregate much more around amyloid-containing NP than DP [7, 43, 44, 46], and there is little evidence

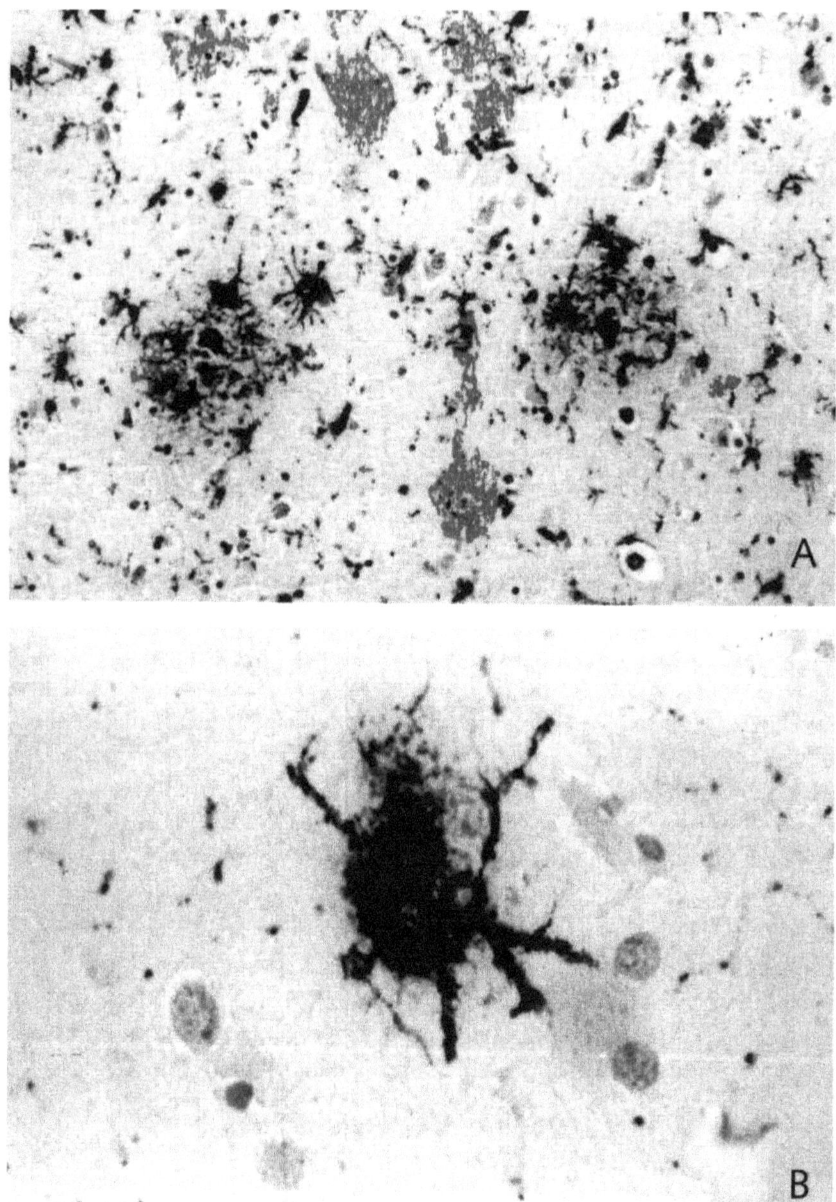

Figure 1

(A) Alzheimer's disease brain tissue with numerous activated microglial cells, expressing MHC II (MHC II immunohistochemistry).

(B) Activated microglia aggregate in and around senile plaques (MHC II/Aβ double immunohistochemistry).

of microglial activity when only DP are present [7]. Although these findings make it unlikely that microglia are an important primary source of Aβ, once they become activated microglia may affect Aβ production indirectly through the production of IL-1 [23–27].

Virtually all NP are physically associated with activated microglia [7, 43, 44]. This is not only true in AD but in other human conditions where NP are found, including Down's syndrome [46], dementia with Lewy bodies [37] and pathological aging [7, 10]. This relationship suggests that microglia are either involved in the formation of amyloid-containing neuritic SP or that pre-established NP elicit a microglial response. One way in which microglia could be involved in the formation of NP is by converting nonfibrillar Aβ protein (derived from some other source, such as neurons) into amyloid fibrils – a role similar to that ascribed to peripheral macrophages in systemic amyloidosis [58]. Shigematsu found that reactive microglia phagocytose APP produced by damaged neurons following the injection of kainic acid into rat brain [59] and Wisniewski has shown ultrastructural evidence suggesting that microglia produce and secrete amyloid fibrils in AD [60]. In a less direct fashion, activated microglia could promote amyloid fibril formation through the production of substances that are known to accelerate fibrillogenesis, such as C1q and interleukins [61, 62].

In comparing non-demented individuals with different subtypes of SP, we found a significant increase in the number of microglia associated with DP when NP are also present; suggesting that microglia might be involved in converting diffuse into neuritic plaques [7]. Griffin et al. have studied the relationship of IL-1 immunoreactive microglia with different plaque subtypes in both AD and normal aging [21, 23]. $IL-1^{+}$ cells were present in DP but were most abundant in the "early" (primitive) form of NP; those with APP-immunoreactive neurites but no compact central amyloid core. Their interpretation was that the local production of IL-1 by activated microglia is a key step in transforming diffuse into neuritic SP. IL-1 could promote this transformation either by accelerating amyloid fibril formation or by initiating a sequence of events that result in the formation of dystrophic neurites.

The final possibility is that microglia only become associated with SP once they mature to the NP stage, perhaps in an attempt to remove the amyloid from the tissue. This role is supported by the finding that microglia, both *in vivo* and in culture, phagocytose exogenous Aβ. Several studies have shown that cultured microglia remove soluble Aβ from the culture medium and that they can also bind and internalize aggregated fibrillar Aβ from the surface of the culture dish [63–65]. The ability of these cells to degrade the internalized material appears to be limited, however [65]. Frautschy et al. reported an interesting study in which amyloid cores isolated from AD tissue were injected into the brains of rats [66]. Within one week, many of the cores had been ingested by phagocytes and by one month, many of these phagocytic cells had transported the amyloid to blood vessels, possibly in an attempt to clear the material from the CNS.

Recent studies of transgenic mice that overexpress mutant human APP have generally confirmed the observations in human material [67, 68]. In these animals, activated microglial cells are found to cluster in and around most SP that contain amyloid fibrils but show little association with deposits of nonfibrillar Aβ. In one study, ultrastructural investigation revealed bundles of amyloid fibrils within the cytoplasm of microglial cells; however, it could not be determined whether this represented cellular production of amyloid or phagocytosis [68]. Such animal models may provide a way of more fully understanding the relationship between microglia and SP and will undoubtedly be useful in the investigation of therapies designed to modulate microglial activity.

SP attract and stimulate microglia

Regardless of whether microglia are instrumental in transforming DP into NP or respond to the presence of pre-existing NP, either process would be facilitated by the fact that various components of SP are chemotactic to microglia. As previously mentioned, microglia express receptors for several of the inflammatory mediators which accumulate in SP, including some complement fragments and cytokines [32–35, 69]. In addition, Aβ itself may attract microglia [70]. This effect is maximal with fibrillar Aβ and may involve an interaction with class A scavenger receptors [71]. Immunohistochemical studies indicate that SP amyloid or some other plaque-associated protein undergoes glycation and that SP with dense amyloid cores contain more advanced glycation end-products (AGE) than DP [72]. This glycation may also contribute to the recruitment and activation of microglia that posses specific receptors for AGE (RAGE) [73].

Many of the same SP components that provide chemotactic signalling for microglia also stimulate them to produce a variety of pro-inflammatory mediators that could initiate or help sustain the inflammatory process. Exposure of microglia to Aβ results in a dose-dependent increase in the production of cytokines and complement [13, 15, 74–76]. AGEs may also stimulate cytokine production [77, 78]. Consistent with these observations, immunohistochemical and *in situ* hybridization studies of AD brain tissue reveal SP-associated microglia expressing cytokines IL-1α, IL-1β, IL-6, TNFα, MCP-1 [21, 79, 80], and chemokine receptors CCR3 and CCR5 [69].

Reactive microglia produce neurotoxins

Once they become activated, microglia produce several potentially neurotoxic substances that could contribute to localized or more widespread CNS injury [2, 8, 28, 76, 81–83]. These include several of the previously mentioned inflammatory mediators, such as complement, cytokines and proteolytic enzymes. Consistent with their monocyte lineage, microglia are capable of respiratory burst activity that can generate reactive oxygen species (ROS) [8, 71, 81, 84, 85]. Although rodent microglia are also capable of producing nitric oxide [83, 86], it is uncertain whether human microglia share this property [87]. Finally, excitatory neurotoxicity could result from the production of high levels of glutamate and quinolinic acid by microglia [88–90].

The production of many of these neurotoxins may be amplified in the presence of SP. Several studies have indicated that Aβ is particularly potent at stimulating cultured microglia to produce complement, TNFα, ROS and nitric oxide [13, 15, 28, 71, 76, 82, 83, 85, 91–94]. AGEs may also stimulate microglia to produce cytokines (IL-1β and TNFα) [77, 78] and to induce oxidant stress [73]. Finally, activated microglia associated with SP express complement receptors and may be attempting to phagocytose opsonized SP amyloid. Inadvertent opsonization of neurites in the vicinity of SP could therefore result in microglia causing bystander damage to neurons [2].

Possible therapeutic implications

Consideration of the roles microglia may play in AD pathophysiology suggests that treatments to specifically manipulate microglial activity might be useful. Several epidemiological studies [4] and the results of a single clinical trial [95] suggest that non-steroidal anti-inflammatory drugs (NSAID) may reduce the risk or slow the progression of AD. Although these agents could affect the inflammatory process of AD at multiple steps, some of the studies suggest that NSAIDs may directly alter the activity of microglial cells. For example, we recently compared postmortem brain tissue from non-demented elderly individuals with a history of chronic NSAID use and tissue from age-matched controls [96]. The two groups showed a similar degree of age-related SP and neurofibrillary tangle (NFT) pathology. However, NSAID use was associated with significantly fewer SP-associated activated microglia. In a comparable study using an animal model, Netland et al. infused Aβ into the lateral ventricles of rats for two weeks and found extracellular deposits of the protein to be surrounded by activated microglia [97]. Concurrent treatment with indomethacin significantly attenuated this microglial response. The results of these studies suggest that some NSAIDs may be effective in suppressing the microglial activation associated with Aβ deposition. Klegeris et al. recently reported on the effect of various NSAIDs on cultures of the human monocyte cell line THP-1, which shares many properties with microglia [98]. The supernatant from stimulated cell cultures was found to kill cultured human neuroblastoma cells. This neuronal killing was reduced when the THP-1 cells were pre-incubated with NSAIDs. Importantly, this study demonstrates significant variation in the protective effect of different NSAIDs, indicating the need to evaluate the efficacy of these drugs individually.

Glucocorticoid steroids have a more potent anti-inflammatory effect than NSAIDs. The potential benefit of steroids in the treatment of AD is supported by a number of cell culture studies that suggest that these agents can reduce the microglial proliferation and activation that occurs in response to a variety of stimuli [99–101] and may suppress the production of some neurotoxic substances by microglia [102]. The epidemiological evidence for a protective effect of steroids against AD is somewhat less convincing, however, than it is for NSAIDs. Of the four case-control studies reviewed by McGeer [4], only the twin study of Breitner [103] had an odds ratio considered to be statistically significant. Meta-analysis of the combined results of the steroid studies yielded an odds ratio that just reached significance. A multicenter AD intervention trial with oral prednisone by the Alzheimer's Disease Collaborative Study (ADCS) group [104] failed to find any significant therapeutic benefit.

Propentofylline (PPF) is a xanthine derivative that may modulate glial cell activity by reinforcing or mimicking the effects of adenosine. PPF has been shown to inhibit the proliferation of microglia and to reduce the formation of ROS and the release of cytokines by microglia in culture [105, 106]. PPF may also restore proliferative astrocytes to a differentiated state and stimulate their release of NGF [107]. In rodents exposed to ischemic brain injury, pretreatment with PPF reduced the microglial response [108] and animals subjected to basal forebrain lesions showed improved learning and memory with PPF treatment [109]. The effect of PPF in patients with AD and/or vascular dementia has been examined in Europe in a small number of double-blind, placebo-controlled, randomized trials ranging in duration from six months to more than a year [105]. AD patients treated with PPF demonstrated significant improvements in global function, cognitive performance and activities of daily living compared with the placebo-treated group. In one study by Karlsson et al. (in [105]), the treatment difference was still present eight weeks after withdrawal of PPF, suggesting that the drug does not simply relieve symptoms but may actually slow the progression of disease. Although these reports are encouraging, additional trials are needed to confirm the results and establish whether the beneficial effects of PPF persist for a longer period of time.

Summary of the role of microglia in AD pathogenesis

Most evidence suggests that the inflammatory response in AD brain tissue is triggered by the accumulation of Aβ and subsequent activation of the complement cascade [28–30]. Once SP begin to accumulate and mature, various plaque components attract and stimulate microglial cells to produce pro-inflammatory mediators [13, 15 ,32–35, 69–76]. The production of complement and cytokines by activated microglia helps to sustain the inflammatory process and amplify it by recruiting other cells such as astrocytes. These cells, in turn, provide additional stimulation to

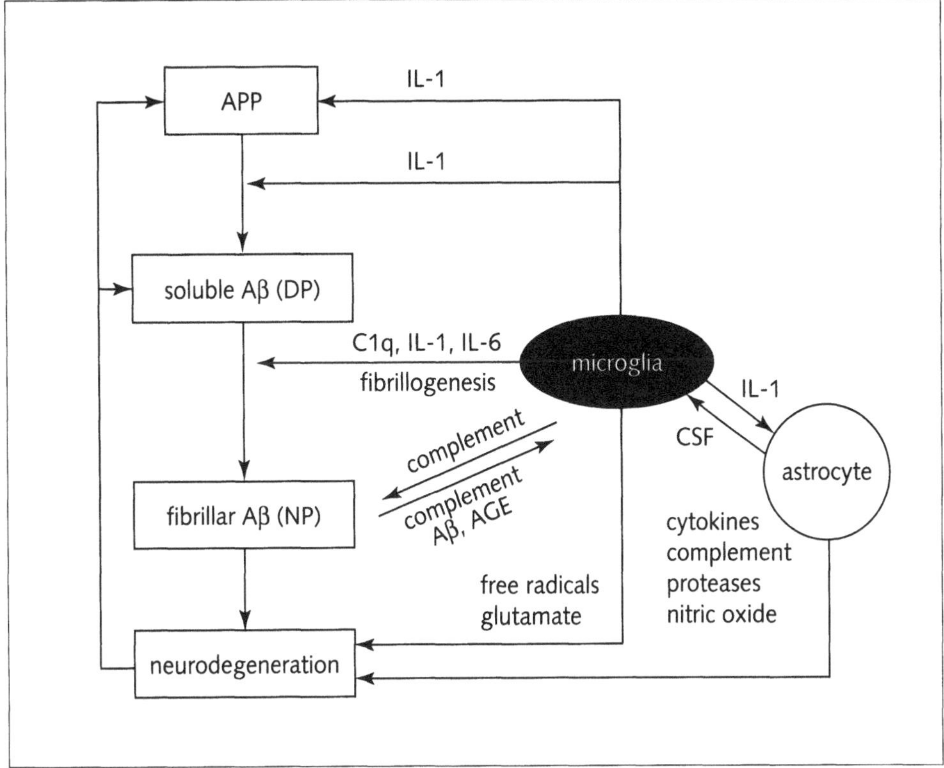

Figure 2
Possible roles and interactions of activated microglial cells in the pathogenesis of Alzheimer's disease.

microglia [19, 20]. The activity of microglia may promote further SP formation by affecting APP metabolism [23–27], and may influence the maturation of SP by accelerating amyloid fibrillogenesis [61, 62] and dystrophic neurite formation [21–23]. As the number of mature SP increases, greater numbers of microglia and astrocytes become stimulated. In addition to propagating the inflammatory process, these cells also produce a variety of potentially neurotoxic substances [2, 8, 13, 15, 28, 71, 76, 81–85, 88–94]. The combined effects of Aβ and these neurotoxins could result in neurodegeneration that may then promote further SP formation. Thus, activated microglia are at the center of three inter-related processes, SP formation, chronic inflammation and neurodegeneration, that may progressively amplify one another, resulting in sufficient neuronal damage to produce the clinical manifestation of AD (Fig. 2). Therapies that modulate the activity of microglial cells may have a beneficial effect in AD by slowing disease progression.

References

1 McGeer P, Akiyama H, Itagaki S, McGeer E (1989) Immune system response in Alzheimer's disease. *Can J Neurol Sci* 16: 516–527
2 McGeer P, McGeer E (1995) The inflammatory response system of brain: implications for therapy of Alzheimer and other neurodegenerative diseases. *Brain Res Rev* 21: 195–218
3 McGeer P, Rogers J, McGeer E (1994) Neuroimmune mechanisms in Alzheimer disease pathogenesis. *Alz Dis Ass Disord* 8: 149–158
4 McGeer P, Schulzer M, McGeer E (1996) Arthritis and anti-inflammatory agents as possible protective factors for Alzheimer's disease: a review of 17 epidemiologic studies. *Neurology* 47: 425–432
5 Davis E, Foster T, Thomas W (1994) Cellular forms and functions of brain microglia. *Brain Res Bull* 34: 73–78
6 Ling E, Wong W (1993) The origin and nature of ramified and amoeboid microglia: a historical review and current concepts. *Glia* 7: 9–18
7 Mackenzie I, Hao C, Munoz D (1995) The role of microglia in senile plaque formation. *Neurobiol Aging* 16: 797–804
8 Banati R, Gehrmann J, Schubert P, Kreutzberg G (1993) Cytotoxicity of microglia. *Glia* 7: 111–118
9 McGeer P, Itagaki S, Tago H, McGeer E (1987) Reactive microglia in patients with senile dementia of the Alzheimer type are positive for histocompatibility glycoprotein HLA-DR. *Neurosci Lett* 79: 195–200
10 Styren S, Civin W, Rogers J (1990) Molecular, cellular and pathologic characterization of HLA-DR immunoreactivity in normal elderly and Alzheimer's disease brain. *Exp Neurol* 110: 93–104
11 Tooyama I, Kimura H, Akiyama H, McGeer P (1990) Reactive microglia express class I and class II major histocompatibility complex antigens in Alzheimer's disease. *Brain Res* 523: 273–280
12 Rogers J, Luber-Narod J, Styren C, Civin W (1988) Expression of immune system- associated antigens by cells of the human central nervous system: Relationship to the pathology of Alzheimer's disease. *Neurobiol Aging* 9: 339–349
13 Haga S, Ikeda K, Sato M, Ishii T (1993) Synthetic Alzheimer amyloid beta/A4 peptides enhance production of complement C3 component by cultured microglial cells. *Brain Res* 601: 88–94
14 Sawada M, Konso N, Suzumura A, Marunouchi T (1989) Production of tumour necrosis factor-alpha by microglia and astrocytes in culture. *Brain Res* 491: 394–397
15 Walker D, Kim S, McGeer P (1995) Complement and cytokine gene expression in cultured microglia derived from postmortem human brains. *J Neurosci Res* 1: 478–493
16 Yao J, Keri J, Taffs R, Colton C (1992) Characterization of interleukin-1 production by microglia in culture. *Brain Res* 591: 88–93
17 Strijbos P, Rothwell N (1995) Interleukin-1 beta attenuates excitatory amino acid-

induced neurodegeneration *in vitro*: involvement of nerve growth factor. *J Neurosci* 15: 3468– 3474
18 Hama T, Kushima Y, Miyamato M, Kubota M, Takei N, Hatanaka H (1991) Interleukin-6 improves the survival of mesencephalic catecholaminergic and septal cholinergic neurons from postnatal, two-week-old rats in culture. *Neuroscience* 40: 445–452
19 Akiyama H, Nishimura T, Kondo H, Ikeda K, Hayashi V, McGeer P (1994) Expression of the receptor for macrophage colony stimulating factor by brain microglia and its upregulation in brains of patients with Alzheimer's disease and amyotrophic lateral sclerosis. *Brain Res* 639: 171–174
20 Lee S, Liu W, Brosan C, Dickson D (1994) GM-CSF promotes proliferation of human fetal and adult microglia in primary cultures. *Glia* 12: 309–318
21 Griffin W, Sheng J, Roberts G, Mrak R (1995) Interleukin-1 expression in different plaque types in Alzheimer's disease: significance in plaque evolution. *J Neuropathol Exp Neurol* 54: 276–281
22 Huell M, Strauss S, Volk B, Berger M, Bauer L (1995) Interleukin-6 is present in early stages of plaque formation and is restricted to the brains of Alzheimer's disease patients. *Acta Neuropathol* 89: 544–551
23 Sheng J, Ito K, Skinner R, Mrak R, Rovnaghi C, van Eldick L, Griffin S (1996) *In vivo* and *in vitro* evidence supporting a role for inflammatory cytokine interleukin-1 as a driving force in Alzheimer pathogenesis. *Neurobiol Aging* 17: 761–766
24 Donnelly R, Friedhoff A, Beer B, Blume A, Vitek M (1990) Interleukin-1 stimulates the beta-amyloid precursor protein promoter. *Cell Mol Neurobiol* 10: 485–495
25 Forloni G, Demicheli F, Giorgi S, Bendotti C, Angeretti N (1992) Expression of amyloid precursor protein mRNAs in endothelial, neuronal and glial cells: Modulation by interleukin-1. Mol *Brain Res* 16: 128–134
26 Goldgarber D, Harris H, Hla T, Maciag T, Donnelly R, Jacobsen J, Vitek M, Gajdusek D (1989) Interleukin 1 regulates synthesis of amyloid beta-protein precursor mRNA in human endothelial cells. *Proc Natl Acad Sci USA* 86: 7606–7610
27 Buxbaum J, Oishi M, Chen H, Pinkas-Kramarski R, Jaffe E, Gandy S, Greengard P (1992) Cholinergic agonists and interleukin 1 regulate processing and secretion of the Alzheimer β/A4 amyloid protein precursor. *Proc Natl Acad Sci USA* 89: 10075–10078
28 Cotman C, Tenner A, Cummings B (1996) β-amyloid converts an acute phase injury response to chronic injury responses. *Neurobiol Aging* 17: 723–731
29 Eikelenboom P, Veerhuis R (1996) The role of complement and activated microglia in the pathogenesis of Alzheimer's disease. *Neurobiol Aging* 17: 673–680
30 Rogers J, Cooper N, Webster S, Schultz J, McGeer P, Styren S, Civin W, Brachova L, Bradt B, Ward P et al (1992) Complement activation by beta-amyloid in Alzheimer disease. *Proc Natl Acad Sci USA* 89: 10016–10020
31 Johnson S, Lampert-Etchells M, Pasinerri G, Rozovsky I, Finch C (1992) Complement mRNA in the mammalian brain: responses to Alzheimer's disease and experimental brain lesioning. *Neurobiol Aging* 13: 641–648
32 Korotzer A, Watt J, Cribbs D, Tenner A, Burkick D, Glabe C, Cotman C (1995) Cul-

tured rat microglia express C1q and receptor for C1q: implications for amyloid effects on microglia. *Exp Neurol* 134: 214–221

33 Akiyama H, McGeer P (1990) Brain microglia constitutively express β2 integrins. *J Neuroimmunol* 30: 81–93

34 Gasque P, Singhrao S, Neal J, Gotze O, Morgan B (1997) Expression of the receptor for complement C5a (CD88) is up-regulated on reactive astrocytes, microglia and endothelial cells in the inflamed human nervous system. *Am J Pathol* 150: 31–41

35 Yao J, Harvarth L, Gilbert D, Colton C (1990) Chemotaxis by a CNS macrophage, the microglia. *J Neurosci Res* 27: 36–42

36 Kawamata T, Akiyama H, Yamada T, McGeer P (1992) Immunologic reactions in amyotrophic lateral sclerosis brain and spinal cord. *Am J Pathol* 140: 691–707

37 Mackenzie I (1998) Activated microglia in dementia with Lewy bodies. *Neurobiol Aging* 19: S202

38 McGeer P, Itagaki S, Boyes B, McGeer E (1988) Reactive microglia are positive for HLA- DR in the substantia nigra of Parkinson's and Alzheimer's disease brains. *Neurology* 38: 1285–1291

39 Paulus W, Bancher C, Jellinger K (1993) Microglial reaction in Pick's disease. *Neurosci Lett* 161: 89–92

40 Sasaki A, Hirato J, Nakazato Y (1993) Immunohistochemical study of microglia in the Creutzfeldt-Jakob diseased brain. *Acta Neuropathol* 86: 337–344

41 Cras P, Kawa M, Siedlak S, Mulvihill P, Gambetti P, Lowery D, Gonzalez-DeWhitt P, Greenberg G, Perry G (1990) Neuronal and microglial involvement in β-amyloid protein deposition in Alzheimer's disease. *Am J Pathol* 137: 241–246

42 Haga S, Akai K, Ishii T (1989) Demonstration of microglial cells in and around senile (neuritic) plaques in the Alzheimer brain: an immunohistochemical study using a novel monoclonal antibody. *Acta Neuropathol* 77: 569–575

43 Itagaki S, McGeer P, Akiyama H, Zhu S, Selkoe D (1989) Relationship of microglia and astrocytes to amyloid deposits of Alzheimer disease. *J Neuroimmunol* 24: 173–182

44 Ohgami T, Kitamoto T, Shin R, Kaneko Y, Ogomori K, Tateishi J (1991) Increased senile plaques without microglia in Alzheimer's disease. *Acta Neuropathol* 81: 242–247

45 Perlmutter L, Scott S, Barron E, Chui H (1992) MHC class II-positive microglia in human brain: associated with Alzheimer lesions. *J Neurosci Res* 33: 549–558

46 Rozemuller J, Eikelenboom P, Stam F, Beyreuther K, Masters C (1989) A4 protein in Alzheimer's disease: primary and secondary cellular events in extracellular amyloid deposition. *J Neuropathol Exp* Neurol 48: 674–691

47 Joachim C, Selkoe D (1992) The seminal role of β-amyloid in the pathogenesis of Alzheimer disease. *Alzheimer Dis Assoc Disord* 6: 7–34

48 Selkoe D (1991) The molecular pathology of Alzheimer's disease. Neuron 6: 487–498

49 Mackenzie I (1994) Senile plaques do not progressively accumulate with normal aging. *Acta Neuropathol* 87: 520–525

50 Mann D, Esiri M (1989) The pattern of acquisition of plaques and tangles in the brains of patients under 50 years of age with Down's syndrome. *J Neurol Sci* 89: 169–179

51 Motte J, Williams R (1989) Age-related changes in the density and morphology of plaques and neurofibrillary tangles in Down syndrome brain. *Acta Neuropathol* 77: 535–546
52 Spargo E, Luthert K, Jonata I, Lantos P (1992) βA4 deposition in the temporal cortex of adults with Down's syndrome. *J Neurol Sci* 111: 26–32
53 Wang D, Munoz D (1995) Qualitative and quantitative differences in senile plaque dystrophic neurites of Alzheimer's disease and normal aged brain. *J Neuropathol Exp Neurol* 54: 548–556
54 Mirra S, Heyman A, McKeel D, Sumi S, Crain B, Brownlee L, Vogel F, Hughes J, van Belle G, Berg L et al (1991) The consortium to establish a registry for Alzheimer's disease (CERAD). Part II. Standardization of the neuropathologic assessment of Alzheimer's disease. *Neurology* 41: 479–486
55 Bauer J, Konig G, Strauss S, Jonas U, Ganter U, Weidemann A, Monning U, Masters C, Volk B, Berger M et al (1991) *In-vitro* matured human macrophages express Alzheimer's beta A4-amyloid precursor protein indicating synthesis in microglial cells. *FEBS Lett* 282: 335–340
56 Haass C, Hung A, Selkoe D (1991) Processing of beta-amyloid precursor protein in microglia and astrocytes favors an internal localization over constitutive secretion. *J Neurosci* 11: 3783–3793
57 Scott S, Johnson S, Zarow C, Perlmutter L (1993) Inability to detect beta-amyloid protein precursor mRNA in Alzheimer plaque-associated microglia. *Exp Neurol* 121: 113–118
58 Shirahama T, Miura K, Ju S, Kisilevsky R, Gruys E, Cohen A (1990) Amyloid enhancing factor-loaded macrophages in amyloid fibril formation. *Lab Invest* 62: 61–68
59 Shigematsu K, McGeer P, Walko D, Ishii T, McGeer E (1992) Reactive microglia/macrophages phagocytose amyloid precursor protein produced by neurons following neuronal damage. *J Neurosci Res* 31: 443–453
60 Wisniewski H, Wegiel J, Wang K, Kujawa M, Lach B (1989) Ultrastructural studies of the cells forming amyloid fibers in classical plaques. *Can J Neurol Sci* 16: 535–542
61 Webster S, Glabe C, Rogers J (1995) Multivalent binding of complement protein C1q to the amyloid β-peptide (Aβ) promotes the nucleation phase of Aβ aggregation. *Biochem Biophys Res Comm* 217: 869–875
62 Webster S, O'Barr S, Rogers J (1994) Enhanced aggregation and β structure of amyloid β peptide after co-incubation with C1q. *J Neurosci Res* 39: 448–456
63 Ard M, Cole G, Wei A, Mehrle A, Fratkin J (1996) Scavenging of Alzheimer's amyloid β-protein by microglia in culture. *J Neurosci Res* 43: 190–202
64 Paresce D, Chung H, Maxfield F (1997) Slow degeneration of aggregates of the Alzheimer's disease amyloid beta-protein by microglial cells. *J Biol Chem* 272: 29390–29397
65 Shaffer L, Dority M, Gupta-Bansal R, Federickson R, Younkin S, Brunden K (1995) Amyloid β protein (Aβ) removal by neuroglial cells in culture. *Neurobiol Aging* 16: 737–745

66 Frautschy S, Cole G, Baird A (1992) Phagocytosis and deposition of vascular beta-amyloid in rat brains injected with Alzheimer beta-amyloid. *Am J Pathol* 140: 1389–1399
67 Frautschy S, Yang F, Irrizarry M, Hyman B, Saido T, Hsiao K, Cole G (1998) Microglial response to amyloid plaques in APPsw transgenic mice. *Am J Pathol* 152: 307–317
68 Stalder M, Phinney A, Probst A, Sommer B, Staufenbiel M, Jucker M (1999) Association of microglia with amyloid plaques in brains of APP23 transgenic mice. *Am J Pathol* 154: 1673–1684
69 Xia M, Qin S, Wu L, Mackay C, Hyman B (1998) Immunohistochemical study of the β-chemokine receptors CCR3 and CCR5 and their ligands in normal and Alzheimer's disease brains. *Am J Pathol* 153: 31–37
70 Davis J, McMurray H, Schubert D (1992) The amyloid beta-protein of Alzheimer's disease is chemotactic for mononuclear phagocytes. *Biochem Biophys Res Comm* 189: 1096–1100
71 El Khoury J, Hickman S, Thomas C, Cao L, Silverstein S, Loike J (1996) Scavenger receptor-mediated adhesion of microglia to beta-amyloid fibrils. *Nature* 382: 716–719
72 Dickson D, Sinicropi S, Yen S, Ko L, Mattice L, Bucala R, Vlassara H (1996) Glycation and microglia reaction in lesions of Alzheimer's disease. *Neurobiol Aging* 17: 733–743
73 Yan S, Chen X, Fu J, Chen M, Shu H, Roher A, Slattery T, Zhao L, Nagashima M, Morser J et al (1996) RAGE and amyloid-β peptide neurotoxicity in Alzheimer's disease. Nature 382: 685–691
74 Araujo D, Cotman C (1992) Beta-amyloid stimulates glial cells *in vitro* to produce growth factors that accumulate in senile plaques in Alzheimer's disease. *Brain Res* 569: 141–145
75 Meda L, Cassatella M, Szendrei G, Otvos L, Baron P, Villalba M, Ferrari D, Rossi F (1995) Activation of microglial cells by β-amyloid protein and interferon-γ. *Nature* 374: 647–650
76 Klegeris A, Walker D, McGeer P (1997) Interacttion of Alzheimer β-amyloid peptide with the human monocytic cell line THP-1 results in a protein kinase C-dependent secretion of tumor necrosis factor-α. *Brain Res* 747: 114–121
77 Vlassara H, Brownlee M, Manogue K, Dinarello C, Pasagian A (1988) Cachectin/TNF and IL-1 induced by glucose modified proteins: role in normal tissue remodeling. *Science* 240: 1546–1548
78 Vlassara H, Bucala R, Striker L (1994) Pathogenic effects of advanced glycosylation: biochemical, biologic and clinical implications for diabetes and aging. *Lab Invest* 70: 138–151
79 Dickson D, Lee S, Mattice L, Yen S, Brosnan C (1993) Microglia and cytokines in neurological disease, with special reference to AIDS and Alzheimer's disease. *Glia* 7: 75– 83
80 Ishizuka K, Kimura T, Igata-Yi R, Katuragi S, Takamatsu J, Miyakawa T (1998) Identification of monocyte chemoattractant protein-1 in senile plaques and reactive microglia of Alzheimer's disease. *Neurobiol Aging* 19: S110
81 Colton C, Gilbert D (1987) Production of superoxide anion by a CNS macrophage, the microglia. *FEBS Lett* 223: 284–288

82 Giulian D, Haverkamp L, Yu J, Karshin W, Tom D, Li J, Kirkpatrick J, Kuo Y, Roher A (1996) Specific domains of β-amyloid from Alzheimer plaque elicit neuron killing in human microglia. *J Neurosci* 16: 6021–6037
83 Goodwin J, Uemura E, Cunnick J (1995) Microglial release of nitric oxide by the synergistic action of β-amyloid and IFN-γ. *Brain Res* 692: 207–214
84 Klegeris A, McGeer P (1994) Rat brain microglia and peritoneal macrophages show similar responses to respiratory burst stimulants. *J Neuroimmunol* 53: 83–90
85 McDonald D, Brunden K, Landreth G (1997) Amyloid fibrils activate tyrosine kinase-dependent signaling and superoxide production in microglia. *J Neurosci* 17: 2284–2294
86 Boje K, Arora P (1992) Microglial-produced nitric oxide and reactive oxides mediate neuronal cell death. *Brain Res* 587: 250–256
87 Lee S, Dickson D, Liu W, Brosnan C (1993) Induction of nitric oxide synthase activity in human astrocytes by interleukin-1 beta and interferon-gamma. *J Neuroimmunol* 46: 19–24
88 Espey M, Chernyshev O, Reinhard J, Namboodiri M, Colton C (1997) Activated human microglia produce the excitotoxin quinolinic acid. *Neuroreport* 8: 431–434
89 Klegeris A, Walker D, McGeer P (1997) Regulation of glutamate in cultures of human monocytic THP-1 and astrocytoma U-373 MG cells. *J Neuroimmunol* 78: 152–161
90 Piani D, Frei K, Do K, Cuenod M, Fontana A (1991) Murine brain macrophages induce NMDA receptor mediated neurotoxicity *in vitro* by secreting glutamate. *Neurosci Lett* 133: 159–162
91 Behl C, Davis J, Lesley R, Schubert D (1994) Hydrogen peroxide mediates amyloid β protein toxicity. *Cell* 77: 817–827
92 Guilian D, Haverkamp L, Li J, Karshin W, Yu J, Tom D, Li X, Kirkpatrick J (1995) Senile plaques stimulate microglia to release a neurotoxin found in Alzheimer brain. *Neurochem Int* 27: 119–137
93 Ii M, Sunamoto, Ohnishi K, Ichimori Y (1996) β-Amyloid protein-dependent nitric oxide production from microglial cells and neurotoxicity. *Brain Res* 720: 93–100
94 Klegeris A, Walker D, McGeer P (1994) Activation of macrophages by Alzheimer β amyloid peptide. *Biochem Biophys Res Commun* 199: 984–991
95 Rogers J, Kirby L, Hempielman S, Berry D, McGeer P, Kaszniak Q, Zalinski J, Cofield M, Mansukhani L, Wilson P et al (1993) Clinical trial of indomethacin in Alzheimer's disease. *Neurology* 43: 1609–1611
96 Mackenzie I, Munoz D (1998) Nonsteroidal anti-inflammatory drug use and Alzheimer-type pathology in aging. *Neurology* 50: 986–990
97 Netland E, Newton J, Majocha R, Tate B (1998) Indomethacin reverses the microglial response to amyloid-beta protein. *Neurobiol Aging* 19: 201–204
98 Klegeris A, Walker D, McGeer E, McGeer P (1998) Non-steroidal anti-inflammatory drugs (NSAIDs) partially protect neuron-like cells from the toxic products of activated THP-1 monocytic cells. *Neurobiol Aging* 19: S258
99 Ganter S, Northoff H, Mannel D, Gebicke-Harter P (1992) Growth control of cultured microglia. *J Neurosci Res* 33: 218–230

100 McRae A, Bona E, Hagberg H (1996) Microglia-astrocyte interactions after cortisone treatment in a neonatal hypoxia-ischemia model. *Brain Res* 94: 44–51
101 Vijayan V, Cotman C (1987) Hydrocortisone administration alters glial reaction to entorhinal lesion in the rat dentate gyrus. *Exp Neurol* 96: 307–320
102 Colton C, Chernyshev O (1996) Inhibition of microglial superoxide anion production by isoproterenol and dexamethasone. *Neurochem Int* 29: 43–53
103 Breitner J, Gau M, Welsh K, Plassman B, McDonald W, Helms M, Anthony J (1994) Inverse association of anti-inflammatory treatments and Alzheimer's disease: initial results of a co-twin control study. *Neurology* 44: 227–232
104 Aisen P, Altstiel L, Marin D, Davis K (1995) Treatment of Alzheimer's disease with prednisone: results of pilot study and design of multicenter trial. *J Am Geriatric Soc* 43: SA27
105 Rother M, Erkinjuntti T, Roessner M, Kittner B, Marcusson J, Karlsson I (1998) Propentofylline in the treatment of Alzheimer's disease and vascular dementia: a review of phase III trials. *Dementia* 9 (suppl 1): 36–43
106 Schubert P, Rudolphi K (1998) Interfering with the pathologic activation of microglial cells and astrocytes in dementia. *Alz Dis Assoc Disord* 12 (suppl 2): S21–28
107 Shinoda I, Furukawa Y, Furukawa S (1990) Stimulation of nerve growth factor synthesis/secretion by propentofylline in cultured mouse astroglial cells. *Biochem Pharmacol* 39: 1813–1816
108 McRae A, Ling E, Schubert P, Rudolphi K (1998) Properties of activated microglia and pharmacologic interference by propentofylline. *Alz Dis Assoc Disord* 12 (suppl 2): S15–20
109 Fuji K, Hiramatsu M, Kameyama T, Nabeshima T (1993) Effects of repeated administrations of propentofylline on memory impairment produced by basal forebrain lesion in rats. *Eur J Pharmacol* 236: 411–417

Neurons

Haruhiko Akiyama

Tokyo Institute of Psychiatry, 2-1-8, Kamikitazawa, Setagaya-ku, Tokyo, 156-8585, Japan

Introduction

It is often thought that microglia and astrocytes are the major players in brain inflammation. Microglia, the brain representatives of the mononuclear phagocyte system, express a variety of cell surface molecules that are involved in inflammation and immune reactions. Astrocytes also express a number of immune-associated molecules such as intercellular adhesion molecule (ICAM)-1. Both microglia and astrocytes transform themselves to become reactive in response to brain lesions. Pro-inflammatory factors that these cell types have been shown to produce include cytokines, eicosanoids, complement components and other proteases of the host defense systems. In fact, microglia and astrocytes at the site of inflammation appear analogous to macrophages and fibroblasts, respectively, in the peripheral organs. Neurons, on the other hand, are regarded as cells that are highly specialized for neural functions such as excitation and synaptic transmission. Therefore, it is natural to consider that neurons perform only passive roles in inflammation. Neurons may become bystander victims of the immune attack and, as a result, fuel the inflammatory processes by providing cell debris, which has to be removed by phagocytic cells and triggers further activation of these cells. The present chapter, however, describes somewhat surprising results of recent studies that suggest that neurons play active roles in brain inflammation. Evidence indicates that, in addition to microglia and astrocytes, neurons synthesize a number of inflammatory mediators.

Complement production by neurons

It has been thought that the liver is the primary site of complement synthesis, with hepatocytes producing over 90% of blood plasma complement. In the peripheral organs, local production of complement proteins also takes place in association with inflammation and tissue injuries, where macrophages and fibroblasts are considered

Neuroinflammatory Mechanisms in Alzheimer's Disease: Basic and Clinical Research,
edited by Joseph Rogers

to synthesize the majority of locally-produced complement components. There is a growing body of evidence that, similar to other organs, brain is capable of producing complement components [1]. This may be particularly significant since normal brain is separated from blood by the blood-brain barrier. *In vitro* studies using primary cultures and cell lines have shown that astrocytes and microglia express both mRNAs and proteins of complement components (see chapters on complement in this volume). A variety of techniques have been employed to investigate the production of complement proteins by neurons. They include *in situ* localization of complement mRNAs and proteins to neurons in brain tissues as well as detection of these components in primary cultured neurons and neuronal cell lines.

An *in situ* hybridization study of the developing rat brain has revealed that neurons express mRNA for complement C4 as early as embryonic day 14 [2]. Neuronal C4 expression shows little change in abundance through 6 weeks postnatal. Another study has demonstrated that mouse pyramidal neurons express mRNA for C3 and factor B (FB) following induction of bacterial meningitis or intraperitoneal injection of tumor necrosis factor α (TNFα) [3]. In the meningitis model, neuronal expression of C3 and FB precedes massive infiltration of leukocytes into the brain, which infers that these complement components promote evolution of the inflammatory processes.

Results obtained in postmortem human brain may not be as conclusive as those in experimental animals or cultured cells because of the inherent limitation of experimental conditions. Nevertheless, evidence indicates that neurons produce a variety of complement components in human brain. In postmortem brain tissues, pyramidal neurons are labeled for both the mRNAs [4, 5] and proteins [6, 7] of complement components. The labeling is enhanced in Alzheimer's disease (AD) compared with controls, suggesting upregulation of complement production by neurons in the AD brain.

Neuronal production of complement components has been confirmed in a number of *in vitro* experiments. Complement mRNAs and proteins have been detected in some human neuroblastoma cell lines [8–10] and rat primary cultured neurons [4, 11]. ELISA of the culture supernatant has indicated that neuroblastoma cells secrete complement proteins and the release is upregulated upon stimulation by certain cytokines [10].

Because complement activation is a non-selective process, cells that synthesize and utilize the complement system usually express complement regulatory molecules to protect themselves from bystander attack. Such regulatory molecules include clusterin, CD59, and C1-inhibitor. Both *in situ* and *in vitro* studies have shown that neurons and neuronal cell lines express clusterin [11–15], CD59 [9, 14, 15] and C1-inhibitor [14, 16, 17].

In summary, it seems evident that neurons are capable of producing a number of complement components. However, controversies still exist over complement expression by neurons. Some investigators reported failure to detect the mRNA for complement C3 in neurons [18]. Others described relatively low expression of C1q by neurons compared with other cell types such as microglia and astrocytes [2, 4]. In *in vitro* studies, discrepancies may be attributed, at least in part, to the difference in cell lines employed in each experiment. In one study, C4 mRNA was detected in three neuroblastoma cell lines, IMR-32, SK-SH and SK-MC, while C3 mRNA was detected only in SK-SH and SK-MC cells, and C9 mRNA expression was limited to SK-MC cells [8]. A neuroblastoma cell line, SH-SY5Y, expresses CD59 [9] whereas NTera2 teratocarcinoma cells, differentiated to post-mitotic neuronal cells, lack CD59 [19]. A neuroblastoma cell line, SK-N-SH, expresses C1-inhibitor but IMR-32 does not [17]. Upregulation of complement production in response to cytokine stimulation also differs among cell lines [10]. In addition, techniques used in each study may affect the results. As mentioned above, the mRNA for C1-inhibitor was not detected in IMR-32 cells by Northern blotting [10] but it was detected in the same cell line after amplification by RT-PCR [16]. It has to be noted that any combination of currently available techniques and materials can provide only limited information in terms of sensitivity, specificity and relevance to the situation in human brain.

Non-lethal effects of complement activation

Major roles of the complement system include opsonization of microbials and tissue debris for phagocytosis, promotion of inflammation by releasing the anaphylatoxins, C3a and C5a, and lytic attack on target cells through formation of the membrane attack complex (MAC). In addition to these classic functions, a number of non-inflammatory effects of complement activation are known. Some of them are mediated by cell surface receptors for complement fragments and others are mediated by non-lethal MAC attack on cells.

There is evidence for non-inflammatory effects of C5 on neurons in brain. Injection of C5a into rat hypothalamus elicits food intake in sated rats [20]. The effect is suppressed by treating rats with a tyrosine hydroxylase inhibitor, suggesting that C5a modulates release of catecholamines at hypothalamic presynaptic terminals [21]. A mouse strain deficient in C5 shows altered synaptic transmission in the glutamatergic system, as well as enhanced neurodegenerative responses to kainic acid [22]. Such results indicate that C5 also modulates excitatory amino acid neurotransmission. Recently, there have been reports on the expression of a C5a receptor (C5aR) by rat neurons [23] and a human neuroblastoma cell line [24]. In rats, neuronal expression of the C5aR is upregulated after traumatic brain injuries [23]. Human neuroblastoma cells exhibit transient increase in intracellular calcium upon stimulation by C5a [24]. Treatment of the same cells with a C5aR ligand, a fragment peptide of C5a, induces DNA fragmentation and apoptotic cell death [24]. These reports, taken together, suggest that C5aR-mediated signaling is likely to be involved in multiple biological events under both physiological and pathological conditions.

Many nucleated cells are resistant to lysis by MAC attack [25]. The MAC is inserted into the plasma membrane to form a stable pore, which causes permeability defects. Cells attacked by the MAC survive only if they can remove the MAC immediately from the membrane. Two modes of removal are known, vesiculation and endocytosis. Vesiculation is a major route of MAC removal in neutrophils, platelets and synoviocytes attacked by non-lethal amounts of homologous complement. Neutrophils remove a small proportion of the cell-bound MAC by endocytosis and subsequent intracellular degradation. In the blood coagulation system, vesiculation of the platelet plasma membrane following MAC attack augments procoagulant activity at the site of inflammation [26]. Prothrombin activation, a key step of the blood coagulation cascade, is catalysed by an enzyme complex (prothrombinase) formed on the plasma membrane. Removal of the MAC by vesiculation from the platelet surface results in the formation of many membrane-derived microparticles ("platelet dusts") which dramatically increases the area of plasma membrane that provides a catalytic surface for assembly and activation of the prothrombinase complex.

The earliest detectable intracellular event caused by MAC attack is a rise in intracellular free calcium ion concentration [25]. This is mediated by both influx *via* the MAC pore and release from intracellular stores. The rise in calcium ion concentration results in the phosphorylation of the substrates of protein kinase C and other intracellular kinases. In neutrophils and macrophages, non-lethal amounts of the MAC stimulate synthesis and release of proinflammatory products such as reactive oxygen species, metabolites of arachidonic acid and some cytokines [25, 27]. These observations indicate that non-lethal MAC attack mediates membrane signaling to certain cell types. Whether the MAC-induced membrane vesiculation or an increase in intracellular calcium ions occurs in neurons and plays a role in neuronal functions has yet to be studied.

Certain cytokines such as TNFα, interferon-γ (IFNγ) and interleukin (IL)-1α/β have been shown to enhance neuronal expression of complement proteins and complement regulatory molecules [10, 17, 23]. Similar upregulation occurs in AD brain [4–7] as well as following introduction of model lesions in animal brain [3, 15]. Enhanced expression in brain lesions or upon cytokine stimulation infers that the neuron-derived complement components are engaged in some pathological processes and, presumably, in inflammation.

Cyclooxygenase (COX)-2

A number of epidemiological studies have consistently shown a protective effect of non-steroidal anti-inflammatory drugs (NSAIDs) against occurrence and/or progression of AD. Long-term administration of NSAIDs is expected to attenuate neuronal damage by reducing the inflammatory responses in the AD brain. NSAIDs are presumed to act by inhibiting cyclooxygenase (COX), the rate-limiting enzyme in the conversion of arachidonic acid to prostanoids. Two isoforms of COX are known, COX-1 as the constitutive, and COX-2 as the inducible form of the enzyme. In fact, both COX-1 and COX-2 are constitutively expressed but the expression of COX-2 is more readily upregulated during inflammation [28].

COX-2 has long been considered to be a pro-inflammatory enzyme and a target of anti-inflammatory drug development. However, recent evidence suggests that the functions of COX-2 are more complicated than have been believed [29, 30]. In a rat inflammation model induced by carrageenin, upregulation of COX-2 expression is biphasic [29]. The profile of prostaglandins produced in the lesion changes from a pro-inflammatory, prostaglandin E2-dominated eicosanoid profile during the development of inflammation to an anti-inflammatory, cyclopentone-dominated eicosanoid profile during the resolution of inflammation. In the resolution phase, inhibition of COX-2 rather exacerbates inflammation with reduction of the cyclopentone-dominated eicosanoids. Other investigators have reported that, in mice, the gut COX-2-dependent arachidonic acid metabolites suppress T cell proliferation in response to a dietary antigen, thereby inhibiting the occurrence of intestinal inflammation [30].

In brains, COX-2 is expressed primarily by neurons [28, 31, 32]. The expression is enhanced under such pathological conditions as AD [28, 33, 34] and ischemia [35, 36]. So far, there seems to be little evidence to indicate a pro-inflammatory role for neuronal COX-2. In experimental animals, neuronal COX-2 expression is upregulated quickly by excitotoxin treatment or sustained seizure, suggesting COX-2 expression is modulated by synaptic activity [31, 37]. Localization of COX-2 to the dendritic spines appears to support the notion that COX-2 is involved in the postsynaptic signaling of excitatory neurons [38]. Some investigators, on the other hand, suggest that COX-2 activity is accompanied by free radical generation and that COX-2 contributes to neuronal oxidative stress, which then induces neuronal damage or delayed neuronal cell death [35, 36]. COX-2 expression is also reported to precede apoptosis of dentate granule cells following exposure to colchicine [39]. In culture, stimulation by β amyloid peptide (Aβ) induces COX-2 expression in SH-SY5Y neuroblastoma cells [34]. A number of hypotheses have been proposed on the mechanism of Aβ neurotoxicity in AD. These include oxidative stress, excitotoxicity of glutamatergic neurotransmission, and apoptosis. In any of these cases, COX-2 might play a significant role for Aβ-induced neuronal damage [40]. A report that treatment with a NSAID attenuates Aβ neurotoxicity to PC12 cells [41] appears to support this idea. Other investigators, however, report that NSAIDs inhibit the IL-1β-induced IL-6 release by astrocytes cultured from postmortem human brain [42] and that NSAIDs reduce the microglial responses to Aβ infused into rat brain [43]. The mechanism of the apparent NSAID action against AD needs further clarification.

Cytokines

Neurons synthesize a number of cytokines, some of which are known to have pro- or anti-inflammatory actions in the periphery. The roles of these cytokines in the central nervous system (CNS) may not be simple, however. Cytokines form complex networks in which both neurons and glial cells are involved. Cytokines act both directly on cells and indirectly through the networks. In addition, a single cytokine has multiple effects (pleiotrophy), and a number of cytokines have a common effect (redundancy). It is therefore difficult to predict the final effects of even a single cytokine *in vivo*.

Pro-inflammatory cytokines that neurons have been reported to synthesize include interferon-γ (IFNγ), interleukin (IL)-1, IL-6, tumor necrosis factor-α (TNFα) and macrophage-colony stimulating factor (M-CSF). IFNγ-like immunoreactivity was first identified in neurons in the rat dorsal root ganglia [44]. Subsequently, a molecule that shared both immunoreactivity and bioactivity with, but was distinct from, lymphocyte-derived (i.e. classic) IFNγ was extracted from rat sensory trigeminal ganglia [45]. More recently, mRNA for classic IFNγ has also been identified in primary cultures of fetal rat dorsal root ganglia neurons [46]. Whether the neuron-derived IFNγ and an IFNγ-like molecule are involved in brain inflammation or not remains unclear. Neurons express a receptor for IFNγ, suggesting the action of IFNγ in an autocrine fashion. *In vitro* studies have shown that IFNγ affects differentiation and survival of neuronal cells. IFNγ also suppresses neuronal degeneration that is caused by nerve growth factor (NGF) withdrawal and facilitates NGF-induced differentiation [47–49].

IL-6 production has been demonstrated in primary culture of rat cortical neurons [50]. Stimulation of cultured neurons with IL-1β and TNFα upregulates the expression of mRNA for IL-6. Transgenic mice overexpressing IL-6 under the control of the glial fibrillary acidic protein (GFAP) promoter exhibit enhanced expression of other inflammatory cytokines such as IL-1α, IL-1β and TNFα in brain, together with the activation of astrocytes and microglia. These mice show a chronic progressive neurodegenerative disorder [51]. Transgenic mice overexpressing IL-6 under the control of the neuron-specific enolase promoter also show upregulated IL-1β and TNFα in brain and activation of glial cells. However, no neuronal damage is observed in the latter mice [52]. Such a result infers that the same cytokine may act differently depending on the cell type that expresses the cytokine.

There are reports on the immunohistochemical localization of IL-1β [53, 54] and TNFα [55] to neurons and neuronal processes in brain tissues. The action of TNFα in the CNS appears to be complicated. Unlike IL-6 transgenic mice, TNFα transgenic mice in which TNFα is overexpressed either in astrocytes under the control of the GFAP promoter or in neurons under control of the neurofilament promoter both exhibit CNS inflammation and a neurological disorder [56]. On the other hand, the mice deficient in TNF develop much more extensive inflammation and demyelination than control animals after immunization with the myelin oligodendrocyte glycoprotein to induce experimental autoimmune encephalomyelitis (EAE) [57]. The exacerbation of EAE in the TNF-deficient mice is reversed by TNF administration. The authors suggest that TNF acts to limit the extent of CNS inflammation [57].

A study has shown that neurons are stained positively for M-CSF in brain tissues and that the expression of both M-CSF transcripts and the protein is detected in SK-N-SH neuroblastoma cells [58]. In the same study, the authors have demonstrated the upregulation of M-CSF expression by SK-N-SH cells upon stimulation by Aβ and claimed that neuron-derived M-CSF activates microglia and increases inflammation in the AD brain. Another study suggests that TNFα and IFNγ increase the inflammatory responses in AD brain, but more indirectly. These two cytokines, when administered together to SK-N-SH neuroblastoma cells, alter the metabolism of amyloid precursor protein (APP), reducing non-amyloidgenic APPα and increasing production of Aβ [59], which then activates microglia and the complement system.

In summary, neurons are likely to be a potential source of a number of inflammatory cytokines but actions of these cytokines in brain may not be easy to determine. A number of cytokines are involved in the proliferation, survival and phenotypic differentiation of neural cells during CNS development. They also modulate neurite outgrowth, synaptic plasticity and neurotransmitter expression. For example, IL-1β increases endogenous adenosine production and suppresses glutamate transmission in hippocampal CA1 pyramidal neurons [60]. IL-1β, IL-2, IL-6 and IFNα enhance release of arginine vasopressin in slices of the rat hypothalamus [61]. It is noteworthy, however, that cytokine expression in brain is generally at a very low level until a damaging stimulus occurs. This infers that certain cytokines, though they are implicated in a variety of physiological processes under normal conditions, play significant roles in the CNS lesions [49].

Other molecules involved in inflammation

Inflammation leads to the activation of multiple host defense systems that were originally discovered in the blood plasma but were later disclosed to be produced in many extravascular tissues. Four major humoral host defense mechanisms are known: the complement, contact activation, blood coagulation and fibrinolysis systems. These systems all involve cascade-like activation of multiple serine proteases and thus are regulated by serine protease inhibitors (serpins). Neurons secrete, in addition to complement inhibitors, serpins that inhibit plasminogen activators (PA) [62, 63]. The expression of neuronal serpins is upregulated upon inflammatory stimuli [62]. The PA/plasmin system plays important roles for neuronal migration and neurite outgrowth in the developing brain. Whether the regulation of the PA/plasmin system by neurons affects brain inflammation is unknown.

The inflammatory process involves a number of cell surface receptors by which inflammatory cells communicate with each other. They include the major histocompatibility complex (MHC) antigens and cell adhesion molecules such as integrins and selectins. Immunohistochemistry for these molecules have shown that neurons lack them. Microglia are the principal cells that express these cell surface receptors in brain [64]. Astrocytes and vascular endothelial cells also express some of them. Recently, a β2-integrin, leukocyte function associated antigen (LFA)-1, has been reported to bind to telencephalin, a cell adhesion molecule that belongs to the immunoglobulin superfamily and is expressed specifically and abundantly by neurons [65]. The major ligand of LFA-1 in the brain parenchyma is considered to be ICAM-1, which is expressed by reactive astrocytes. The expression of LFA-1 and ICAM-1 is sharply upregulated in inflammatory lesions such as AD senile plaques. This contrasts with the decline in the telencephalin expression in the AD brain [66]. Neuronal telencephalin might compete with astrocytic ICAM-1 to suppress the LFA-1/ICAM-1 pathway so that neurons could regulate inflammatory state in normal brain.

Conclusion

Neurons might play an active role in brain inflammation. Currently available evidence, however, is limited to the expression of molecules that potentially enhance or suppress inflammation. Stimulation by certain cytokines enhances neuronal production of a number of inflammatory molecules. Similar upregulation occurs in model lesions induced in experimental animal brains as well as in lesions of human neurological diseases. These facts appear to favor the presence of neuronal modulation of inflammatory processes, even if neurons may not be the principal cells that govern brain inflammation. On the other hand, many ‘classic’ inflammatory molecules are now known to be involved in a variety of non-inflammatory events, which include differentiation, growth and survival of CNS cells, synaptogenesis, neurotransmission, and neuronal cell death. Obviously, the relevance of the neuron-derived pro- and anti-inflammatory molecules to brain inflammation is an issue for further investigation.

References

1 Barnum SR (1995) Complement biosynthesis in the central nervous system. *Crit Rev Oral Biol Med* 6: 132–146

2 Johnson SA, Pasinetti GM, Finch CE (1994) Expression of complement C1qB and C4 mRNAs during rat brain development. *Dev Brain Res* 80: 163–174

3 Stahel PF, Kossmann T, Morganti-Kossmann MC, Hans VHJ (1997) Experimental dif-

fuse axonal injury induces enhanced neuronal C5a receptor mRNA expression in rat. *Mol Brain Res* 50: 205–212

4 Johnson SA, Lampert-Etchells M, Pasinetti GM, Finch CE (1992) Complement mRNA in the mammalian brain: responses to Alzheimer's disease and experimental brain lesioning. *Neurobiol Aging* 13: 641–648

5 Shen Y, Li R, McGeer EG, McGeer PL (1997) Neuronal expression of mRNAs for complement proteins of the classical pathway in Alzheimer brain. *Brain Res* 769: 391–395

6 Afagh A, Cummings BJ, Cribbs DH, Cotman CW, Tenner AJ (1996) Localization and cell association of C1q in Alzheimer's disease brain. *Exp Neurol* 138: 22–32

7 Terai K, Walker DG, McGeer EG, McGeer PL (1997) Neurons express proteins of the classical complement pathway in Alzheimer disease. *Brain Res* 769: 385–390

8 Walker DG, McGeer PL (1993) Complement gene expression in neuroblastma and astrocytoma cell lines of human origin. *Neurosci Lett* 157: 99–102

9 Shen Y, Sullivan T, Lee CM, Meri S (1998) Induced expression of neuronal membrane attack complex and cell death by Alzheimer's β-amyloid peptide. *Brain Res* 796: 187–197

10 Veerhuis R, Janssen R, De Groot CJA, Van Muiswinkel FL, Hack CE, Eikelenboom P (1999) Cytokines associated with amyloid plaques in Alzheimer's disease brain stimulate human glial and neuronal cell cultures to secrete early complement proteins, but not C1-inhibitor. *Exp Neurol* 160: 289–299

11 Rozovsky I, Morgan TE, Willoughby DA (1994) Selective expression of clusterin (SGP-2) and complement C1qB and C4 during responses to neurotoxins *in vivo* and *in vitro*. *Neurosci* 62: 741–758

12 McGeer PL, Kawamata T, Walker DG (1992) Distribution of clusterin in Alzheimer brain tissue. *Brain Res* 579: 337–341

13 Dragunaw M, Preston K, Dodd J, Young D (1995) Clusterin accumulates in dying neurons following status epilepticus. *Mol Brain Res* 32: 279–290

14 Gasque P, Thoams A, Fontaine M, Morgan BP (1996) Complement activation on human neuroblastoma cell lines *in vitro*: route of activation and expression of functional complement regulatory proteins. *J Neuroimmunol* 66: 29–40

15 Mattosson P, Morgan BP, Svensson M (1998) Complement activation and CD59 expression in the motor facial nucleus following intracranial transection of the facial nerve in the adult rat. *J Neuroimmunol* 91: 180–189

16 Walker DG, Yasuhara O, Patston PA, McGeer EG, McGeer PL (1995) Complement C1 inhibitor is produced by brain tissue and is cleaved in Alzheimer disease. *Brain Res* 675: 75–82

17 Veerhuis R, Janssen I, Hoozemans JJM, De Groot CJA, Hac CE, Eikelenboom P (1998) Complement C1-inhibitor expression in Alzheimer's disease. *Acta Neuropathol* 96: 287–296

18 Barnum SR, Jones JL, Muller-Ladner U, Samimi A, Campbell IL (1996) Chronic complement C3 gene expression in the CNS of transgenic mice with astrocyte-targeted interleukin-6 expression. *Glia* 18: 107–117

19 Agoropoulou C, Wing MG, Wood A (1996) CD59 expression and complement susceptibility of human neuronal cell line (NTera2). *Neuroreport* 7: 997–1004
20 Williams CA, Schupf N, Hugli TE (1985) Anaphylatoxin C5a modulation of an α-adrenergic receptor system in the rat hypothalamus. *J Neuroimmunol* 9: 29–40
21 Schupf N, Williams CA, Berkman A, Cattell WS, Kerper L (1989) Binding specificity and presynaptic action of anaphylatoxin C5a in rat brain. *Brain Behav Immun* 3: 28–38
22 Pasinetti GM, Tocco G, Sakhi S, Musleh WD (1996) Hereditary deficiencies in complement C5 are associated with intensified neurodegenerative responses that implicate new roles for the C-system in neuronal and astrocytic functions. *Neurobiol Dis* 3: 197–204
23 Stahel PF, Frei K, Fontana A, Eugster HP (1997) Evidence for intrathecal synthesis of alternative pathway complement activation proteins in experimental meningitis. *Am J Pathol* 151: 897–904
24 Farkas I, Baranyi L, Takahashi M, Fukuda A, Liposits AS, Yamamoto T, Okada HA (1998) A neuronal C5a receptor and an associated apoptotic signal transduction pathway. *J Physiol* 507: 679–687
25 Morgan BP (1989) Complement membrane attack on nucleated cells: resistance, recovery and non-lethal effects. *Biochem J* 264: 1–14
26 Sims PJ, Wiedmer T (1991) The response of human platelets to activated components of the complement system. *Immunol Today* 12: 338–342
27 Nicholson-Weller A, Halperin JA (1993) Membrane signaling by complement C5b-9, the membrane attack complex. *Immunol Res* 12: 244–257
28 Yasojima K, Schwab C, McGeer EG, McGeer PL (1999) Distribution of cyclooxygenase-1 and cyclooxygenase-2 mRNAs and proteins in human brain and peripheral organs. *Brain Res* 830: 226–236
29 Gilroy DW, Colville-Nash PR, Willis D, Chivers J, Paul-Clark MJ, Willoughby DA (1999) Inducible cyclooxygenase may have anti-inflammatory properties. *Nature Med* 5: 698–701
30 Newberry RD, Stenson WF, Lorenz RG (1999) Cyclooxygenase-2-dependent arachidonic acid metabolites are essential modulators of the intestinal immune response to dietary antigen. *Nature Med* 5: 900–906
31 Yamagata K, Andreasson KI, Kaufmann WE, Barnes CA, Worley PF (1993) Expression of a mitogen-inducible cyclooxygenase in brain neurons: regulation by synaptic activity and glucocorticoids. *Neuron* 1: 371–386
32 Tocco G, Freire-Moar J, Schreiber SS, Sakhi SH, Aisen PS, Pasinetti GM (1997) Maturational regulation and regional induction of cyclooxygenase-2 in rat brain: implications for Alzheimer's disease. *Exp Neurol* 144: 339–349
33 Oka A, Takashima S (1997) Induction of cyclo-oxygenase 2 in brains of patients with Down's syndrome and dementia of Alzheimer type: specific localization in affected neurons and axons. *Neuroreport* 8: 1161–1164
34 Pasinetti GM, Aisen PS (1998) Cyclooxygenase-2 expression is increased in frontal cortex of Alzheimer's disease brain. *Neurosci* 87: 319–324

35 Nogawa S, Zhang F, Ross ME, Iadecola C (1997) Cyclo-oxygenase-2 gene expression in neurons contributes to ischemic brain damage. *J Neurosci* 17: 2746–2755

36 Sairanen T, Ristimaki A, Karjalainen-Lindsberg ML, Paetau A, Kaste M, Lindsberg PJ (1998) Cyclooxygenase-2 is induced globally in infarcted human brain. *Ann Neurol* 43: 738–747

37 Adams J, Collaco-Moraes Y, de Belleroche J (1996) Cyclooxygenase-2 induction in cerebral cortex: an intracellular response to synaptic excitation. *J Neurochem* 66: 6–13

38 Kaufmann WE, Worley PF, Pegg J, Bremer M, Isakson P (1996) COX-2, a synaptically induced enzyme, is expressed by excitatory neurons at postsynaptic sites in rat cerebral cortex. *Proc Natl Acad Sci USA* 93: 2317–2321

39 Ho L, Osaka H, Aisen PS, Pasinetti GM (1998) Induction of cyclooxygenase (COX)-2 but not COX-1 gene expression in apoptotic cell death. *J Neuroimmunol* 89: 142–149.

40 Pasinetti GM (1998) Cyclooxygenase and inflammation in Alzheimer's disease: Experimental approaches and clinical interventions. *J Neurosci* Res 54: 1–6

41 Fagarasan MO, Aisen PS (1996) IL-1 and anti-inflammatory drugs modulate Aβ cytotoxicity in PC12 cells. *Brain Res* 723: 231–234

42 Blom MAA, van Twillert MGH, de Vries SC, Engels F, Finch CE, Veerhuis R, Eikelenboom P (1997) NSAIDS inhibit the IL-1β-induced IL-6 release from human postmortem astrocytes: the involvement of prostaglandin E2. *Brain Res* 777: 210–218

43 Netland EE, Newton JL, Majocha RE, Tate BA (1998) Indomethacin reverses the microglial response to amyloid beta-protein. *Neurobiol Aging* 19: 201–204

44 Kiefer R, Kreutzberg GW (1990) Gamma interferon-like immunoreactivity in the rat nervous system. *Neurosci* 37: 725–734

45 Olsson T, Kelic S, Edlund C, Bakhiet M, Hojeberg B, Meide PH van der, Ljungdahl A, Kristensson K (1994) Neuronal interferon-γ immunoreactive moelcule: bioactivities and purification. *Eur J Immunol* 24: 308–314

46 Neumann H, Schmidt H, Wilharm E, Behrens L, Wekerle H (1997) Interferon-γ gene expression in sensory neurons: evidence for autocrine gene regulation. *J Exp Med* 186: 2023–2031

47 Chang JY, Martin DP, Johnson Jr EM (1990) Interferon suppresses sympathetic neuronal cell death caused by nerve growth factor deprivation. *J Neurochem* 55: 436–445

48 Jonakait GM, Wei R, Sheng ZL, Hart RP (1994) Interferon-γ promotes cholinergic differentiation of embryonic septal nuclei and adjacent basal forebrain neurons. *Neuron* 12: 1149–1159

49 Zhao B, Schwartz JP (1998) Involvement of cytokines in normal CNS development and neurological diseases: recent progress and perspectives. *J Neurosci Res* 52: 7–16

50 Ringheim GE, Burgher KL, Heroux JA (1995) Interleukin-6 mRNA expression by cortical neurons in culture: evidence for neuronal sources of interleukin-6 production in the brain. *J Neuroimmunol* 63: 113–123

51 Campbell IL, Abraham CR, Masliah E, Kemper P, Inglis JD (1993) Neurologic disease induced in transgenic mice by cerebral overexpression of interleukin 6. *Proc Natl Acad Sci USA* 90: 10061–10065

52 Fattori E, Lazzaro D, Musiani P, Modesti A (1995) IL-6 expression in neurons of transgenic mice causes reactive astrocytosis and increase in ramified microglial cells but not neuronal damage. *Eur J Neurosci* 7: 2441–2449
53 Breder CD, Dinarello CA, Saper CB (1988) Interleukin-1 immunoreactive intervation of the human hypothalamus. *Science* 240: 321–324
54 Lechan RM, Toni R, Clark BD, Cannon JG (1990) Immunoreactive interleukin-1β localization in the rat forebrain. *Brain Res* 514: 135–140
55 Breder CD, Tsujimoto M, Terano Y, Scott DW (1993) Distribution and characterization of tumor necrosis factor-α-like immunoreactivity in the murine central nervous system. *J Comp Neurol* 337: 543–567
56 Probert L, Akassoglou K, Kassiotis G, Pasparakis M (1997) TNF-α and knockout models of CNS inflammation and degeneration. *J Neuroimmunol* 72: 137–141
57 Liu J, Marino MW, Wong G, Grail D, Dunn A, Bettadapura J, Slavin AJ, Old L, Bernard CCA (1998) TNF is a potent anti-inflammatory cytokine in autoimmune-mediated demyelination. *Nature Med* 4: 78–83
58 Yan SD, Zhu H, Fu J, Yan SF, Roher A, Tourtellotte WW (1997) Amyloid-β peptide-receptor for advanced glycation endproduct interaction elicits neuronal expression of macrophage-colony stimurating factor: a proinflammatory pathway in Alzheimer disease. *Proc Natl Acad Sci USA* 94: 5296–5301
59 Blasko I, Marx F, Steiner E, Hartmann T (1999) TNFα plus IFNγ induce the production of Alzheimer β-amyloid peptides and decrease the secretion of APPs. *FASEB J* 13: 63–68
60 Luk WP, Zhang Y, White TD, Lue FA, Wu C, Jiang CG, Zhang L, Moldofsky H (1999) Adenosine: a mediator of interleukin-1β-induced hippocampal synaptic inhibition. *J Neurosci* 19: 4238–4244
61 Raber J, Sorg O, Horn TFW, Yu N, Koob GF (1998) Inflammatory cytokines: putative regulators of neuronal and neuro-endocrine function. *Brain Res Rev* 26: 320–326
62 Reddington M, Haas C, Kreutzberg GW (1994) The plasminogen activator system in neurons and glia during motoneuron regeneration. *Neuropathol Appl Neurobiol* 20: 188–190
63 Osterwalder T, Cinelli P, Baici A, Pennella A (1998) The axonally secreted serine proteinase inhibitor, nueroserpin, inhibits plasminogen activators and plasmin but not thrombin. *J Biol Chem* 273: 2312–2321
64 McGeer PL, McGeer EG (1995) The inflammatory response system of brain: implications for therapy of Alzheimer and other neurodegenerative diseases. *Brain Res* Rev 21: 195–218
65 Mizuno T, Yoshihara Y, Inazawa J, Kagamiyama H, Mori K (1997) cDNA cloning and chromosomal localization of the human telencephalin and its distinctive interaction with lymphocyte function-associated antigen-1. *J Biol Chem* 272: 1156–1163
66 Hino H, Mori K, Yoshihara Y, Iseki E, Akiyama H, Nishimura T, Ikeda K, Kosaka K (1997) Reduction of telencephalin immunoreactivity in the brain of patients with Alzheimer's disease. *Brain Res* 753: 353–357

The gero-inflammatory manifold

Caleb E. Finch and Valter D. Longo

Andrus Gerontology Center and Department of Biological Sciences, University of Southern California, Los Angeles, CA 90089-0191, USA

Introduction

Inflammatory processes during Alzheimer's disease (AD) may be considered as part of a larger manifold of oxidative and inflammatory processes that slowly develop during aging in many tissue beds throughout the organism as well as in the brain. Other chapters in this volume have described the many cellular and molecular interactions between aggregates of amyloid β-peptide (Aβ) and inflammatory system components. In considering whether inflammatory processes are primary or secondary during AD and in aging, we discuss evidence that inflammatory processes are associated with amyloid formation in many tissues. We also point out similarities and differences between AD and brain aging changes in humans and in various laboratory models. Moreover, some experimental and clinical interventions of aging in the brain and in non-neural tissues may work by modulating oxidative and inflammatory processes through systemic physiological factors. Thus, inflammatory processes during AD could be considered in a larger systemic context of age-related pathobiology which we designate the gero-inflammatory manifold (Fig. 1).

The classical hallmarks of inflammatory processes (rubor, tumor, calor, dolor) are not found in AD brains. Thus, AD may be considered in the main as an atrophic process, without increased blood flow or tissue swelling; pain would not be expected in any case because the brain has limited nociception. By these criteria, AD stands in great contrast to the painful inflammatory components of joint diseases that are common in the elderly. Another instructive counter-example is multiple sclerosis, which shows extensive microglial/monocytic activation, but which, unlike AD, additionally has autoreactive T cells. Nonetheless, AD lesions have long been associated with the robust activation of glial cells [1–3], including microglia, which are ultimately bone marrow-derived. The absence of recombinatorial immune cell functions in AD and the expression of many cytokine and complement factors by resident brain cells [4, 5] are characteristics of the primitive host defense mechanisms that were present in early vertebrates and in invertebrates [6, 7]. This feature

Neuroinflammatory Mechanisms in Alzheimer's Disease: Basic and Clinical Research,
edited by Joseph Rogers

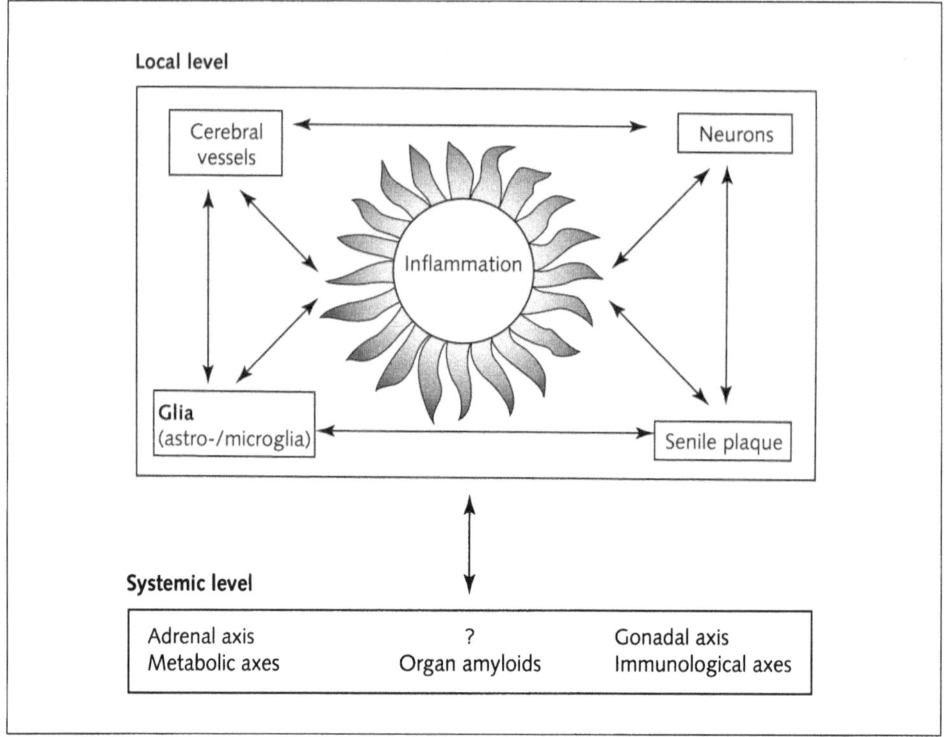

Figure 1
The gero-inflammatory manifold: Cross-talk between inflammatory processes within the brain during aging and Alzheimer disease (upper box), and systemic interactions with peripheral inflammatory processes of aging in other organ systems (lower box). Microglia in the brain are considered to be of bone marrow origin which enter the brain as monocytes. Hormones include secretions of the endocrine and autonomic systems and other acute phase factors as well as cytokines. The importance of systemic nutrients to brain aging is shown by the attenuation of glial activation during aging through caloric restriction (Fig. 2). Blood glucose and other metabolites modify the rate of oxidation of proteins and lipids through non-enzymatic glycation (glycoxidation) (Fig. 3). We speculate on the possibility, indicated as (?), that age-related accumulations of peripheral organ "senile amyloids" (distinct from the amyloid β-peptide) may interact with brain aging processes. Original drawing from Caleb E. Finch and Chris P. Anderson.

may allow general therapeutic approaches to AD as part of the gero-inflammatory manifold. The evidence that some anti-inflammatory drugs (NSAIDS) being used to treat peripheral conditions [8] may also protect against AD supports the concept of general interventions.

Inflammatory features of brain aging

Emerging evidence indicates that subsets of the inflammatory mechanisms observed in AD also arise during normal aging, but in the absence of clinical disease (Tab. 1). In particular, an age-related activation of microglia and astrocytes occurs during middle-age, but without evidence of overt neurodegeneration such as neuron loss. For example, we observed a three-fold increase in the numbers of activated microglia in the myelinated cortico-striatal bundles in middle-aged rats [9] (Fig. 2). A growing literature documents the activation of microglia and astrocytes throughout aging brains and other rodent genotypes [10–15]. Although astrocytes are widely considered as supportive cells for neurons, astrocytes can also produce superoxide and other reactive oxygen species (ROS) [16, 17]. Whether production of ROS changes with age-related glial activation in the brain is not known. The significance of glial activation to neurodegeneration during aging is suggested by two examples. Infusion of aggregated Aβ into old primate brains caused greater microglial activation and neuron damage than in young primate brains [18], whereas we observed that microglia from middle-aged rats were resistant to down-regulation of LPS-induced nitric oxide generation by TGF-β_1 [19].

Glial fibrillary acidic protein (GFAP), an intermediate filament of astrocytes that is associated with fibrous transformation in reactive astrocytes, shows robust progressive increases in expression during normal aging in rodents and humans. Using *in situ* hybridization it has been shown that GFAP mRNA increases progressively during aging at an average rate of about five mRNA copies per astrocyte per month [13]. Depending on brain region, astrocyte GFAP mRNA reaches levels that are two- to four-fold above those in young adults by the end of their lifetime [9, 20]. The increased GFAP expression can be attributed to increased transcription as shown by measurement of intron RNA [9, 20], although post-translational changes have not been evaluated. The increase of GFAP per cell is not associated with age changes in the *total* numbers of astrocytes, which are modest to imperceptible, e.g. in the hippocampus [9, 21]. In humans, GFAP mRNA [22] and numbers of fibrous astrocytes [23] also increase progressively during aging in the absence of neuropathology. GFAP is the first example of a gene in any tissue to show progressive activation during aging in the absence of specific pathological changes. Because GFAP transcription is also activated by oxidative stress [20], we hypothesized that the age-related increases of GFAP transcription are stimulated by oxidative components of inflammatory processes during aging. We showed that the upstream rat GFAP promoter has an NF-κB binding element that mediates GFAP responses to hydrogen peroxide [24], as well as induction by IL-1 [25]. Moreover, Aβ and hydrogen peroxide treatment of astrocytes induces nuclear proteins that bind to this element [24].

There are many indications of oxidative stress during aging. Oxidized groups of proteins increase during aging in rodents and human brains (reviewed in [9]), as well as in peripheral tissues, as described below. In the case of rodents, we can rule

Table 1 - Neuroinflammatory changes in Alzheimer and aging

	AD senile plaques[a]	Normal aging rodent[b]	Normal aging human
astrocytes, activated	↑	↑ (GFAP)	↑ (GFAP)[c]
microglia, activated	↑	↑ (OX-6,-42)	↑
neurite abnormalities	↑	↑ (no NFT)	↑
Aβ	↑		↑
APP	↑X		
α1-antichymotrypsin	↑		
α2-macroglobulin	↑		
apoE	↑	↑ (mRNA)	
apoJ (clusterin)	↑	↑ (mRNA)	↑ corpora amylacea[d]
CRP	↑		
heme oxygenase-1	↑	↑ (ICC)	
complement factors			
C1q	↓ CSF[e]	↑ (mRNA)	↑ corpora amylacea[d]
C3	↑		↑ increase in CSF[f]
C9	↑		
cytokines			
IL-1	↑		↑ plasma
IL-6	↑		
TGF-β_1	↑	↑ (mRNA)	
TNFγ	↑		

AD, relative to healthy elderly brains; normal aging, relative to young
[a][2, 6, 8, 18, 91]; [b][1, 6, 9, 15, 91]; [c][15, 23]; [d][29, 30]; [e][32]; [f][31]

out Aβ amyloids as a factor since aging laboratory rodent brains do not accumulate Aβ peptides. Some types of fibrils are found in granules within astrocytes, which are immunoreactive for proteoglycans and laminin, but not for those Aβ peptides tested [26].

In addition to these indications of activated glia during aging, we note that a subset of the same inflammatory factors associated with AD also increase during brain aging. Readers should be aware, however, that the subject of "gero-inflammation"

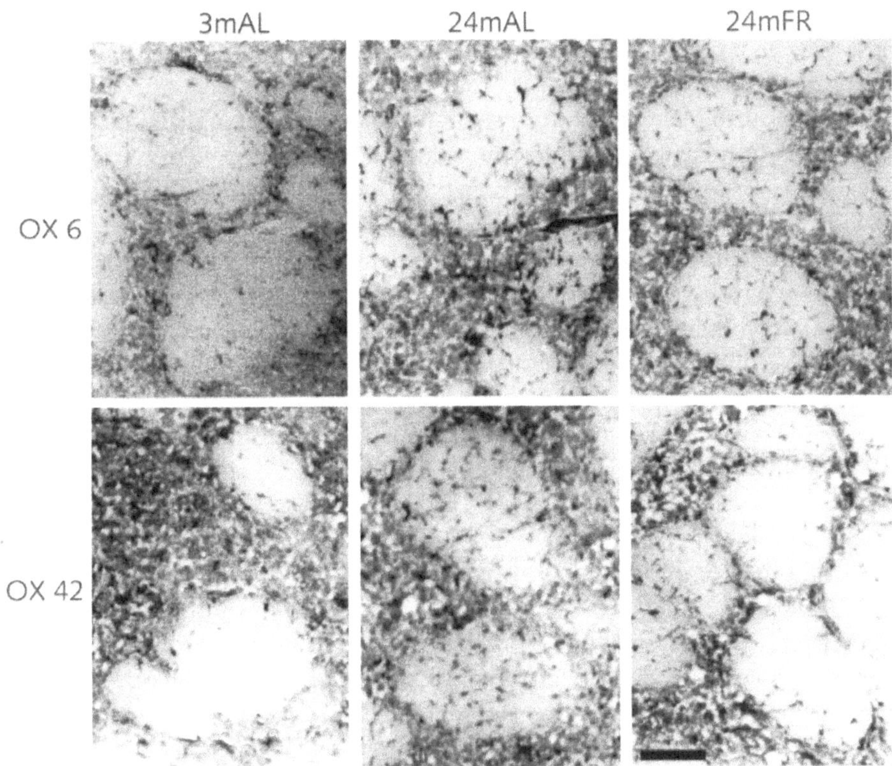

Figure 2
Microglial activities in cortico-striatal bundles, as identified by immunohistochemistry for OX6 (Mhc class II antigen) and OX42 (complement receptor C3). The numbers of activated microglia increase three-fold during aging in 3 vs 24 month old male rats (F1 hybrids (BN × F344)); rats aged 24 months in this genotype may be considered as middle-aged because the mean life span is 32 months. Caloric restriction by –35% of the ad libitum *intake attenuates microglial activation, particularly in myelinated tracts. From the authors' laboratory [9].*

is in an early state and findings have not been shown to broadly generalize among rodent genotypes. For example, in aging rat striatum of the F344, but not in an F1 hybrid, we showed modest increases of mRNAs for C1q, apoJ (clusterin), and TGF-β_1 by blot hybridization; GFAP mRNA increased at the same rate in both genotypes, however [13]. In one study of aging rats, hippocampal IL-1β increased [27], whereas another showed loss of response of glutamate release by IL-1β [28], two findings which are not contradictory. Corpora amylacea are not usually discussed by molecular neurobiologists in the context of aging, although these microscopic structures with inflammatory factors are well known to neuropathologists. However, normal aging brains commonly have abundant corpora amylacea that show immunopositivity for many complement factors [29, 30]. In AD, the numbers of corpora amylacea increase further above control-age brains. In the CSF, complement factor C3a increases with normal aging, but does not show further changes with AD [31]; however, CSF C1q decreases during AD, suggesting consumption of activated complement [32].

In summary, glial activation occurs during aging in the absence of obvious neuron loss or synaptic regression. This conclusion is based on studies of laboratory rodents in which brain amyloid is not found. Similar findings are indicated in dogs and primates which, like humans, accumulate brain amyloid during aging. Thus, glial activation during aging can be independent of brain amyloid. Glial activation during middle-age, like vascular wall thickening and loss of elasticity (see below), may be considered a canonical feature of aging.

Gero-inflammation in non-neural tissues

Atherosclerosis is increasingly recognized as a chronic inflammatory process [33]. Various subsets of inflammatory mediators (e.g. cytokines, chemokines, growth factors) are secreted during acute responses to infections or wounds and are also found in atherosclerotic lesions. Moreover, inflammatory mediators have major roles in many other age-related conditions [34], including degenerative bone and joint diseases and abnormal growths. In turn, cytokines (IL-1, IL-6, TNFα) can induce other acute-phase proteins (C-reactive protein, serum amyloid A) [35] and ROS. In view of the major successes in understanding the mechanisms in chronic inflammatory diseases of aging (vascular disease, joint disease), it is striking how little is known about associations between inflammation and cell dysfunctions in tissues during "normal" aging, in the absence of, or independent of, specific diseases of aging. This issue is germane to how inflammatory activities during normal brain aging may or may not be related to the specific inflammatory changes of AD.

The primary inflammatory cells (macrophages, neutrophils) that mediate the phagocytosis and death of invading organisms and the clearance of cellular debris are also potentially harmful to normal tissues throughout the body. These phagocytes release cytokines, chemokines, growth factors and ROS that contribute to focal necrosis and to the formation of the fibrous tissue associated with atherosclerosis, rheumatoid arthritis, and other inflammatory diseases. These roles parallel those of brain microglia/macrophages that are associated with amyloid deposits.

In general, the mitochondrial electron transport chain generates most of the ROS. However, phagocytes also utilize cytosolic NADPH oxidases to generate high doses of ROS during the oxidative burst. Phagocyte-mediated damage has been linked to many diseases including atherosclerosis, rheumatoid arthritis, and vasculitis by arachidonic acid metabolites and ROS. For example, phagocyte-derived ROS is associated with myocardial damage by increasing the atherogenicity of LDL, by modulating extracellular matrix degradation, and by increasing thrombin generation and thrombosis [36]. Other chapters in this volume have considered the activation of brain microglia and the generation of ROS as mediators of Aβ-peptide neurotoxicity. However, we do not yet know the roles of inflammatory-oxidative responses in aging of peripheral tissues that may be independent of specific diseases.

A scattered literature on age changes in peripheral macrophage activity merits a brief survey. We note that the common distinction between neural and non-neural can be misleading because of the extensive autonomic innervation throughout the body which can directly regulate inflammatory gene expression, e.g. sympathetic regulation of IL-6 mRNA in liver [37]. It is hard to evaluate reports on changes in non-neural inflammatory changes during aging because of the diverse animal and cell models studied. Nonetheless, IL-6 has shown relatively consistent increases during aging in the absence of specific diseases in several animal models and human populations [38]. Moreover, IL-6 production is increased in macrophages from older donors, measured as basal secretion or after stimulation with LPS or PHA [38, 39].

However, the extent of IL-6 increase varies widely between individuals. For example, several community-based studies of generally healthy older men and woman show that elevations of IL-6 are restricted to subgroups [40, 41]. A subpopulation of particular interest is type-2 diabetes, which is characterized by elevated IL-6 and serum amyloid A (SAA) [42]. Type-2 diabetes is commonly associated with obesity, hypertension, and accelerated atherogenesis (metabolic syndrome-X). In centenarians with high levels of lipoprotein(a), a risk factor for coronary heart disease, IL-6 plasma levels are four-fold higher than in young controls; however, those with low lipoprotein(a) also had low IL-6 [43]. Thus, the increase in IL-6 in some elderly subgroups may represent intensification of vascular diseases or other conditions associated with inflammation. Moreover, sex steroids can influence cytokine production, e.g. cultured bone marrow cells from women on estrogen replacement had a decreased IL-6 production [39].

Longitudinal studies of inflammatory markers have great promise in identifying individuals with distinct outcomes of aging. In rats, blood levels of T kininogen, an acute phase protein, are elevated several months before death [44]. In community-based samples, progressive increases of plasma IL-6 were associated with a two-fold higher risk of disability [45]. Similarly, TNFα elevations are associated with a two-fold higher risk for increased insulin-resistance [46], a characteristic of type-2 diabetes. On the other hand, IL-6 and other cytokines did not show changes in CSF or serum in AD during a phase of major cerebral atrophy [47]. We anticipate valuable findings from human and rodent population-based studies that will identify peripheral inflammatory markers for risks of changes in brain functions.

Does aging alter the generation of ROS by phagocytic cells? On one hand, several studies with peripheral blood cells from older humans and rodents report that untreated phagocytes generate increased cytokines [15, 41] and ROS [48, 49], suggesting that peripheral blood monocytes may be in a chronically activated state. However, stimulation of rodent and human monocytes by PMA or chemotactic peptides is variously reported to show either no change in ROS induction [49] or slight decreases [50,51]. Studies are needed of aging rodents under well-defined conditions, which include analysis of organ pathology and immunological status in *individuals* from which cells are obtained. Few animal model experimenters would be enthusiastic about such clinically-minded strategies.

In summary, in old rodents and humans, macrophage-like cells appear to be in a low but chronic activation state that tends to generate more ROS and certain cytokines. Overall, we have the impression of extensive variability in inflammatory manifestations during aging, e.g. in plasma levels of IL-1β, IL-6, IFNγ and TNFα, or in their production per cell under basal or stimulated conditions. However, these individual variations are not surprising in view of the well recognized individual courses of inflammatory processes, e.g. differences of cytokine expression during fevers [35] and the greatly variable course of tuberculosis. Provisionally, we conclude that peripheral blood levels of cytokines and other inflammatory mediators represent multiple processes, rather than a single unified aging process. Further studies are needed to understand the role of phagocyte-derived oxidants in inflammatory diseases as well as in normal aging.

Amyloids and aging

Amyloid deposits have been identified as chronic inflammatory stimulants in AD, and many studies, some dating from early in this century, amply document that "senile amyloids" are common in non-neural tissues of aging individuals, humans and animal models [52–55]. By amyloids we mean the extracellular aggregates of fibrillar proteinaceous materials that bind Congo red or Thioflavin-S and which may be formed from about 20 different proteins [54, 56, 57]. Several amyloid-forming proteins are acute phase proteins, e.g. C-reactive protein and serum amyloid (SAA), which have roles in antimicrobial defense and tissue repair [6]. A new role for serum amyloid P (SAP) is the clearance of nucleoprotein debris from apoptotic cells [58], which should be examined in neural tissues in view of the presence of SAP in senile plaques. In addition, many other aggregated proteins that do not meet the classical criteria for tissue amyloids should be further considered in reaction to alternate pathways of aggregation. A distinction is made in the larger field of amyloid pathobiology between systemic (primary) vs. localized (secondary) amyloid deposits [54, 57]. The brain deposits of Aβ peptide in AD, for example, are not associated with systemic amyloids and would be considered as a secondary amyloidosis. However, these distinctions may blur when one considers that certain familial forms of AD are associated with increased cellular production and body fluid levels of the Aβ peptide in many locations [59]. Moreover, deposits of the Aβ peptide in skin are more common in AD than in cognitively normal age-matched controls [60, 61].

In the heart and aorta, several types of amyloids become increasingly common after 50 years [55, 62, 63]. Myocardial amyloids include atrial natriuretic peptide (α-ANP) [64] and transthyretin, particularly in African-American carriers of a mutant transthyretin [65]. Myocardial amyloids can accumulate sufficiently to modify heart structure and function, causing arrhythmias and conduction disturbances, which may be a significant cause of heart failure in the elderly. The aorta accumulates different (and unidentified) amyloids, particularly in the medial layer [62]. Pancreatic amyloid forms in type-2 diabetics from amylin, which is co-secreted with insulin. "Senile" amyloids accumulate in other vital organs to varying degrees. There is a need for a thorough study of non-neural amyloids in individuals whose brains are characterized for the neuropathology of AD. This major project might identify a new relationship between the peripheral and central inflammatory processes of aging, in which amyloid deposits could be a variable outcome, for example, in the skin of AD patients as noted above.

Senile amyloids are also common in domestic animals. Aging dogs have well characterized accumulations of the Aβ peptide in cerebral vessels and as senile plaques [66, 67], as well as other (not identified) amyloids in heart, lung, and intestine [68]. As in humans, amyloid accumulations vary widely between individual animals during aging [67, 69]. Laboratory mice are well known to lack brain amyloid during aging unless engineered with certain familial AD transgenes. However, senile amyloid deposits commonly increase during aging in kidney and other non-neural tissues in widely-used strains of mice [70, 71]. The over-expression of TGF-β_1 in transgenic mice caused age-related deposits of the Aβ peptide in cerebral vessels [72], which suggests the importance of TGF-β_1 and other cytokines in tissue amyloid deposits.

Of much interest, inflammation also promotes amyloid formation in non-neural tissues [6, 57, 73, 74]. For example, tuberculosis with major host inflammatory responses frequently leads to systemic amyloidosis [57, 75]. Renal dialysis, through little understood processes that lead to the accumulation of inflammatory cells, is also associated with tissue amyloids [74, 76]. The mechanisms are still a mystery. We speculate that the polypeptide conformations that favor aggregation of certain proteins as amyloids [56] might be enhanced by decreased levels of tissue antioxidants during inflammatory processes, e.g. glutathione. Many examples of aging changes in protein structure are associated with oxidation of amino acids [56].

Molecular oxidation, a basic process in aging

Many of the inflammatory changes described above could be considered as epiphenomena to specific diseases, e.g. the presence of amyloid deposits in Alzheimer brains might activate complement, leading to further recrutiment of microglia by anaphylactic peptides. However, we must consider yet another level in these complex processes: the spontaneous chemistry of oxidative aging in long-lived proteins. For example, the oxidation of collagen and elastin is a progressive ongoing extracellular process from birth onwards, which is caused in part by the spontaneous chemical addition of glucose to the ε-amine groups of lysine (non-enzymatic autooxidative glycation or glycoxidation). Pentosidine is among a variety of complex condensation products designated as AGEs (advanced glycation endproducts), which are formed, for example, through free radical intermediates [56, 77–80]. In addition to glucose, other common metabolites also avidly form AGEs, including ascorbate, glucose-6-phosphate, and glyceraldehyde-3-phosphate. Increased carbonyl content is another marker of oxidized proteins that can arise during the formation of AGEs, but that can be generated by other oxidative processes as well [56]. The chemically-based oxidative changes of aging are highly complex with many different outcomes depending, for example, on microenvironmental variations in the extracellular concentrations of transition metals or of reducing agents, or electrical activity of neuron terminals projecting from other brain regions that are under stress.

Most tissues show robust, progressive age-related increases of pentosidine from birth onwards, e.g. skin collagen of mammals ranging from dogs to humans [79] (Fig. 3). AGEs also accumulate on senile plaque amyloids in AD, as would be expected for any long-lived proteins, because of the inescapable exposure to glucose in interstitial fluids (reviewed in [9, 77]). Cerebral vessels also accumulate AGEs and there may be brain parenchymal AGEs independent of those in senile plaques. Pentosidine and other AGEs also can form covalent bridges that can cross-link neighboring peptides. The age-related decrease in elasticity of blood vessels associated with AGE formation is accelerated by chronic hyperglycemia, as in type-2 diabetes, and is a factor in hypertension (see for example [79, 80]).

The rate of formation of AGEs is thought to be mainly driven by the concentration of glucose in the fluids surrounding the reactive protein groups, but may also be influenced by many other pro- and antioxidants. In addition to this basic chemistry, macrophages and vascular endothelial cells can become involved, since their scavenger receptors are activated by AGEs, and can result in local production of ROS (see for example [77, 78, 81, 82]). The increase of pentosidine in plasma and synovial fluid of patients with various inflammatory diseases [83] implies an important contribution from cellular ROS to AGE formation, in addition to that from glucose and other sugars. Since inflammation is responsible for a considerable portion of the ROS released extracellularly, phagocytes may play a major role in glycoxidation during aging. Thus, the accumulation of AGEs can trigger a cascade of further oxidative damage which could be considered as part of the broad manifold of the gero-inflammatory process.

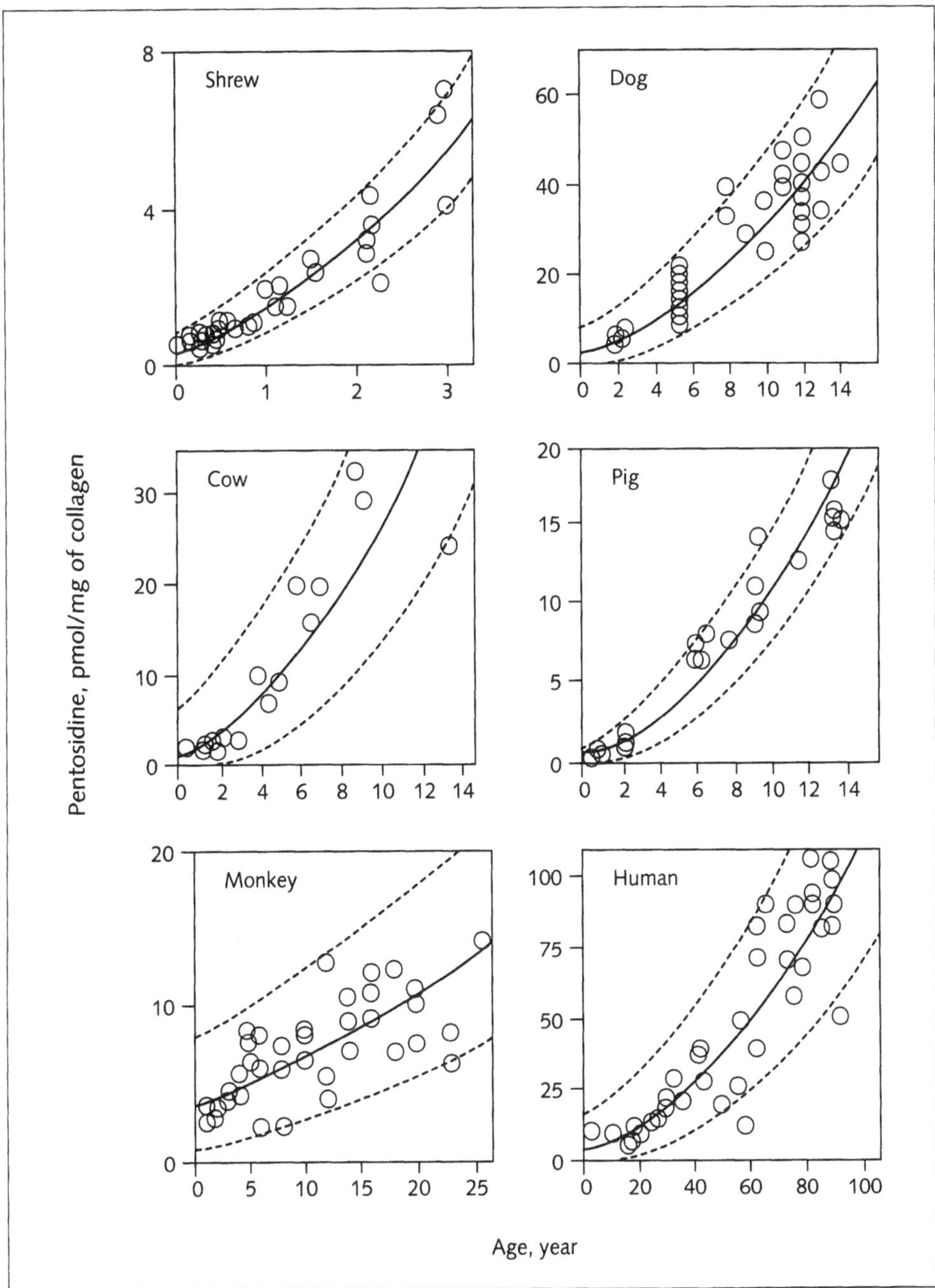

Figure 3
Age-related increase in skin collagen pentosidine, which is a marker of protein glycoxidation [79, 80]. The increases in these six species are progressive from birth onwards and show acceleration at later ages. From [79] with permission of author.

Modulations of gero-inflammatory processes by diet and hormones

Many of the gero-inflammatory processes described above can be slowed or even reversed. For example, we showed [9, 20] that the activation of microglia in white matter of aging rats is attenuated by chronic caloric restriction, in which *ad libitum* food intake is reduced by 35% during the adult life span, but without deficits in micronutrients (Fig. 1). These effects extend to other glial activities and regional populations, including the attenuation of GFAP transcription [20]. Caloric restriction is well-established to increase the rodent life span in association with the slowing of molecular aging changes, e.g. oxidation of proteins and the attenuation of diverse organ specific diseases, such as glomerulosclerosis and lymphomas [84, 85]. Of great interest to our thesis, caloric restriction decreased peripheral amyloid deposits in a strain of mouse with accelerated senescence [71]. Ongoing studies may reveal if caloric restriction modifies brain amyloid deposits in mice carrying human AD transgenes.

The physiology of caloric restriction may be as complex as that of diabetes. Among the major effects observed in rodents are the lowering of blood glucose and insulin, in association with increased glucocorticoids. The lowering of blood glucose would be expected to slow AGE formation in the brain, as in other tissues. Consistent with this hypothesis, caloric restriction decreases the load of oxidized proteins and lipids in the brain (reviewed in [9, 77]). The regulation of GFAP transcription by oxidative stress (see above) is the basis for a working hypothesis that caloric restriction attenuates glial activities by reducing local oxidative stimuli associated with AGE *via* the activation of scavenger receptors and further ROS production. In view of its attenuation of glial activation during aging, it is of great interest that caloric restriction of young rodents also attenuated a peripheral inflammatory response, the carragheenin-induced foot pad swelling, which is a classical model for evaluating anti-inflammatory drugs [86].

In addition, AGE formation may be reversible. ALT-711, a small heterocyclic molecule that interacts with AGEs, reversed the loss of elasticity associated with diabetes in a rat model [80]. It would be of interest to know if NSAID treatments that decreased microglial activation in AD and control brains [87] also decreased the load of AGE in brain parenchyma or cerebrovasculature.

We briefly note some complex issues about steroids in relation to glial activation and brain aging. Chronic elevations of glucocorticoids are associated with neuron degeneration and glial activation [11, 12, 88, 89]. On the other hand, caloric restriction, which attenuates many of these changes, causes increased plasma glucocorticoids. There is no easy explanation of this paradox. Another puzzle concerns estradiol. On one hand, the activation of hypothalamic microglia and astrocytes during aging in rodents is attenuated by aging in the absence of the ovary [88, 90]; reciprocally, chronic exposure to elevated estradiol in rodents rapidly induces astrocytic hyperactivity in association with oxidative stress [91]. However, IL-6 production by bone marrow cells is much less in women using estrogen replacement therapy [39], as noted above. Thus estrogen may be anti-inflammatory in some situations, but pro-inflammatory in others. Postmortem studies are not yet available to evaluate if estrogen replacement therapy modifies neurodegeneration during aging or AD.

Conclusion

We have argued that the neuroinflammatory processes observed in AD should be considered in the context of similar, but less intense, changes in the brain during normal aging, particularly with regard to the activation of astrocytes and microglia. The occurrence of glial activation during aging in rodents clearly dissociates glial activation of aging from the accumulation of amyloid deposits, which are not normally found in rodent brains. Moreover, non-neural tissues show many manifestations of inflammatory processes during aging. We place the accumulation of oxidized proteins (AGEs) in this context because macrophages and endothelia have scavenger receptors that respond to AGEs.

Thus, we can consider two domains of the gero-inflammatory manifold: processes that are widespread throughout the body (AGE accumulation; macrophage activation) compared to focal processes in particular tissues (astrocyte activation). Further studies are needed to determine the contribution of ROS from microglia, astrocytes, and neurons to increased oxidative damage to macromolecules.

In non-neural tissues the role of inflammation in cellular damage during "normal aging" is unclear, although local inflammatory mechanisms are well recognized in atherogenesis. Systemically, blood IL-6 is often elevated during aging; however, the wide individual differences may represent degrees of underlying disease processes, e.g. atherosclerosis or rheumatoid arthritis. Systemic inflammation can modify outcomes of aging by promoting the chronic increase of inflammatory proteins known to form amyloids, such as CRP and SAA. These deposits could, in turn, perpetuate inflammatory responses by activating phagocytes. The factors that govern individual accumulations of amyloid are unknown. The sporadic occurrence of amyloids during aging suggests a chaotic process with transients that escape overall homeostatic regulation.

The oxidants generated during inflammation may also contribute to the damage of non-neural tissue by increasing the formation of extracellular amyloid deposits and of glycoxidized proteins. However, the role of non-neural amyloids in tissue damage has not been proven experimentally and may prove to be as complex as the issue of amyloid neurotoxicity in AD. In any case, there is a remarkable general association of inflammatory processes of aging with amyloid formation in many tissues besides the brain. The specific mechanisms by which aging processes are pro-amyloidogenic are likely to vary widely between tissues and be sensitive to the genotype.

At a more fundamental level, spontaneous oxidative processes occur through the non-enzymatic addition of glucose and other sugars to amino groups of long-lived proteins, resulting in the accumulation of pentosidine and other AGEs. These processes are progressive in most tissues from birth onwards and may have profound importance to brain aging because AGEs activate microglia/macrophages through scavenger receptors. A fundamental chemical aspect of aging may be the basic substrate for inflammatory epiphenomena which, depending on the tissue and the genotype, results in specific pathogenic pathways.

In conclusion, during "normal aging" human and rodent brains consistently show general features of chronic inflammation. Similar, but much more specific, age-dependent inflammatory changes are also observed in non-neural tissues. In essence, we propose a convergence of the inflammatory and oxidative damage hypotheses of aging. While the role of inflammation in diseases ranging from AD to atherosclerosis is becoming clarified, our understanding of whether and how inflammation contributes to age-dependent changes is at an earlier stage. The study of the longevity and inflammatory features of transgenic and knockout mice with altered expression of cytokines and other proteins that mediate inflammation should provide better tools to test the role of inflammation in aging. We may consider a global hypothesis of aging in which chronic, initially low grade, inflammatory processes progress during aging to become proamyloidogenic in different tissues. Individual outcomes of aging may depend on how smouldering gero- inflammatory processes are fanned by the external environment, according to the genotype and species, but also by physiological influences of hormones and metabolism (Fig. 1).

References

1. Alzheimer A (1907) Uber eine einartige Erkrankung der Hindrinde. In: E Schultze, O Snell (eds): *Allgemeine Zeitschrift für Psychiatrie und Psychisch-Gerichtliche Medizin.* 64: 146–148. Translated as "A characteristic disease of the cerebral cortex". In: K Bick, L Amaducci, G Pepeu (eds): *The early story of Alzheimer's disease.* Livonia Press, Padova Italy, distributed through Raven Press, New York
2. Akiyama H, Barger S, Barnum S, Bradt B, Bauer J, Cole GM, Cooper NR, Eikelenboom P, Emmerling M, Fiebich BL et al (2000) Inflammation and Alzheimer's disease. *Neurobiol Aging* 21: 383–421
3. Terry RD, Gonatas NK, Weiss M (1964) Ultrastructural studies in Alzheimer's presenile dementia. *Am J Pathol* 44: 269–297
4. Goldsmith SK, Wals P, Rozovsky I, Morgan TE, Finch CE (1997) Kainic acid and decorticating lesions stimulate the synthesis of C1q protein in adult rat brain. *J Neurochem* 68: 2046–2052

5 Johnson SA, Pasinetti GM, Finch CE (1994) Expression of complement C1qB and C4 mRNAs during rat brain development. *Devel Brain Res* 80: 163–174
6 Finch CE, Marchalonis J (1996) An evolutionary perspective on amyloid and inflammatory features of Alzheimer disease. *Neurobiol Aging* 17: 809–815
7 Hoffman JA, Kafatos FC, Janeway Jr CA, Ezekowitz RAB (1999) Phylogenetic perspectives in innate immunity. Science 284: 1313–1318
8 Yasojima K, Schwab C, McGeer EG, McGeer PL (1999) Up-regulated production and activation of the complement system in Alzheimer's disease brain. *Am J Pathol* 154: 927–936
9 Morgan TE, Xie Z, Goldsmith S, Yoshida T, Lanzrein A-S, Stone D, Rozovsky I, Perry G, Smith MA, Finch CE (1999) The mosaic of brain glial hyperactivity during normal aging and its attenuation by food restriction. *Neuroscience* 89: 687–699
10 Gordon MN, Schreier WA, Ou X, Holcomb LA, Morgan DG (1997) Exaggerated astrocyte reactivity after nigrostriatal deafferentation in the aged rat. *J Comp Neurol* 388: 106–119
11 Landfield PW (1994) The role of glucocorticoids in brain aging and Alzheimer's disease: an integrative physiological hypothesis. *Exp Gerontol* 29: 3–11
12 Lindsay JD, Landfield PW, Lynch G (1979) Early onset and topographical distribution of hypertrophied astrocytes in hippocampus of aging rats: a quantitative study. *J Gerontol* 34: 661–671
13 Pasinetti GM, Hassler M, Stone D, Finch CE (1999) Glial gene expression during aging in rat striatum and in long-term responses to 6-OHDA lesions. *Synapse* 31: 278–284
14 Perry VH, Matyszak M, Fearn S (1993) Altered antigen expression of microglia in aged rodent CNS. Glia 7: 60–67
15 Finch CE, Morgan TE, Rozovsky I, Xie Z, Weindruch R, Prolla T (2001) Microglia and aging in the brain. In: WJ Streit (ed): *Microglia in the degenerating and regenerating CNS.* Springer Verlag, New York (*in press*)
16 Bolaños JP, Medina JM (1996) Induction of nitric oxide synthase inhibits gap junction permeability in cultured rat astrocytes. *J Neurochem* 66: 2091–2099
17 Tolias CM, McNeil CJ, Kazlauskaite J, Hillhouse EW (1999) Superoxide generation from constitutive nitric oxide synthase in astrocytes *in vitro* regulates extracellular nitric oxide availability. *Free Rad Biol Med* 26: 99–106
18 Geula C, Wu CK, Saroff D, Lorenzo A, Yuan M, Yankner BA (1998) Aging renders the brain vulnerable to amyloid beta-protein neurotoxicity. *Nat Med* 4:827–831
19 Rozovsky I, Finch CE, Morgan TE (1998) Age-related activation of microglia and astrocytes: *in vitro* studies show persistence of phenotypes of aging, increased proliferation, and resistance to down-regulation. *Neurobiol Aging* 19: 97–103
20 Morgan TE, Rozovsky I, Goldsmith SK, Stone DJ, Yoshida T, Finch CE (1997) Increased transcription of the astrocyte gene GFAP during middle-age is attenuated by food restriction: implications for the role of oxidative stress. *Free Rad Biol Med* 23: 524–528
21 Long JM, Kalehua AN, Muth NJ, Calhoun ME, Jucker M, Hengemihle JM, Ingram DK,

Mouton PR (1998) Stereological analysis of astrocyte and microglia in aging mouse hippocampus. *Neurobiol Aging* 19: 497–503

22 Nichols NR, Day JR, Laping NJ, Johnson SA, Finch CE (1993) GFAP mRNA increases with age in rat and human brain. *Neurobiol Aging* 14: 421–429

23 Hansen L.A., Armstrong, D.M., and Terry, R.D. (1987) An immunohistochemical quantification of fibrous astrocytes in the aging human cerebral cortex. *Neurobiol Aging* 8: 1–6

24 Wei M, Rozovsky I, Lopez LM, Morgan TE, Finch CE (1999) Oxidative stress and the GFAP promoter. *Soc Neurosci Abstr* 25: 1317

25 Krohn K, Rozovsky I, Wals P, Teter B, Anderson CP, Finch CE (1999) Glial fibrillary acidic protein (GFAP) transcription responses to TGF-β1 and IL-1β are mediated by an NF-1 like site in the near-upstream promoter. *J Neurochem* 72: 1353–1361

26 Jucker M, Walker LC, Kuo H, Tian M, Ingram DK (1994) Age-related fibrillar deposits in brains of C57BL/6 mice. A review of localization, staining characteristics, and strain specificity. *Mol Neurobiol* 9: 125–133

27 Takao T, Nagano I, Tojo C, Takemura T, Makino S, Hashimoto K, De Souza EB (1996) Age-related reciprocal modulation of interleukin-1beta and interleukin-1 receptors in the mouse brain-endocrine-immune axis. *Neuroimmunomodulation* 3: 205–212

28 Murray CA, McGahon B, McBennett S, Lynch MA (1997) Interleukin-1 beta inhibits glutamate release in hippocampus of young, but not aged, rats. *Neurobiol Aging* 18: 343–348

29 Cavanagh JB (1999) Corpora-amylacea and the family of polyglucosan diseases. *Brain Res Brain Res Rev* 29: 265–295

30 Singhrao SK, Morgan BP, Neal JW, Newman GR (1995) A functional role for corpora amylacae based on evidence from complement studies. *Neurodegeneration* 4: 335–345

31 Loeffler DA, Brickman CM, Juneau PL, Perry MF, Pomara N, Lewitt PA (1997) Cerebrospinal fluid C3a increases with age, but does not increase further in Alzheimer's disease. *Neurobiol Aging* 18: 555–557

32 Smyth MD, Cribbs DH, Tenner AJ, Shankle WR, Dick M, Kesslak JP, Cotman CW (1994) Decreased levels of C1q in cerebrospinal fluid of living Alzheimer patients correlate with disease state. *Neurobiol Aging* 15: 609–614

33 Ross R (1999) Mechanisms of disease: atherosclerosis – an inflammatory disease. *N Engl J Med* 340: 115–126

34 Ballou SP, Kushner I (1997) Chronic inflammation in older people: recognition, consequences, and potential intervention. *Clin Geriatr Med* 13: 653–659

35 Gabay C, Kushner I (1999) Mechanisms of disease: acute-phase proteins and other systemic responses to inflammation. *N Engl J Med* 340: 448–454

36 Ricevuti G (1996) Host tissue damage by phagocytes. *Ann NY Acad Sci* 832: 426–448

37 Song DK, IM YB, Jung JS, Suh HW, Huh SO, Song JH, Kim YH (1999) Central injection of nicotine increases hepatic and splenic interleukin 6 (IL-6) mRNA expression and plasma IL-6 levels in mice: involvement of the peripheral sympathetic nervous system. *FASEB J* 13: 1259–1267

38 Ershler WB, Keller ET (2000) Age-associated increased interleukin-6 gene expression, late-life diseases, and frailty. *Annu Rev Med* 51: 245–270

39 Cheleuitte D, Mizuno S, Glowacki J (1998) *In vitro* secretion of cytokines by human bone marrow: effects of age and estrogen status. *J Clin Endocrinol Metab* 83: 2043–2051

40 Cohen HJ, Pieper CF, Harris T, Rao KM, Currie MS (1997) The association of plasma IL-6 levels with functional disability in community-dwelling elderly. *J Gerontol A Biol Sci Med Sci* 52: M201–M208

41 Roubenoff R, Harris TB, Abad LW, Wilson PW, Dallal GE, Dinarello CA (1998) Monocyte cytokine production in an elderly population: effect of age and inflammation. *J Gerontol A Biol Sci Med Sci* 53: M20–M26

42 Pickup JC, Battock MB, Chusney GD, Burt D (1997) NIDDM as a disease of the innate immune system: association of acute-phase reactants and interleukin-6 with metabolic syndrome X. *Diabetologia* 40: 1286–92

43 Baggio G, Donazzan S, Monti D, Mari D, Martini S, Gabelli C, Dalla Vestra M, Previato L, Guido M, Pigozzo S et al (1998) Lipoprotein(a) and lipoprotein profile in healthy centenarians: a reappraisal of vascular risk factors. *FASEB J* 12: 433–437

44 Walter R, Murasko DM, Sierra F (1998) T-kininogen is a biomarker of senescence in rats. *Mech Ageing Dev* 106: 129–144

45 Ferrucci L, Harris TB, Guralnik JM, Tracy RP, Corti MC, Cohen HJ, Penninx B, Pahor M, Wallace R, Havlik RJ (1999) Serum IL-6 level and the development of disability in older persons. *J Am Geriatr Soc* 47: 639–646

46 Paolisso G, Rizzo MR, Mazziotti G, Tagliamonte MR, Gambardella A, Rotondi M, Carella C, Giugliano D, Varricchio M, D'Onofrio F (1998) Serum levels of insulin-like growth factor-I are related to age and not to body composition in healthy women and men. *J Gerontol A Biol Sci Med Sci* 53: M176–M182

47 Lanzrein AS, Johnston CM, Perry VH, Jobst KA, King EM, Smith AD (1998) Longitudinal study of inflammatory factors in serum, cerebrospinal fluid, and brain tissue in Alzheimer disease: interleukin-1beta, interleukin-6, interleukin-1 receptor antagonist, tumor necrosis factor-alpha, the soluble tumor necrosis factor receptors I and II, and alpha1-antichymotrypsin. *Alzheimer Dis Assoc Disord* 12: 215–227

48 Davila DR, Edwards CK 3rd, Arkins S, Simon J, Kelley KW (1990) Interferon-gamma-induced priming for secretion of superoxide anion and tumor necrosis factor-alpha declines in macrophages from aged rats. *FASEB J* 4: 2906–2911

49 Varga Z, Jacob MP, Robert L, Csongor J, Fulop T Jr (1997) Age-dependent changes of K-elastin stimulated effector functions of human phagocytic cells: relevance for atherogenesis. *Exp Gerontol* 32: 653–662

50 Alvarez E, Conde M, Machado A, Sobrino F, Santa Maria C (1995) Decrease in free-radical production with age in rat peritoneal macrophages. *Biochem J* 312: 555–560

51 Rollo EE, Denhardt DT (1996) Differential effects of osteopontin on the cytotoxic activity of macrophages from young and old mice. *Immunology* 88: 642–647

52 Cornwell GG 3rd, Johnson KH, Westermark P (1995) The age related amyloids: a growing family of unique biochemical substances. *J Clin Pathol* 48: 984–989

53 Kunze WP (1979) Senile pulmonary amyloidosis. Pathol Res Pract 164: 413–422

54 Pepys MB (1988) Amyloidosis. In: Samter M (ed): *Immunological diseases,* vol I. 4th edition Little, Brown and Co, Boston MA, 631–674

55 Schwartz P (1970) *Amyloidosis: Cause and manifestations of senile deterioration.* CC Thomas, Springfield ILL

56 Gafni A (1997) Structural modifications of proteins during aging. *JAGS* 45: 871–880

57 Sipe JD (1994) Amyloidosis. *Crit Rev Clin Lab Sci* 31: 325–354

58 Bickerstaff MC, Botto M, Hutchinson WL, Herbert J, Tennent GA, Bybee A, Mitchell DA, Cook HT, Butler PJ, Walport MJ et al (1999) Serum amyloid P component controls chromatin degradation and prevents antinuclear autoimmunity. *Nat Med* 5: 694–697

59 Price DL, Tanzi RE, Borchelt DR, Sisodia SS (1998) Alzheimer's disease: genetic studies and transgenic models. *Annu Rev Genet* 32: 461–493

60 Joachim CL, Mori H, Selkoe DJ (1989) Amyloid beta-protein deposition in tissues other than brain in Alzheimer's disease. *Nature* 341: 226–230

61 Wen GY, Wisniewski HM, Blondal H, Benedikz E, Frey H, Pirttila T, Rudelli R, Kim KS (1994) Presence of non-fibrillar amyloid beta protein in skin biopsies of Alzheimer's disease (AD), Down's syndrome and non-AD normal persons. *Acta Neuropathol (Berlin)* 88: 201–206

62 McCarthy RE 3rd, Kasper EK (1998) A review of the amyloidoses that infiltrate the heart. *Clin Cardiol* 21: 547–552

63 Westermark P, Mucchiano G, Marthin T, Johnson KH, Sletten K (1995) Apolipoprotein A1-derived amyloid in human aortic atherosclerotic plaques. *Am J Pathol* 147: 1186–1192

64 Kawamura S, Takahashi M, Ishihara T, Uchino F (1995) Incidence and distribution of isolated atrial amyloid: histologic and immunohistochemical studies of 100 aging hearts. *Pathol Int* 45: 335–342

65 Jacobson DR, Pastore RD, Yaghoubian R, Kane I, Gallo G, Buck FS, Buxbaum JN (1997) Variant-sequence transthyretin (isoleucine 122) in late-onset cardiac amyloidosis in black Americans. *N Engl J Med* 336: 466–473

66 Tekirian TL, Cole GM, Russell MJ, Yang F, Wekstein DR, Patel E, Snowdon DA, Markesbery WR, Geddes JW (1996) Carboxy terminal of beta-amyloid deposits in aged human, canine, and polar bear brains. *Neurobiol Aging* 17: 249–257

67 Wegiel J, Wisniewski HM, Dziewiatkowski J, Tarnawski M, Dziewiatkowska A, Morys J, Soltysiak Z, Kim KS (1996) Subpopulation of dogs with severe brain parenchymal beta amyloidosis distinguished with cluster analysis. *Brain Res* 728: 20–26

68 Uchida K, Okuda R, Yamaguchi R, Tateyama S, Nakayama H, Goto N (1993) Double-labeling immunohistochemical studies on canine senile plaques and cerebral amyloid angiopathy. *J Vet Med Sci* 55: 637–642

69 Head E, Callahan H, Muggenburg BA, Cotman CW, Milgram NW (1998) Visual- dis-

crimination learning ability and beta-amyloid accumulation in the dog. *Neurobiol Aging* 19: 415–425
70 Higuchi K, Kitagawa K, Naiki H, Hanada K, Hosokawa M, Takeda T (1991) Polymorphism of apolipoprotein A-II (apoA-II) among inbred strains of mice. Relationship between the molecular type of apoA-II and mouse senile amyloidosis. *Biochem J* 279: 427–433
71 Kohno A, Yonezu T, Matsushita M, Irino M, Higuchi K, Higuchi K, Takeshita S, Hosokawa M, Takeda T (1985) Chronic food restriction modulates the advance of senescence in the senescence accelerated mouse (SAM). *J Nutr* 115:1259–1266
72 Wyss-Coray T, Masliah E, Mallory M, McConlogue L, Johnson-Wood K, Lin C, Mucke L (1997) Amyloidogenic role of cytokine TGF-beta1 in transgenic mice and in Alzheimer's disease. *Nature* 389: 603–606
73 Kisilevsky R (1994) Inflammation-associated amyloidogenesis: Lessons for Alzheimer's amyloidogenesis. *Mol Neurobiol* 8: 65–66
74 Buxbaum JN, Tagoe CE (2000) The genetics of the amyloidoses. *Annu Rev Med* 51: 543–569
75 Urban BA, Fishman EK, Goldman SM, Scott WW Jr, Jones B, Humphrey RL, Hruban RH (1993) CT evaluation of amyloidosis: spectrum of disease. *Radiographics* 13: 1295–1308
76 Ehlerding G, Schaeffer J, Drommer W, Miyata T, Koch KM, Floege J (1998) Alterations of synovial tissue and their potential role in the deposition of beta2-microglobulin-associated amyloid. *Nephrol Dialysis Transplant* 13: 1465–1475
77 Finch CE, Cohen DM (1996) Aging, metabolism, and Alzheimer disease: review and hypotheses. *Exp Neurol* 143: 82–102
78 Kristal BS, Yu BP (1992) An emerging hypothesis: synergistic induction of aging by free radicals and Maillard reactions. *J Gerontol* 47: B107–B114
79 Sell DR, Lane MA, Johnson WA, Masoro EJ, Mock OB, Reiser KM, Fogarty JF, Cutler RG, Ingram DK, Roth GS et al (1996) Longevity and the genetic determination of collagen glycoxidation kinetics in mammalian senescence. *Proc Natl Acad Sci USA* 93: 485–490
80 Wolffenbuttel BH, Boulanger CM, Crijns FR, Huijberts MS, Poitevin P, Swennen GN, Vasan S, Egan JJ, Ulrich P, Cerami A, Levy BI (1998) Breakers of advanced glycation end products restore large artery properties in experimental diabetes. *Proc Natl Acad Sci USA* 95: 4630–4634
81 Li JJ, Dickson D, Hof P, Vlassara H (1998) Receptors for advanced glycosylation end-products in human brain: role in brain homeostasis. *Mol Med* 4: 46–60
82 Mackic JB, Stins M, McComb JG, Calero M, Ghiso J, Kim KS, Yan SD, Stern D, Schmidt AM, Frangione B et al (1998) Human blood-brain barrier receptors for Alzheimer's amyloid-beta 1–40. Asymmetrical binding, endocytosis, and transcytosis at the apical side of brain microvascular endothelial cell monolayer. *J Clin Invest* 102: 734–743
83 Miyata T, Ishiguro N, Yasuda Y, Ito T, Nangaku M, Iwata H, Kurokawa K (1998)

Increased pentosidine, an advanced glycation end product, in plasma and synovial fluid from patients with rheumatoid arthritis and its relation with inflammatory markers. *Biochem Biophys Res Commun* 244: 45–49

84 Masoro EJ (1998) Hormesis and the antiaging action of dietary restriction. *Exp Gerontol* 33: 61–66

85 Sohal RS, Weindruch R (1996) Oxidative stress, caloric restriction, and aging. *Science* 273: 59–63

86 Klebanov S, Diais S, Stavinoha WB, Suh Y, Nelson JF (1995) Hyperadrenocorticism, attenuated inflammation, and the life-prolonging action of food restriction in mice. *J Gerontol A Biol Sci Med Sci* 50: B79–82

87 MacKenzie IRA, Munoz DG (1998) Nonsteroidal anti-inflammatory drug use and Alzheimer-type pathology in aging. *Neurology* 50: 986–990

88 Finch CE, Felicio LS, Mobbs CV, Nelson JF (1984) Ovarian and steroidal influences on neuroendocrine aging processes in female rodents. *Endocr Rev* 5: 467–497

89 Sapolsky RM (1992) *Stress, the aging brain, and the mechanisms of neuron death.* MIT Press

90 Schipper H, Brawer JR, Nelson JF, Felicio LS, Finch CE (1981) Role of the gonads in the histologic aging of the hypothalamic arcuate nucleus. *Biol Reprod* 25: 413–419

91 Schipper HM (1996) Astrocytes, brain aging, and neurodegeneration. *Neurobiol Aging* 17: 467–480

Index

The PIR-Series
Progress in Inflammation Research

Homepage: http://www.birkhauser.ch

Up-to-date information on the latest developments in the pathology, mechanisms and therapy of inflammatory disease are provided in this monograph series. Areas covered include vascular responses, skin inflammation, pain, neuroinflammation, arthritis cartilage and bone, airways inflammation and asthma, allergy, cytokines and inflammatory mediators, cell signalling, and recent advances in drug therapy. Each volume is edited by acknowledged experts providing succinct overviews on specific topics intended to inform and explain. The series is of interest to academic and industrial biomedical researchers, drug development personnel and rheumatologists, allergists, pathologists, dermatologists and other clinicians requiring regular scientific updates.

Available volumes:

T Cells in Arthritis, P. Miossec, W. van den Berg, G. Firestein (Editors), 1998
Chemokines and Skin, E. Kownatzki, J. Norgauer (Editors), 1998
Medicinal Fatty Acids, J. Kremer (Editor), 1998
Inducible Enzymes in the Inflammatory Response, D.A. Willoughby, A. Tomlinson (Editors), 1999
Cytokines in Severe Sepsis and Septic Shock, H. Redl, G. Schlag (Editors), 1999
Fatty Acids and Inflammatory Skin Diseases, J.-M. Schröder (Editor), 1999
Immunomodulatory Agents from Plants, H. Wagner (Editor), 1999
Cytokines and Pain, L. Watkins, S. Maier (Editors), 1999
In Vivo *Models of Inflammation*, D. Morgan, L. Marshall (Editors), 1999
Pain and Neurogenic Inflammation, S.D. Brain, P. Moore (Editors), 1999
Anti-Inflammatory Drugs in Asthma, A.P. Sampson, M.K. Church (Editors), 1999
Novel Inhibitors of Leukotrienes, G. Folco, B. Samuelsson, R.C. Murphy (Editors), 1999
Vascular Adhesion Molecules and Inflammation, J.D. Pearson (Editor), 1999
Metalloproteinases as Targets for Anti-Inflammatory Drugs, K.M.K. Bottomley, D. Bradshaw, J.S. Nixon (Editors), 1999
Free Radicals and Inflammation, P.G. Winyard, D.R. Blake, C.H. Evans (Editors), 1999
Gene Therapy in Inflammatory Diseases, C.H. Evans, P. Robbins (Editors), 2000
New Cytokines as Potential Drugs, S. K. Narula, R. Coffmann (Editors), 2000
High Throughput Screening for Novel Anti-inflammatories, M. Kahn (Editor), 2000
Immunology and Drug Therapy of Atopic Skin Diseases, C.A.F. Bruijnzeel-Komen, E.F. Knol (Editors), 2000
Novel Cytokine Inhibitors, G.A. Higgs, B. Henderson (Editors), 2000
Inflammatory Processes. Molecular Mechanisms and Therapeutic Opportunities, L.G. Letts, D.W. Morgan (Editors), 2000

Cellular Mechanisms in Airways Inflammation, C. Page, K. Banner, D. Spina (Editors), 2000
Inflammatory and Infectious Basis of Atherosclerosis, J.L. Mehta (Editor), 2001
Muscarinic Receptors in Airways Diseases, J. Zaagsma, H. Meurs, A.F. Roffel (Editors), 2001
TGF-β and Related Cytokines in Inflammation, S.N. Breit, S. Wahl (Editors), 2001
Nitric Oxide and Inflammation, D. Salvemini, T.R. Billiar, Y. Vodovotz (Editors), 2001

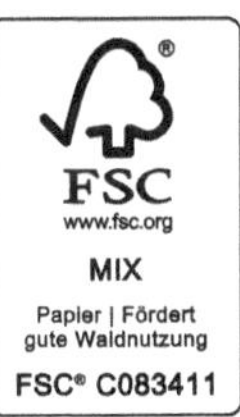

Zeitfracht Medien GmbH
Ferdinand-Jühlke-Straße 7
99095 Erfurt, Deutschland
produktsicherheit@kolibri360.de